C000115688

# Hypertension
# for the
# Clinician

# Hypertension for the Clinician

J. Ian S. Robertson

*BSc, MB, BS, FRCP (Lond); MD (Hons Causa, Free University of Brussels); F Inst Biol; FRCP (Glas); FRS (Edin)*
*Formerly Visiting Professor of Medicine, Prince of Wales Hospital, Chinese University of Hong Kong.*

Stephen G. Ball

*MA, MB, BChir (Cantab); PhD (Leeds); FRCP (Lond)*
*Professor of Cardiovascular Studies, University of Leeds, UK.*

W.B. SAUNDERS COMPANY LTD

London   Philadelphia   Toronto   Sydney   Tokyo

W. B. Saunders Company Ltd   24-28 Oval Road
London NW1 7DX

The Curtis Center
Independence Square West
Philadelphia, PA 19106-3399, USA

Harcourt Brace & Company
55 Horner Avenue
Toronto, Ontario, M8Z 4X6, Canada

Harcourt Brace & Company, Australia
30–52 Smidmore Street
Marrickville
NSW 2204, Australia

Harcourt Brace & Company, Japan
Ichibancho Central Building
22–1 Ichibancho
Chiyoda-ku, Tokyo 102, Japan

© 1994 W. B. Saunders Company Limited

This book is printed on acid-free paper

All rights reserved. No part of this publication may be reproduced, stored in a retrieval
system or transmitted, in any form or by any other means, electronic, mechanical, photocopying
or otherwise, without the prior permission of W. B. Saunders Company Ltd, 24–28 Oval Road,
London NW1 7DX, England.

A catalogue record for this book is available from the British Library

ISBN 0-7020-1812-0

Typeset by Paston Press Ltd, Loddon, Norfolk
Printed and bound in Great Britain by The Bath Press, Bath, Avon

# —Contents—

# Section Three—Treating essential hypertension

# Section Four—Secondary forms of hypertension

# Section Five—Hypertension in pregnancy

# ──Preface──

The medical care of high blood pressure, both in primary and hospital practice, continues to gain in importance. The value of prophylactic therapy, not least in elderly subjects, is now beyond doubt; we have learned much recently of the aetiological aspects of essential (primary) hypertension; and there is increasing understanding and expertise in the diagnosis and treatment of the diverse forms of secondary hypertension.

There is no dearth of books dealing in detail with virtually all aspects of hypertension. Briefer texts are scarcer. This deficiency became evident as we were preparing the section on hypertension for the second edition of *Diseases of the Heart* (1), and whilst one of us was engaged in editing two much larger works (2, 3).

The present book is an attempt to meet this perceived need. It is intended, in succinct form, to provide severally for the primary care physician, the post-graduate student, and the hospital specialist. The layout has been designed with these various aims in mind.

Section 1 (chapters 1–3) deals with basic principles. In particular, in chapter 1, the nature of hypertension, its pathogenesis and management are summarized.

Section 2 then enters in more detail into the epidemiology, development and pathological effects of essential (primary) hypertension (chapters 4–20). We have herein not attempted to evade controversies, and the bibliography is fairly extensive.

Section 3 (chapters 21–25) concerns the treatment of essential hypertension. Again, contentious issues are expounded, with appropriate accompanying bibliography. However, where aspects are extensively referenced elsewhere, for example as for antihypertensive drugs, we have economised on space by directing the reader as necessary to alternative review articles and books.

Section 4 (chapters 26–46) considers, often in detail, the very varied secondary forms of hypertension. It is not expected that the average reader will wish to study all of these at length. However, it is intended that these chapters will aid especially the hospital doctor encountering such problems. Accordingly, references here have again been limited. In particular we have relied extensively upon, and have directed these seeking more information especially to, two much larger texts (2, 3).

Section 5 (chapter 47) concerns hypertension in pregnancy. Primary sources, as well as reviews, are quoted extensively.

Appendix 1 details antihypertensive drugs. Appendix 2 sets out a series of 23 illustrative test cases of hypertension. These progress sequentially from common, but important, examples through to rarities. All are based on patients known personally to the authors. It is hoped that the reader will find these problems stimulating and informative. Appendix 3 is a reprinted critical appraisal written by one of us (4) of current treatment guidelines.

Stephen G. Ball
*Leeds*

J. Ian S. Robertson
*Hong Kong, Beerse and Glasgow*

## References to Preface

1. Robertson JIS, Ball SG, Hypertension. In *Diseases of the Heart*, 2nd edn (eds DG Julian, AJ Camm, KM Fox, RJC Hall and PA Poole-Wilson). London: WB Saunders, 1995.
2. *Handbook of Hypertension*, Vol. 15: *Clinical Hypertension* (ed. JIS Robertson). Amsterdam: Elsevier, 1992.
3. *The Renin–Angiotensin System* (eds JIS Robertson and MG Nicholls). London/New York: Gower Medical Publishing/Mosby Yearbook, 1993.
4. Robertson JIS. Guidelines for the treatment of hypertension: a critical review. *Cardiovascular Drugs & Therapy* 1994; **8**: 91–98.

# Acknowledgements

We are indebted to the editor of *Cardiovascular Drugs and Therapy* and to the publishers, Kluwer, Dordrecht, for permission to reprint the article which appears here as appendix 3.

We are grateful to Elsevier Science Publishers, Amsterdam, and to Gower/Mosby Yearbook, London/New York for allowing us to draw upon material which appeared in *Clinical Hypertension*, Handbook of Hypertension, Volume 15, 1992 (edited by JIS Robertson); and *The Renin–Angiotensin System*, 1993 (edited by JIS Robertson and MG Nicholls) respectively. We thank especially the many contributors to those volumes. We appreciate also the kindness of the authors and publishers who have allowed us to reproduce various figures, and who are acknowledged individually in the text.

We are grateful to Gill Robinson and Claire Gilman of W B Saunders, to Lidi Van Gool for secretarial help, and to Mignon for assiduous checking of references.

# Glossary

We give here a short list of alternative names for certain substances, and of American synonyms for English words used in the text.

## Alternative terms

Angiotensinogen–also known as renin substrate.
Vasopressin–also known as arginine vasopressin, antidiuretic hormone, ADH.

| English term | American term |
|---|---|
| adrenaline | epinephrine |
| frusemide | furosemide |
| isoprenaline | isoproterenol |
| liquorice | licorice |
| noradrenaline | norepinephrine |

# Section 1
## Basic principles

# 1

# Introduction: Hypertension in outline

The height of arterial blood pressure is a powerful indicator of the risks of a range of cardiac and vascular complications, namely the malignant phase of hypertension, hypertensive encephalopathy, hypertensive heart failure, stroke, coronary artery disease and its consequences, and progressive impairment of renal function. Cardiovascular risk is associated with both systolic and diastolic hypertension, although their relative importance remains controversial (pages 102–103 and 146–147). Appropriate blood pressure reduction, by pharmacological or other means, may correct, prevent or delay the appearance of many of these hypertension-related disorders. Thus, there is a strong case for identifying people with even symptomless and mild blood pressure elevation.[1]

This book is intended to provide a succinct, although reasonably comprehensive, account of the problems posed by hypertension. As such, it is written primarily, but not exclusively, for the needs of the practising doctor, whether primary care physician or hospital-based clinician. We begin, therefore, with a summary chapter, which provides in outline an account of the nature of hypertension, the reasons why it can cause cardiovascular diseases, how these maladies can be prevented or corrected, and especially how therapy should be addressed in practice. This is conceived not simply as an introductory precis; the summary chapter should also serve as a rapid reference source for the clinician in need of speedy advice. The deliberately brief account herein is extensively cross-referenced to those sections of the book which provide a full account of the respective topics, and to which the reader can readily turn.

## Hypertension in outline: a summary account of its problems and their treatment

### Hypertension: definitions

The term 'hypertension', as usually applied clinically, means simply 'raised arterial pressure'. Hypertension is not capable of definition in absolute terms (page 9), since there is no threshold level at which blood pressure ceases to be normal and high blood pressure begins (see Figure 2.1). Moreover, arterial pressure within an individual is continually varying, according to diurnal and physiological circumstances. Thus clinical concern with the blood pressure of a particular person or patient centres on its tessitura, that is, the range in which the pressure predominantly lies.

### Blood pressure measurement

Most clinical measurements of blood pressure are made indirectly, employing a mercury, or less often aneroid, sphygmomanometer and an inflatable occluding cuff applied round the upper arm. An account of the technique, and especially of the prevalent likely inaccuracies, and precautions necessary to limit them, are given in Chapter 23, page 133.

Less often, more detailed or more accurate information can be obtained by making continuous measurements over, say, 24 h (see Figure 3.1), or by means of an intra-arterial catheter and suitable pressure transducer. Further information on these procedures is given on pages 12 and 136.

Despite the very limited information provided by most blood pressure measurements, and the numerous inaccuracies, it is remarkable how extensive and relevant the epidemiological, clinical and therapeutic studies derived from them have been.

### Changes of blood pressure with age

In Western or Westernized populations, the prevailing levels of systolic and diastolic change with age. Systolic pressure usually rises throughout life, with often a fairly steep increase in the teenage years (see Figure 4.1). Diastolic pressure also increases up to about the fifth decade, again fairly steeply during the teenage years. However, in later life, unlike systolic pressure, the diastolic pressure levels off, or can even fall slightly (see Figure 4.1).

This Western pattern of blood pressure change is not universal. Some, usually small and isolated, communities show modest or little increase in arterial pressure with ageing and thus in them the prevailing level of blood pressure is low (Table 4.1). The low blood pressure is imposed by environmental, not genetic, influences, because migration from such communities is usually accompanied by the more typical age-related increase in pressure. The implications of these observations are discussed on pages 17 and 21.

### Causes of raised blood pressure: secondary and primary hypertension

Secondary hypertension is raised blood pressure due to an identifiable and potentially correctable cause (Table 1.1). Only some 1–5% of cases of hypertension, however defined, are secondary. Nevertheless, identification of secondary hypertension is important, because correction or elimination of the cause can alleviate hypertension; since many of the underlying conditions require therapy in their own right; and because study of the mechanisms involved in hypertension of known causation may provide more general insight into the pathogenesis of other forms of hypertension. Secondary forms of hypertension are listed in Table 1.1, and are considered in detail in Chapters 26–47.

It should be noted that the phrase 'hypertension due to a secondary cause', occasionally used in medical writing, is internally contradictory and betrays confusion of thought; the phrase should be eschewed.

The diversity of secondary hypertension embraces aortic coarctation; a wide range of drug-induced forms of hypertension, especially that due to the oestrogen–progestogen oral contraceptive pill; numerous renal and renal arterial lesions; various adrenocortical disorders; phaeochromocytoma; thyroid gland diseases; the porphyrias; cerebral tumours; and a variety of very rare conditions. Pregnancy-induced hypertension ('pre-eclampsia/eclampsia') is an important but separate form of secondary hypertension; it is considered in detail in Chapter 27.

Primary ('essential') hypertension was traditionally defined as raised blood pressure without evident cause. However, in recent years, increasing recognition of the environmental, especially dietary, influences leading to the expression of essential hypertension have made this definition less apt. There is a clear inherited predisposition to essential hypertension (see Figure 5.1) as discussed in Chapter 5. This genetic substrate requires to react with a range of environmental influences for essential hypertension to develop. The existence of communities with low blood pressure, already mentioned above (see also Table 4.1), and considered in more detail in Chapter 4, shows clearly that genetic factors alone are insufficient. The environmental contributions include the total food consumption and hence increased body weight (see Figure 7.2) (Chapter 7), and high alcohol intake (see Figure 7.7) (Chapter 7). Less clearly implicated are a high intake of sodium salts and a low intake of salts of potassium, magnesium and calcium (Chapter 7). Certain incompletely characterized dietary changes associated with, but not dependent upon, vegetarianism can limit hypertension (see Figure 7.8) (Chapter 7). Exposure to noise appears to elevate arterial pressure (Chapter 6). Conversely, seclusion from society can markedly limit the normal increase of blood pressure with age (see Figure 6.2) (page 23).

**Table 1.1.** Secondary forms of hypertension

Coarctation of the aorta
Drug-induced hypertension
Renal or renovascular diseases
    Unilateral
    Bilateral
Mineralocorticoid-induced hypertension
    Aldosterone excess: Conn's syndrome and related disorders
    Carcinoma secreting corticosterone or deoxycorticosterone
    Apparent idiopathic deoxycorticosterone excess
    $17$-$\alpha$-Hydroxylase deficiency
    $11$-$\beta$-Hydroxylase deficiency
    $11$-$\beta$-Hydroxysteroid dehydrogenase deficiency
Cushing's syndrome
Liddle's syndrome
Gordon's syndrome
Phaeochromocytoma
Acromegaly
Thyroid disease
    Hypothyroidism
    Hyperthyroidism
Angiotensinogen-secreting tumour
Endothelin-secreting tumour
Intracranial tumour
Guillain–Barré neuropathy
Autonomic epilepsy
Porphyria
Pre-eclampsia/eclampsia: pregnancy-induced hypertension

There is an increasingly evident, but still imperfectly defined, association between non-insulin-dependent diabetes mellitus, hyperinsulinaemia, obesity and primary hypertension (see Figure 9.2) (Chapter 9). Other endocrine, autocrine and paracrine mechanisms involved in primary hypertension are also described in Chapter 9.

It should be noted that by far the majority of hypertension encountered clinically is primary (essential) hypertension.

### Complications of hypertension

The vascular and cardiac implications of hypertension increase in frequency in proportion to the height of the arterial pressure, systolic or diastolic.

Therapy, by lowering blood pressure, or by limiting its rise with age, is directed towards the correction or prevention of these complications.

The complications of hypertension (Table 21.1) comprise the malignant ('accelerated') phase (Figure 13.6) (Chapter 13); hypertensive encephalopathy (Chapter 13); overt hypertensive heart failure (Chapter 17); stroke (Figure 15.1) (Chapter 15); progressive renal impairment (Chapter 16); and coronary artery disease (Chapter 17).

Of these, malignant hypertension, hypertensive encephalopathy, hypertensive heart failure and haemorrhagic stroke (Figure 15.1) can be taken as direct complications of high blood pressure *per se*; they are hence found particularly with more severe blood pressure elevation. The atheromatous associations (Figure 13.1), notably infarctive stroke and coronary artery disease, are less directly, although still clearly, associated with hypertension. These atheromatous complications can be seen with more modest elevation of arterial pressure. Numerically they predominate.

### Compounding the risks of hypertension

The risks of elevated arterial pressure are modified substantially by a wide range of other influences (Chapter 20).

Advancing age predisposes to stroke, cardiac failure, coronary artery disease and renal impairment. Intracerebral Charcot–Bouchard aneurysms (Figure 13.5) and arterial endothelial lesions are more prevalent in older persons. Alone amongst the complications of hypertension, the malignant phase (Figure 13.6) is more likely to occur before the age of 60 years.

The complications of hypertension are more frequent in men than in women (Figure 20.1); in persons less socially privileged; in blacks than in whites; in cold weather (Figure 20.2); with high serum total cholesterol and with higher ratios of LDL:HDL cholesterol (at least in subjects below about the age of 60); with concomitant diabetes mellitus; with excessive alcohol consumption; and more especially, with cigarette smoking (Figure 20.6) (pages 38 and 90). Whether or not modestly raised plasma concentrations of renin and angiotensin II predispose to certain complications, such as myocardial infarction, is controversial (page 92).

### Benefits of antihypertensive drug therapy

The use of antihypertensive drugs has been clearly shown to correct the malignant phase, hypertensive encephalopathy and overt hypertensive heart failure. Controlled trials (Figure 21.1) have demonstrated undoubted prophylactic benefit in diminishing the incidence of stroke. These advantages (Table 21.4) concern those complications of hypertension related most nearly to raised blood pressure *per se* (page 108).

Despite the evident association between atheromatous (atherosclerotic) arterial disease and hypertension, drug treatment has made less inroads into these aspects (Table 21.4). Whilst there is some evidence that prophylactic therapy can limit hypertension-associated coronary artery disease and its consequences, this remains a major unsolved problem, especially because coronary disease is the most prevalent complication accompanying modest blood pressure elevation (page 107). Some extravagant claims for benefit in limiting coronary events by treating hypertension have depended on the selective inclusion of some questionable trials (pages 103–107) and on controversial definitions of myocardial infarction.

Antihypertensive treatment, the malignant phase apart, has not been clearly shown to slow the rate of decline of renal function. In part this deficiency is probably because the brevity of intervention trials has precluded evaluation of this usually slowly developing complication (page 301).

### Investigation of hypertension

Investigations are directed towards identifying secondary forms of hypertension, the detection of hypertensive organ damage, and the evaluation of risk factors additional to hypertension (Tables 24.1–24.3). The extent of investigation, and especially the search for secondary hypertension, will usually be more detailed in young subjects and those in certain occupations (e.g. airline pilots) (Table 24.7).

Thus history (Table 24.4) should always include enquiries concerning drug intake, especially of non-steroidal anti-inflammatory agents and oral contraceptives; of body weight and its changes; of alcohol or liquorice consumption; of any previous blood pressure measurements (e.g. for insurance purposes or military service); of family history; of features of past or present cardiac, vascular or renal problems; and an account of any pregnancies.

Clinical examination (Table 24.5) should note obesity and any features of endocrine disease (e.g. Cushing's syndrome, acromegaly, or thyroid disease); should seek and exclude aortic coarctation by simultaneous palpation of the radial and femoral pulses; and should comprise full clinical evaluation of cardiac, vascular, ophthalmological and renal features.

Investigations (Table 24.6) should as a minimum include urine testing; measurement of plasma concentrations of urea, creatinine, sodium, potassium, cholesterol and uric acid; and ECG. Echocardiography, both cardiac and renal, is highly desirable. As necessary, more detailed testing is pursued as indicated by the initial assessment (Table 24.7) (page 141).

### Drug treatment

So far as possible, treatment should be accomplished with a single daily antihypertensive drug. If a drug of one class is not effective, or is not tolerated, it should usually be withdrawn and replaced by another as monotherapy (page 148). However, it must be recognized that probably more than 50% of all patients require two and sometimes three drugs given together for adequate blood pressure control (page 148).

Suitable initial drug classes include, in modest dose, a thiazide diuretic in fixed combination with a potassium-conserving agent; a β-blocker; an angiotensin-converting enzyme (ACE) inhibitor; or a calcium antagonist. As necessary, a diuretic can be combined with a β-blocker or an ACE inhibitor; or a calcium antagonist with an ACE inhibitor, a β-blocker or (controversially) a diuretic (Table 22.2).

Alternative second- or third-step agents include α-blockers, hydralazine, or the centrally acting drugs methyldopa, reserpine or clonidine (Table 22.2).

### Urgent treatment; parenteral therapy

Urgent treatment is only rarely needed (page 151). Even rarer is the requirement for parenteral therapy, which can be dangerous (Figure 15.2). Oral atenolol 50 or 100 mg, or oral nifedipine 5 mg will usually suffice to achieve rapid control of blood pressure. Should parenteral treatment be justified, sodium nitroprusside, hydralazine, tri-metaphan or labetalol are recommended (Figure 25.2) (page 152).

### Non-pharmacological blood pressure reduction

Various methods of lowering blood pressure without the administration of antihypertensive drugs have been developed.

Dietary approaches include weight reduction, restriction of alcohol intake, vegetarian diets, the addition of fish oils, restriction of sodium and caffeine, supplementation of potassium and magnesium, and ingestion of fibre (Chapter 7). Physical exercise, independently of weight reduction, can lower blood pressure (page 21). Psychological approaches include yoga, transcendental meditation, relaxation training and 'biofeedback' methods (page 129).

It must be emphasized that none of these non-pharmacological methods has been demonstrated to limit hypertension-associated morbidity. Moreover their side-effects and safety remain largely unassessed (page 129).

Many authorities recommend non-pharmacological means of blood pressure reduction both to precede and to accompany drug therapy.

### Objective of treatment

The objective of treatment should be a diastolic pressure of 80–90 mmHg with a systolic of 120–140 mmHg in the absence of unacceptable side-effects (page 152). The problem of resistant hypertension is discussed on page 150.

Excessively rapid reductions of pressure and very low diastolic pressures should be avoided (pages 73 and 151).

### Cessation of smoking

Although habitual cigarette-smoking does not directly affect pressure (Chapter 8), it has severe deleterious effects on the heart and arteries, and thus greatly compounds the complications of hypertension. Smoking can also interfere with the ability of drug therapy to lower blood pressure (page 38).

All patients should therefore be strongly enjoined to avoid smoking.

### Indications for the investigation and treatment of hypertension: comparative urgency (Table 25.1) (page 145)

Malignant ('accelerated') hypertension, with retinal haemorrhages and exudates, irrespective of the presence of papilloedema, requires admission to hospital forthwith for urgent treatment and subsequent investigation.

Hypertension encephalopathy, in which confusion, clouding of consciousness or coma, with or without epileptiform convulsions, are present, is usually superimposed on malignant hypertension. Hypertensive encephalopathy requires most immediate treatment, followed rapidly by transfer to hospital.

Severe hypertension, with a fifth phase diastolic pressure above 120 mmHg, especially when accompanied by cardiac or renal impairment, proteinuria, other evidence of hypertensive arterial or organ damage, or diabetes mellitus, requires prompt and thorough investigation, and early antihypertensive drug therapy.

Mild hypertension is by far the most often encountered, and the majority of such subjects will be symptom-free. In many of these persons, the pressure will subside with subsequent visits, or may not be raised on 24-h recording. Treatment should not therefore be started prematurely.

Antihypertensive drugs are recommended if, on repeated measurements over 1–2 weeks, the fifth phase diastolic pressure remains at or above 110 mmHg and/or the systolic remains at or above 160 mmHg (the latter is more likely in subjects over 60).

Drugs should be started in subjects whose diastolic remains at 100–109 mmHg on three or more occasions over days or weeks and who show evidence of hypertensive organ damage or who possess cardiovascular risk factors additional to hypertension (glucose intolerance, previous cigar-

ette smoking, hypercholesterolaemia, male gender, family history of hypertension or its complications (Chapter 20)). Requiring emphasis, however, despite statements to the contrary, is that antihypertensive treatment limits complications less effectively in the presence of other risk factors (page 300).

With diastolic at 100–109 mmHg, but without organ damage or other risk factors, the patient should be observed weekly initially and thereafter monthly. If, after 3 months, the pressure remains in this range, drug treatment should be started. With diastolic pressures either initially, or with repeated measurement, at 90–99 mmHg, annual or semi-annual review is recommended. In such persons, treatment should more readily be begun if there are additional cardiovascular risk factors, or sinister family history.

### Follow-up

Once adequate reduction of blood pressure is achieved, review is recommended every 3–6 months. This is to reinforce advice and encouragement, to ensure good blood pressure control, and may be used to check for any changes in plasma potassium or in renal function (page 152).

### Screening for hypertension

Every doctor should take every opportunity to screen for hypertension. All practitioners should record the blood pressures of all patients on their list, and the measurements should be repeated at regular intervals (Chapter 23).

No woman should be on oral contraceptive treatment without prior and subsequent regular blood pressure checks (page 160).

---

### Reference

1. Robertson JIS. The nature of hypertension. In *Handbook of Hypertension*, Vol. 15: *Clinical Hypertension* (ed. JIS Robertson). Amsterdam: Elsevier, 1992: 1–13.

# 2
# Distribution of blood pressure in populations

For many years there was vigorous debate as to whether or not the distribution of systolic and diastolic blood pressure values was continuous (i.e. unimodal rather than bimodal) within populations.[1] The arguments appeared eventually to have been settled, since virtually all sufficiently large population samples seemed to show a continuous, roughly bell-shaped curve of blood pressure values, the curve being slightly but definitely skewed towards the upper end if the abscissa was to a linear scale (Figure 2.1).[2] Thus it became widely, if in some quarters reluctantly, accepted that no clear-cut division, other than one quite arbitrary, could be made between normal blood pressure and 'hypertension'.[1,3,4]*

Pickering in particular developed the theme that the unimodal distribution of blood pressures was evidence in favour of a polygenic form of inheritance.[5]

The distribution of cardiovascular risk, although subject to several influences additional to raised arterial pressure, as will be discussed later, is also continuous, there being no point of cut-off at which risk ceases.[6] These notions, therefore, raise crucial issues in the practicalities and economics of preventive antihypertensive therapy. At the highest blood pressure levels, there are small numbers of persons at high risk; as lower, but still above average, blood pressures are considered, there is a very much larger population in which, overall, the

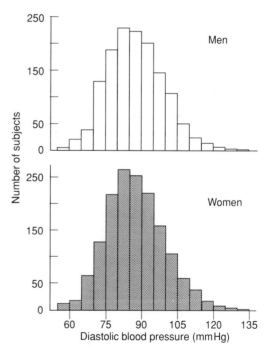

**Figure 2.1.** Pattern of diastolic blood pressures in a population of middle-aged men and women, showing bell-shaped distribution, skewed towards the upper end. Systolic pressures showed a similar distribution at higher absolute blood pressure values. (Reproduced from Ref. 2, with permission.)

---

* In English-speaking countries, people with blood pressures at the lower end of the distribution are not usually regarded as diseased, since constitutional hypotension is taken to be epidemiologically desirable. In some other populations, by contrast, associated symptoms are common; one women in 20 in Germany is undergoing treatment for 'low blood pressure'.[11]

cardiovascular risks, although distinct, are much more modest. The apparent continuous distribution of blood pressure values within populations and the corresponding continuous distribution of the danger of complications are thus central to the principles of preventive antihypertensive therapy,[3] as currently applied. In most cases, hypertension is not a disease in the traditional sense, but rather an indicator of cardiovascular risk. Although hypertension may come to light because of its adverse vascular effects, notably on the arteries, eye, brain, kidney or heart, or, in the case of secondary hypertension, from features of the disease causing the raised pressure (see later), the great majority of cases are largely devoid of clinical symptoms or signs, and hypertension is often discovered at routine blood pressure measurement.

The foregoing concepts, with which many workers are now comfortable, were established only after extensive debate and no little acrimony.[1] The comfort is, however, in part ill-founded. Notwithstanding the seemingly smooth continuous distribution of blood pressures as recorded within a given population, it has long been accepted that concealed within the curve are the blood pressure values of a small number of subjects with secondary forms of hypertension (see later), in whom the causes of any blood pressure elevation are quite distinct from those regulating arterial pressure in the majority of subjects surveyed. In other scientific fields it is recognized that an overall normal frequency distribution can conceal two or more very distinct conditions (Figure 2.2). Cusi and Bianchi[8] have now, moreover, drawn attention to the detailed mathematical analysis performed by McManus[9] on the survey of systolic blood pressures reported by Bøe et al.[10] in 67 976 persons over the age of 14 in Bergen, Norway. Despite the smooth distribution curve apparent on simple inspection of the data, it was shown that a compound log-normal distribution gave a better and more significant fit than did one that was single and log-normal. Moreover, the second distribution was composed of mean systolic blood pressure values above the ordinary range in all the various age-groups examined. This more recent interpretation of the data does not necessarily disturb the epidemiological concepts of a roughly continuous distribution of risk in relation to the height of the arterial pressure, or the corollary concerning present therapeutic intervention. However, it has, as will be discussed shortly, important genetic

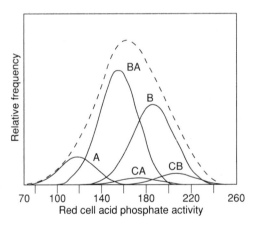

**Figure 2.2.** Distribution of red cell acid phosphatase activities in the general population (dashed line) and divided according to separate isoenzyme activities and frequencies (A, BA, B, CA, CB). (Redrawn from Ref. 7, with permission.)

implications, as well as offering the possibility of more precisely applied drug treatment in the future. There could well exist a limited number of subtypes of primary (essential) hypertension, each with different heritable pathogenetic mechanisms.[8]

## References

1. Swales JD. *Platt versus Pickering: An Episode in Recent Medical History*. London: Keynes Press/BMA, 1985.
2. Hawthorne VM, Greaves DA, Beevers DG. Blood pressure in a Scottish town. *Br. Med. J.* 1974; **3**: 600–3.
3. Gross FH, Robertson JIS (eds). *Arterial Hypertension*. London: Pitman Medical, 1979.
4. Robertson JIS. The nature of hypertension. In *Handbook of Hypertension*, Vol. 15: *Clinical Hypertension* (ed. JIS Robertson). Amsterdam: Elsevier, 1992: 1–13.
5. Pickering GW. *The Nature of Essential Hypertension*. London: Churchill, 1961.
6. Kannel WB. Hypertension and the risk of cardiovascular disease. In *Hypertension: Pathophysiology and Management* (eds JH Laragh and BM Brenner). New York: Raven, 1990: 101–17.
7. Harris H. Enzyme polymorphism in man. *Proc. Roy. Soc. B.* 1966; **164**: 298–310.
8. Cusi D, Bianchi G. Genetic and molecular aspects of primary hypertension. In *Handbook of Hypertension*, Vol. 15: *Clinical Hypertension* (ed. JIS Robertson). Amsterdam: Elsevier, 1992: 63–94.
9. McManus IC. Bimodality of blood pressure levels. *Statist. Med.* 1983; **2**: 253–8.
10. Bøe J, Humerfelt S, Wederwang F. Blood pressure in a population: blood pressure readings and height and weight determinations in the adult population in the city of Bergen. *Acta Med. Scand.* 1957; **257** (suppl. 321).
11. Mann A. Psychiatric symptoms and low blood pressure. *Br. Med. J.* 1992; **304**: 64–5.

# 3
# Single versus repeated or continuous blood pressure measurements

Most of the epidemiological and therapeutic data to be considered herein have derived from single measurements, or from a strictly limited number of measurements, of blood pressure. Such single observations necessarily provide very restricted information on blood pressure patterns.

For example, recordings made over 24-h periods have consistently shown that blood pressure values are highest in the morning, decrease gradually through the day, and are lowest at night (Figure 3.1).[1–5] This pattern is similar whether the subjects are normally ambulant or are kept recumbent over the 24-h period, although in the latter case the blood pressure levels, whilst showing the usual circadian variation, are lower throughout (Figure 3.1). Sensory deprivation, not surprisingly, is accompanied by lower and less variable arterial pressures (Figure 3.1).[4]

Since arterial pressure is normally so variable, it is remarkable how informative epidemiological and interventional studies based on isolated, or on very few, blood pressure readings have been. That such limited observations have shortcomings is perhaps less noteworthy than that they have been, and continue to be, of major value.

Given the substantial variations of blood pressure over a 24-h period, and the increases imposed by physical activity and by sensory stimuli, it is not surprising that where the relevant observations have been made, cardiovascular morbidity has been found to correlate more closely with continuous or repeated blood pressure measurements than with more limited or single readings.[5,6]

In particular, it has been proposed that there is a gradual increase of blood pressure between about 0300 and 0600 h, before the time of wakening, and that this increase could be largely responsible for the considerable incidence of stroke and myocardial infarction found in the early morning.[2]

Others have disputed this, and have provided evidence that the rise in blood pressure early in the day coincides with waking, the different times of waking imposing a more diffuse pattern over the morning hours when groups of individuals are considered.[3,4]

Interpretation is further hindered in that a stroke or heart attack may have occurred during the night, yet be noted or reported only in the morning. Thus there are suggestions, partly counter to those presented above,[2–4] that the low arterial pressures during sleep may predispose to coronary artery thrombosis, especially in treated patients with coronary atheromatous lesions.[7] These concepts are integral with the so-called 'J-curve' hypothesis,[8] which is considered further on pages 79, 81 and 108.

To cite another important issue, 24-h ambulatory monitoring has revealed, with dietary salt restriction, much more modest blood pressure lowering than on single resting measurements[9] (see also pages 29–30).

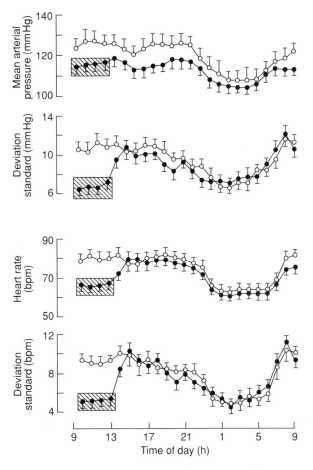

**Figure 3.1.** Hourly changes of blood pressure and heart rate in subjects who were either ambulatory during the day (open circles) or recumbent for 24 h (closed circles). The hatched area represents a period of sensory deprivation. (Redrawn from Ref 1, with permission.)

───────── References ─────────

1. Van den Meiracker AH, Man in't Veld AJ, Ritsema van Eck HJ *et al.* Determinants of short-term blood pressure variability: effects of bed rest and sensory deprivation in essential hypertension. *Am. J. Hypertens.* 1988; **1**: 22–6.

2. Millar-Craig MW, Bishop CN, Raftery EB. Circadian variation of blood pressure. *Lancet* 1978; **i**: 795–7.

3. Littler WA, Watson RDS. Circadian variation of blood pressure. *Lancet* 1978; **i**: 995–6.

4. Pickering TG. Characterization of blood pressure variations with ambulatory monitoring. In *Handbook of Hypertension*, Vol. 14: *Blood Pressure Measurement* (eds E O'Brien and K O'Malley). Amsterdam: Elsevier, 1991: 218–44.

5. Neutel JM, Smith DHG, Weber MA. Diurnal and ambulatory blood pressure monitoring. In *Handbook of Hypertension*, Vol. 15: *Clinical Hypertension* (ed. JIS Robertson). Amsterdam: Elsevier, 1992: 51–62.

6. Perloff D, Sokolow M, Cowan R. The prognostic

value of ambulatory blood pressure. *J. Am. Med. Assoc.* 1983; **299**: 2792–8.

7. Floras JS. Antihypertensive treatment, myocardial infarction, and nocturnal myocardial ischaemia. *Lancet* 1988; **ii**: 994–6.

8. Cruickshank JM. Coronary flow reserve and the J curve relation between diastolic blood pressure and myocardial infarction. *Br. Med. J.* 1988; **297**: 1227–30.

9. Moore TJ, Malarick C, Olmedo A, Klein RC. Salt restriction lowers resting blood pressure but not 24-H ambulatory blood pressure. *Am. J. Hyp.* 1991; **4**: 410–5.

# Section 2
## The development and effects of essential hypertension

# 4
# Epidemiology of essential (primary) hypertension

In Western or Westernized populations, the apparently continuous pattern of systolic and diastolic blood pressure values has already been described, with the upper end of the distribution skewed (page 9). In such populations, blood pressure also typically rises with age. The age-related increase in systolic pressure continues until late in life, whereas diastolic pressure values tend to level off, or even to fall slightly, after 50 years (Figure 4.1).[1]

This characteristic pattern of blood pressure distribution is not universal. Scattered throughout the world are communities in which the rise of blood pressure with age is absent or slight, and in consequence the prevailing level of blood pressure is on average low.[2] These communities have attracted much attention because of the possibility of identifying the factors responsible for the failure of blood pressure to rise with age. Therein could be

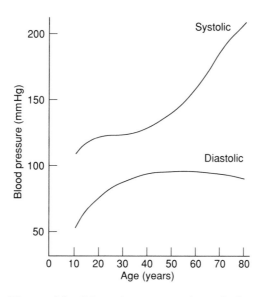

**Figure 4.1.** Schematic representation of the changes of systolic and diastolic blood pressures with age in a Western population. (Reproduced from Ref. 1, with permission.)

**Table 4.1.**   Some characteristics of communities with low blood pressure

Isolated
Small
Simple economy; often no monetary system
Physical activity high
Food supplies low
Low sodium intake
High potassium intake
Often high ambient temperature

important clues to the aetiology and prevention of hypertension in the Western world. The diversity of location of these peoples with low blood pressures deserves emphasis: they are found in Pacific islands, parts of Africa, Asia and New Guinea, the Andean highlands, and the South American jungle. Nevertheless, they share various common features, any or all of which might be relevant to their low blood pressure (Table 4.1). They tend to be isolated, small in population and with a strong intra-communal interdependence. Food supplies are short, often frankly deficient, and generally low in sodium and high in potassium content. Physical activity tends to be high. Economy is usually simple, often having no involvement with a monetary system. In many, but not all of these groups, there is a high ambient temperature.[2,3]

There seems little doubt of environmental influences in the development of high blood pressure; migration from such communities to more Westernized societies tends to be accompanied by a rise in arterial pressure. This was seen for example in Tokelauans, whose blood pressure rose on migrating from their Pacific islands to New Zealand.[3] Although genetic factors are needed, these require to interact with the appropriate environmental stimuli before hypertension develops. Unfortunately, the studies on migrants have been less revealing than might have been supposed, because on movement from a primitive to a more developed culture,

usually more than one, and often many, of the possibly relevant factors change.

Even within the UK, distinct geographic variations of blood pressure are seen. Elford et al.[4] found that men living in the south of England, regardless of where they were born, had lower systolic and diastolic blood pressures than men living in Scotland. The regional differences in blood pressure appeared to be more strongly influenced by where the men had lived for most of their adult lives rather than where they were born and reared.

The genetic and environmental factors responsible for blood pressure elevation will now be considered in more detail.

──────────────── References ────────────────

1. Robertson JIS. The nature of hypertension. In *Handbook of Hypertension*, Vol. 15: *Clinical Hypertension* (ed. JIS Robertson). Amsterdam: Elsevier, 1992: 1–13.
2. Gross FH, Robertson JIS (eds). *Arterial Hypertension.* London: Pitman Medical, 1979.
3. Prior I. Hypertension risk factors: a preventive point of view. In *Mild Hypertension: Natural History and Management* (eds F Gross and T Strasser). London: Pitman Medical. 1979: 127–136.
4. Elford J, Phillips A, Thomson AG, Shaper AG. Migration and geographic variations in blood pressure in Britain. *Br. Med. J.* 1990; **300**: 291–5.

# 5
# Genetic influences in essential hypertension

The importance of genetic factors in the pathogenesis of essential hypertension is indicated by the similarity of blood pressure values between close ('first-degree') relatives, such as between siblings, and between parents and children.[1] These similarities are usually described by correlation coefficients of the order of 0.1–0.3.

In one interesting Swedish study,[2] although the results confirmed significant correlations between the blood pressures of siblings, and of mothers and their children, no such relationship was found between the pressures of children and their putative fathers. This divergence was interpreted as perhaps indicating genetic transmission of the prevailing blood pressure via the distaff line; certainly a more prominent maternal than paternal influence. An alternative explanation derives from the circumstance that maternity is more definitely established than paternity; the differences might simply reflect sometimes aberrant social behaviour in southern Sweden.

For both systolic and diastolic pressures the correlation coefficients of the values recorded for parents and their natural children are about double those between parents and adopted children; this also holds for the correlation between natural siblings when compared with that between adopted siblings (Figure 5.1).[4] These observations again emphasize the aetiological relevance of both genetic and environmental influences.

Although the correlations found between the blood pressures of close relatives are statistically highly significant, the coefficients are low,[1,4] and several interpreters have taken this to indicate a rather modest, albeit distinct, genetic influence on human essential hypertension. It should be remembered, however, that blood pressure varies continuously and also is subject to substantial errors of

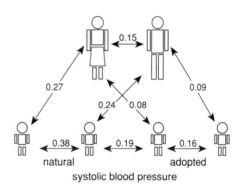

systolic blood pressure

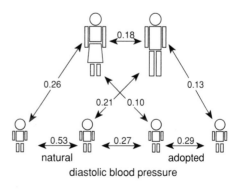

diastolic blood pressure

**Figure 5.1.** Correlation coefficients of blood pressures between family members in the Montreal study. (Redrawn from Ref. 3, with permission.)

measurement. Moreover, hypertension-dependent organ damage (for example to the kidney) can activate additional pressor mechanisms, which can then distort the effects of an initial genetic influence on blood pressure. For such reasons familial associations between blood pressure values are inevitably less close than is the case for other, more stable, measurements, such as height.

In a detailed re-evaluation of the available data, Cusi and Bianchi conclude[4] that there is a strong genetic effect on the phenotypic expression of blood pressure in man. They consider that there are probably several subtypes of hypertension, each with its different pathogenetic mechanisms and different intermediate phenotypes, all leading to the final phenotype 'essential hypertension'. These important concepts have potentially critical implications both for prevention and treatment. Hitherto, therapy for essential hypertension, pharmacological or otherwise, has been implemented largely non-specifically, with little regard to possible pathogenic differences between patients. Such essays as have been attempted in differential therapy, for example by prescribing different classes of drug according to age or to the plasma renin value, have been largely unrewarding.[5,6] The newer interpretations and developments outlined here, albeit so far embryonic, offer the possibility, long delayed, of deploying antihypertensive drugs capable of correcting particular pathophysiological faults. Such therapy should be both more effective and better tolerated. Whilst the concept of a continuous intrapopulation distribution of blood pressures has hitherto served well as a basis for evaluating cardiovascular risk, and as a guide to the initiation of treatment, greater precision and specificity should be possible in future.[4]

## References

1. Gross FH, Robertson JIS (eds). *Arterial Hypertension*. London: Pitman Medical, 1979.
2. Bengtsson B, Thulin T, Schersten B. Familial resemblance in casual blood pressure: a maternal effect? *Clin. Sci.* 1979; **57** (suppl.): 279–81.
3. Mongeau, JG, Biron P, Sing CK. The influences of genetics and household environment upon the variability of normal blood pressure: the Montreal Adoption survey. *Clin. Exp. Hypertens.* 1986; **A8**: 653–66.
4. Cusi D, Bianchi G. Genetic and molecular aspects of primary hypertension. In *Handbook of Hypertension*, Vol. 15: *Clinical Hypertension* (ed. JIS Robertson). Amsterdam: Elsevier, 1992: 63–94.
5. Robertson JIS, Doyle AE, Vanhoutte P. (eds) Age-related effects of antihypertensive therapy: the Corsendonk Symposium. *J. Cardiovasc. Pharm.* 1988; **12** (suppl. 8).
6. Swales JD. The renin–angiotensin system in essential hypertension. In *The Renin–Angiotensin System* (eds JIS Robertson and MG Nicholls). London/New York: Gower Medical, 1993: chapter 62.

# 6
# Environmental influences in essential hypertension

The recognition of a major effect of genetic factors in the pathogenesis of essential hypertension does not depreciate the critical actions of a wide array of environmental influences. The latter, impinging on a susceptible genotype, lead to the phenotypic expression of essential hypertension. Indeed, because various environmental aspects are, at least potentially, open to intervention, they offer more ready preventive and therapeutic opportunities. The strength of environmental factors in elevating arterial pressure was clearly shown by the studies on migrants mentioned above (Chapter 4). Moreover, Cusi and Bianchi, in their article emphasizing the importance of genetics, also point to the distinct influence of extraneous aspects.[1] For example, sojourn in the same household tended to induce similarities of blood pressure, even amongst genetically unrelated children. However, correlations were closer when genetically related subjects shared a habitat. The greater similarity of blood pressure of natural than of adopted siblings, mentioned earlier (Chapter 5), underscores these concepts.

The dietary, behavioural and environmental influences to be outlined in this chapter, and in Chapter 7, are not comprehensive. Nevertheless, they emphasize that, even with a genetic predisposition, the development of hypertension is not inevitable. Thus, although the term 'essential' ('primary') hypertension retains its valuable descriptive role, it should not discourage appropriate preventive or therapeutic efforts.

## Social influences

Social factors are not easily disentangled from other pathogenic influences.[2] Blood pressures are consistently higher in people from the lower socio-economic classes, and stroke and coronary artery disease are accordingly more common.[3] The poorer classes have, however, concurrently higher average body weight, greater consumption of alcohol and tobacco, and more exposure to noise, any or all of which might, as we shall show, raise arterial pressure. In Birmingham, England, blacks of West Indian origin were found to have a greater prevalence of hypertension than were Asians; the extent to which this reflects social or genetic influences is unknown.[4]

An interesting example of social factors was seen in the Tokelauan migrant study mentioned earlier. Those migrants who, in New Zealand, remained involved with their Pacific native culture, showed less of a rise of blood pressure than did their fellow-countrymen who became more integrated into New Zealand society.[5,6]

## Physical activity and fitness

Early studies in this area were handicapped by difficulty in evaluating effects of exercise independently of changes in body weight (page 26). However, Jennings et al.[7] showed that in normal volunteers, bicycle exercise for 30 min, 3 times weekly for 4 weeks, at 65–70% of maximum exercise capacity, lowered systolic blood pressure by

10–12 mmHg as compared with sedentary periods. Similar observations were made in mildly hypertensive subjects, in whom there was an average fall in arterial pressure of 11/9 mmHg with exercise 3 times weekly, and of 16/7 mmHg with exercise 7 times weekly. Most of the blood pressure fall took place in the initial 2 weeks of the exercise periods.[7] The blood pressure changes in these and other studies[8] were independent of changes in body weight (page 26), although with exercise fat was probably replaced by an increase in bulk of skeletal muscle.

In a survey of Danish men aged 40–59 years, in whom evaluation was by maximum oxygen uptake, lower blood pressures were seen to be associated with increased physical fitness, and this was independent of age, obesity or alcohol intake.[9]

## Changes in blood pressure during the normal menstrual cycle

Systolic and diastolic pressures are highest at the onset of menstruation. Diastolic pressure has been found to be higher in the follicular than in the luteal phase of the cycle; blood pressures are lower during days 17–26 than during the remainder of the cycle.[10] Similar patterns have been seen in normotensive and hypertensive women.

## Ambient temperature and seasonal variations in blood pressure

Blood pressure values are consistently higher in colder weather and hence in winter months. Brennan et al.[11] showed in the UK that in subjects with mild hypertension, both systolic and diastolic pressures were higher in winter than in summer. These differences were closely related to the maximum and minimum daily air temperatures but not to rainfall. The variation was greater in older subjects, was found both in men and women, and was seen both with and without antihypertensive drug

treatment. These data were confirmed and extended in a Canadian study (Figure 6.1).[12]

As is discussed on page 89, the incidence of adverse cardiovascular events is higher in cold weather.

## Noise and hypertension

Several epidemiological studies strongly suggest that prolonged exposure to excessive noise can predispose to hypertension in man.[13–16] Loud noise has been found acutely to cause an increase in blood pressure in both healthy subjects and patients with hypertension.[17] In subjects with essential hypertension and in normotensive relatives of essential hypertensives, the rise in pressure was a result of vasoconstriction. The blood pressure response in normotensive subjects without a family history of hypertension was, by contrast, due to an increase in cardiac output.

In patients with essential hypertension, plasma noradrenaline increased in response to noise, while plasma adrenaline and renin were unchanged. No changes in catecholamines or other hormones were seen with noise exposure in normal subjects. The acute rise in blood pressure caused by noise was not affected by either cardioselective or non-selective $\beta$-blockade, or by a combination of $\alpha_1$-blockade with non-selective $\beta$-blockade.

## 'Stress' and hypertension

The quotation marks are deliberate, and emphasize the difficulty in defining stressful stimuli.[18] Almost certainly, such stimuli vary greatly in relevance and potency from person to person and also, equally likely, from time to time. Most epidemiological studies intended to evaluate a connection between supposedly stressful events or psychiatric disturbances and sustained hypertension have been negative or at best inconclusive.[19–21] However, there is some evidence of

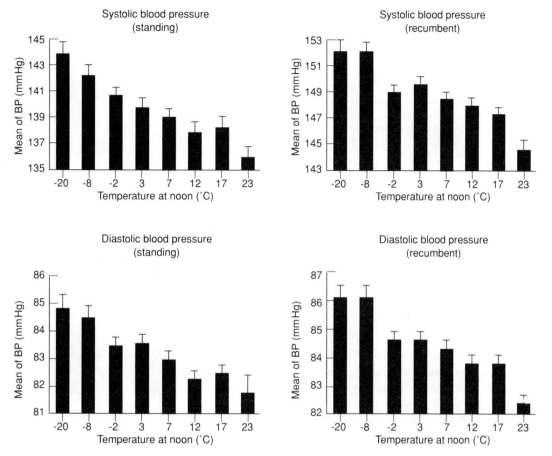

**Figure 6.1.** Systolic and diastolic blood pressures standing and recumbent according to temperature variations. Means ± SEM plotted. (Redrawn from Ref. 12, with permission.)

elevation of blood pressure with suppressed feelings of hostility or with perceived difficulties at the workplace.[22]

Converse therapeutic efforts have been directed to various behavioural interventions, including muscle relaxation training, transcendental meditation, yoga and biofeedback.[23,24] Whilst several trials have reported short-term blood pressure reductions with such procedures, convincing long-term effects have been elusive.[25] Moreover, these methods are, in many societies, unsuitable for broad-scale therapeutic application (see also page 129).

## — Seclusion and low blood pressure —

Masterton *et al.* found[26] blood pressures of 116 female long-stay psychiatric inpatients to be substantially lower than in control subjects in the same city. After a mean incarceration of 19 years in hospital, systolic was on average 28 mmHg and diastolic 12.8 mmHg lower than in the controls (Figure 6.2). Body weight was only slightly lower in the patients.

Timio *et al.*,[27] in a prospective study, found that blood pressures of 144 nuns who spent 20 years in a monastic environment characterized by silence,

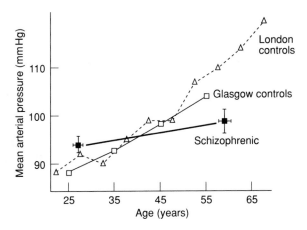

**Figure 6.2.** Mean arterial pressures in 23 schizophrenic women (earliest and latest readings shown) who were continuously in a Glasgow hospital for at least 25 years. Control values are from free-living Glasgow and London women. Bars = 1 SEM. (Redrawn from Ref. 26, with permission.)

meditation and isolation from society showed little or no increase over time. A control group of lay-women had similar blood pressure to the nuns at entry, but their blood pressure rose clearly with age. Body weight and sodium excretion were closely similar in both groups throughout the study.

These papers suggest that some aspect of seclusion from society can prevent or limit the normal rise of blood pressure with age.

## Sleep apnoea, hypoxaemia and snoring

There has been much interest in apnoea and hypoxaemia during sleep, and whether it could contribute to hypertension (see also Chapter 10). In a careful study, it was shown that though systemic blood pressure correlated significantly with overnight hypoxaemia, this was due to the cross-correlation with age, obesity and alcohol consumption. No independent predictive effect of overnight hypoxaemia was found. Snoring was correlated with systemic blood pressure but not significantly so, and

also was not an independent predictor once age, obesity and alcohol consumption had been allowed for.[28]

## References

1. Cusi D, Bianchi G. Genetic and molecular aspects of primary hypertension. In *Handbook of Hypertension*, Vol. 15: *Clinical Hypertension* (ed. JIS Robertson). Amsterdam: Elsevier, 1992: 63–94.
2. Angell M. Privilege and health: what is the connection? *N. Engl. J. Med.* 1993; **329**: 126–7.
3. Ménard J, Degoulet P, Chatellier G *et al.* Influence of educational and sociocultural factors on hypertension care. *J. Hypertens.* 1985; **3** (suppl. 2): 45–9.
4. Cruickshank JK, Beevers DG, Osbourne VL *et al.* Heart attack, stroke, diabetes and hypertension in West Indians, Asians and Whites in Birmingham, England. *Br. Med. J.* 1980; **281**: 1108.
5. Prior I. Hypertension risk factors: a preventive point of view. In *Mild Hypertension: Natural History and Management* (eds F Gross and T Strasser). London: Pitman Medical. 1979: 127–36.

6. Prior I. Primary prevention of hypertension. In *Arterial Hypertension* (eds FH Gross and JIS Robertson). London: Pitman Medical, 1979: 158–64.

7. Jennings G, Nelson L, Nestel P *et al*. The effects of changes in physical activity on major cardiovascular risk factors, hemodynamics, sympathetic function and glucose utilization in man: a controlled study of four levels of activity. *Circulation* 1986; **73**: 30–40.

8. Duncan JJ, Farr JE, Upton SJ *et al*. The effects of aerobic exercise on plasma catecholamines and blood pressure in patients with mild essential hypertension. *J. Am. Med. Assoc.* 1985; **254**: 2609–13.

9. Gyntelberg F, Meyer J. Relationship between blood pressure and physical fitness, smoking and alcohol consumption in Copenhagen males aged 40–59. *Acta Med. Scand.* 1974; **195**: 375–80.

10. Dunne FP, Barry DG, Ferriss JB, Grealy G, Murphy D. Changes in blood pressure during the normal menstrual cycle. *Clin. Sci.* 1991; **81**: 515–18.

11. Brennan PJ, Greenberg G, Miall WE, Thompson SG. Seasonal variation in blood pressure. *Br. Med. J.* 1982; **285**: 919–23.

12. Kunes J, Tremblay J, Bellevance F, Hamet P. Influence of environmental temperature on the blood pressure of hypertensive patients in Montreal. *Am. J. Hypertens.* 1991; **4**: 422–6.

13. Jonsson A, Hansson L. Prolonged exposure to a stressful stimulus (noise) as a cause of raised blood pressure in man. *Lancet* 1977; **i**: 86–9.

14. Parvizpoor D. Noise exposure and prevalence of high blood pressure among weavers in Iran. *J. Occ. Med.* 1976; **18**: 730–1.

15. Knipschild P. Medical effects of aircraft noise. *Int. Arch. Occ. Environ. Health* 1977; **40**: 185–90.

16. Eiff AW, Neus H. Verkehrslärm und Hypertoni-Risiko. *Münch. Med. Wschr.* 1980; **122**: 894–7.

17. Andrén L. Cardiovascular effects of noise. *Acta Med. Scand.* 1982; (suppl. 657): 1–45.

18. Wilkinson G. Stress: another chimera: an unreliable word best used sparingly. *Br. Med. J.* 1991; **302**: 191–2.

19. Greenberg G. Psychosocial factors and hypertension. *Br. Med. J.* 1988; **296**: 591.

20. Mancia G, Tavazzi L. (eds). Mental stress as a trigger for cardiovascular events. *Hypertension* 1991; **17** (suppl. III).

21. Falkner B. Blood pressure response to mental stress. *Am. J. Hypertens.* 1991; **4** (suppl.): 621–3.

22. Light KC, Turner JR, Hinderliter AL. Job strain and ambulatory work blood pressure in healthy young men and women. *Hypertension* 1992; **20**: 214–8.

23. Shapiro AP, Schwartz GE, Redmond DP *et al*. Non-pharmacologic treatment of hypertension. *Ann. NY Acad. Sci.* 1978; **304**: 222–35.

24. Patel C, Marmot M. Can general practitioners use training in relaxation and management of stress to reduce mild hypertension? *Br. Med. J.* 1988; **296**: 21–4.

25. Johnston DW, Gold A, Kentish J *et al*. Effect of stress management on blood pressure in mild primary hypertension. *Br. Med. J.* 1993; **306**: 963–6.

26. Masterton G, Main CJ, Lever AF, Lever RS. Low blood pressure in psychiatric inpatients. *Br. Heart J.* 1981; **45**: 442–6.

27. Timio M, Verdecchia P, Venanzi S *et al*. Age and blood pressure changes: a 20-year follow-up study in nuns in a secluded order. *Hypertension* 1988; **12**: 457–61.

28. Stradling JR, Crosby JH. Relation between systemic hypertension and sleep hypoxaemia on snoring: analysis in 748 men drawn from general practice. *Br. Med. J.* 1990; **300**: 75–8.

# 7

# Dietary aspects of pathogenesis: Implications for prevention and treatment

Epidemiological evidence early directed attention to dietary factors as being perhaps relevant to the pathogenesis, prevention and treatment of hypertension (Figure 7.1). These various aspects interrelate and therefore will be considered together.[1-4]

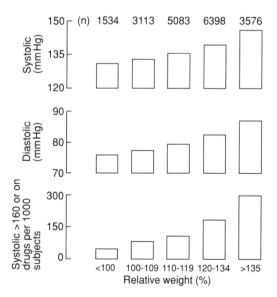

**Figure 7.1.** Data of Chicago Heart Study, showing continuous relationship between relative weight and either measured blood pressure or prevalence of treated hypertension in men aged 18–64 years. (Redrawn from Ref. 1, with permission, from original data of Ref. 83.)

## Body weight and fat

There is extensive epidemiological evidence testifying to an association between body weight and raised blood pressure.[1-5] This has been confirmed by intra-arterial blood pressure recording,[6] and is not an artefact of imprecise blood pressure measurement with too small a sphygmomanometer cuff on a fat arm, although contamination of the data could have arisen in some studies from this cause. The relationship with blood pressure holds throughout the range of body weight; the pressor influence or influences are not confined to the morbidly obese. The effect of body weight on arterial pressure is seen from infancy to old age. Moreover, children who gain weight most rapidly,[7] especially in their teens, show generally the most rapid age-related rise in blood pressure and are likely to have higher pressures in adult life.

Barker et al.[8] found that in the UK, systolic pressures of large samples of children aged 10 years and of adults were inversely related to birth weight. Whincup et al.[9] confirmed that in children aged 5–7½, systolic pressure was inversely correlated with birth weight, but only when standardized for current weight; they speculated that this could reflect the rate of weight gain in infancy.

It has been suggested that fat accumulation predominantly in the upper body ('android' distribution) is more likely to be associated with hypertension than is a predominant accumulation in the lower trunk and thighs ('gynoid' distribution).[10]

Moreover, the extent of blood pressure elevation relates more closely to central body fat than to peripheral fat.[2,11]

The effect of obesity on blood pressure is independent of other factors studied.[1] Further, body weight is additive to pressor influences such as alcohol consumption or the oestrogen–progestogen oral contraceptive.[12,13]

The cause of the higher blood pressures associated with greater body weight is not understood.[77] There is evidence of increased sympathetic activity in obese hypertensive subjects.[2,5,14] Obese hypertensives have been compared with obese normotensives and found to have higher extracellular and interstitial fluid volumes; by contrast, plasma volume, total body water and cardiac output did not differ significantly between the groups.[15] Obese hypertensives have been reported as having an increased pulse wave velocity, and thus probably diminished large arterial compliance.[16]

It has been proposed that congestive heart failure, ventricular arrhythmias and sudden death might be especially frequent in obese hypertensive subjects.[2,14] However, there is no good evidence that obese hypertensives are at greater risk than lighter subjects who have similar levels of blood pressure.[2] The relationship between body weight and hypertension-associated morbidity is thus evidently complex. For example, in the American Hypertension Detection and Follow-up Program (HDFP) study, individuals whose body mass index at entry was either in the highest or lowest groups fared worse in the course of the trial than those with intermediate body weights (Table 7.1).[17] Moreover, heavier subjects did better than lighter ones. This study is discussed further on page 103.

The results of several studies have confirmed an antihypertensive effect of weight reduction, an effect that seems to be independent of dietary sodium restriction (Figure 7.2).[1–5,18–20]

--- Sodium ---

### Dietary sodium intake

The notion that an excessive intake of sodium chloride in the diet might be important in the pathogenesis of hypertension has been a controversial issue for many years.[21–25,78] Further, there are related proposals that sodium restriction could be valuable in both the prevention and treatment of hypertension. It is our view that the pathogenetic and therapeutic aspects should be considered quite

**Table 7.1.** Five-year mortality in HDFP for Stepped Care (SC) and Referred Care (RC) participants according to body mass index (BMI) at entry

| BMI (kg/m$^2$) | Treatment group | Sample size | No. of deaths | Adjusted death rates per 1000 (SE) |
|---|---|---|---|---|
| <23.89 | SC | 1144 | 106 | 90.2 (8.7) |
|  | RC | 1045 | 142 | 127.6 (10.3) |
| 23.89–26.42 | SC | 1107 | 70 | 65.3 (7.5) |
|  | RC | 1061 | 75 | 71.9 (8.0) |
| 26.43–28.78 | SC | 1050 | 52 | 46.4 (6.3) |
|  | RC | 1141 | 84 | 73.1 (7.7) |
| 28.79–32.25 | SC | 1083 | 57 | 54.0 (6.8) |
|  | RC | 1093 | 57 | 52.6 (6.7) |
| >32.25 | SC | 1090 | 62 | 59.7 (7.7) |
|  | RC | 1094 | 59 | 61.8 (8.2) |

*Source:* From Ref. 17.

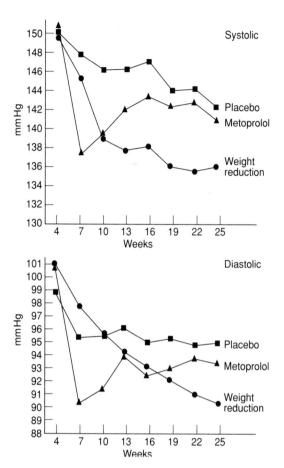

**Figure 7.2.** Changes in systolic and diastolic pressures in hypertensive obese women ($n = 56$) on placebo, metoprolol 200 mg daily, or with weight reduction. (Redrawn from Ref. 20, with permission.)

mentioned previously, in which blood pressure is low overall and shows little tendency to rise with age, generally have a small dietary intake of salt (page 18). Interpretation is difficult, however, because these peoples almost always are exposed to a range of other influences tending to lower arterial pressure.[29] Moreover, on migration from such areas, whilst blood pressure often then rises, several potentially pressor factors usually operate simultaneously, in addition to there being an increase in sodium chloride intake.[29] Thus although comparisons of different population groups have frequently shown differences in blood pressures in proportion to the overall salt intake,[30] the numerous confounding factors prevent ready interpretation.

Studies conducted within populations have usually failed to demonstrate significant correlations between blood pressure and either sodium chloride intake or excretion. There are, however, exceptions. Khaw and Barrett-Connor[31] did find a positive correlation in a Californian survey; this was closer with ageing in men, in women taking oral contraceptives, and with obesity.

One of the largest studies, the worldwide Intersalt Survey,[30] was inconclusive. This analysed blood pressure in relation to sodium excretion, which varied over a very wide range. Correction was made for the effects of age, gender, body weight, and for the intake of alcohol and potassium. The possible confounding effects of climate, physical activity and acculturation remained, however. Four isolated populations with very low urinary sodium excretion rates (0.2 up to 51 mmol/24 h) showed the lowest blood pressures. Statistically significant positive associations between sodium excretion and blood pressure were found in eight centres; insignificant positive associations in 25; and negative associations in 19. Interpretations of the Intersalt results have been varied and often emotional. Such evidence as is provided suggests to the present authors, as well as to other reviewers[2,23,32] that whilst there may be a weak influence of salt intake on blood pressure, this is less than the effects, for example, of body weight or of alcohol intake.

separately. Whilst the evidence that salt intake is relevant to the genesis of essential hypertension is tenuous, restriction of dietary sodium chloride can be a useful adjunct to antihypertensive treatment. If sodium is important in this context, sodium chloride appears to be more potent than other sodium salts, such as the citrate or bicarbonate.[25-27] However, a pressor effect of grossly excessive intake of sodium bicarbonate has been recorded.[28]

Amongst the earliest and most influential evidence was the observation that the communities

## Body sodium content

Particularly germane to this contentious issue are assessments of body sodium content. Important technically is that measurements performed in two quite different ways, of total exchangeable and of total body sodium, have provided concordant results. These studies showed that, although average values for both total exchangeable and total body sodium are normal in untreated essential hypertension, body sodium content is positively and significantly correlated with arterial pressure (Figure 7.3).[33] In mild, and presumably early, hypertension, body sodium is significantly low (Figure 7.4).[33,34] However, with more severe hypertension, and with ageing, body sodium content is increased.[33] These relationships are more marked in men than in women.[33]

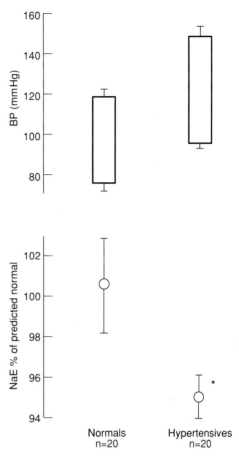

**Figure 7.4.** Systolic and diastolic blood pressure (BP) and exchangeable sodium (NaE) expressed as percentage of predicted normal value in 20 normal subjects and 20 young hypertensives matched for age, sex and leanness index. Means ± SD plotted. Exchangeable sodium is significantly reduced in the hypertensives (P < 0.05). (Redrawn from Ref. 34, with permission.)

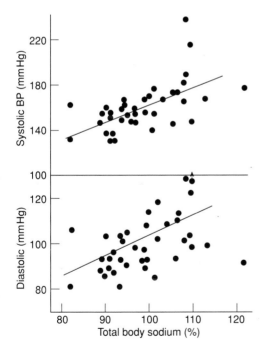

**Figure 7.3.** Relation in hypertensive patients of systolic and diastolic blood pressure (BP) to total body sodium expressed as percentage of predicted normal. Systolic  r = 0.55,  P < 0.001;  diastolic  r = 0.44, P < 0.01. (Redrawn from Ref. 33, with permission.)

Probably, essential hypertension may be initiated by a mechanism that is independent of sodium retention. Later in the course of the disease, perhaps as a consequence of hypertension-induced renal changes, there is a tendency to sodium retention.

The finding of a clear depression of body sodium in young subjects with mild hypertension (Figure

7.4) should be noted;[34] it argues strongly against sodium excess being involved in the initial pathogenesis of the condition. Furthermore, the broad-scale restriction of dietary salt intake in hypertension as a preventive measure cannot be recommended on this and other present evidence. In concordance with these concepts, Overlack et al. have reported[35] that whilst dietary sodium restriction lowered blood pressure in a group of hypertensive subjects with a mean age of 61 years, in younger patients (mean age 43 years) blood pressure was by contrast increased when sodium intake was lowered. Those reacting with a rise in blood pressure to salt restriction had significantly higher plasma renin concentrations at baseline and during sodium deprivation.

The expanded body sodium content of the usually older subjects with more severe hypertension[33] suggests that in these, dietary salt restriction may be useful. Indeed, controlled studies have shown that lowering sodium intake to the range 50–100 mmol/day can significantly lower arterial pressure at least in some patients. The antihypertensive effect of salt restriction is, moreover, more marked in older patients,[35,36] and with more severe hypertension.[37] However, while salt restriction may lower resting blood pressure, the effect on 24-h ambulatory pressure can be very slight.[80]

Although the value of such therapy is more obvious as an adjunct to drug treatment than as a measure which is effective alone, it is often worthy of trial.

Several papers by Law et al.[38–40] purport to show a large influence of salt intake on blood pressure, of substantial public health importance. These analyses gave rise to claims that modest dietary reduction in salt intake could usefully lower arterial pressure and lead to a reduction in cardiovascular morbidity, including lower mortality from coronary artery disease.[40,41] These analyses[38–40] have, however, been severely criticized as being systematically biased by the selective publication and inclusion of inadequately controlled trials, leading to spurious conclusions.[25,42] Moreover, the speculative benefits are largely dependent upon the flawed analysis by Collins et al.[43] (see pages 103 and 301) which in any event claimed a modest reduction only in coronary artery morbidity, not, as Law et al. incorrectly state, coronary mortality, from antihypertensive therapy.[41] The much more rigorous meta-analysis of trials of salt restriction performed by Elliott,[44] which, so far as possible excluded confounded studies,[42] found a very modest average 2.2/1.3 mmHg blood pressure reduction (Figure 7.5).

The contentious issue of whether dietary sodium

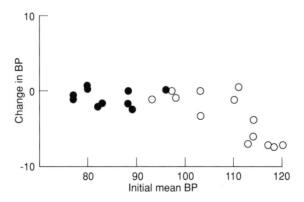

**Figure 7.5.**   Change in mean blood pressure (BP, mmHg) induced in normotensive (●) and hypertensive (○) subjects by salt depletion. Only randomly allocated controlled trials are included. (Redrawn from Ref. 42, with permission.)

restriction elevates serum cholesterol is considered on pages 90 and 304. Salt restriction has also been found to impair glucose tolerance.[82] Of particular concern is among treated hypertensives, a strong and independent association between low sodium intake and increased myocardial infarction and total cardiovascular disease has been reported.[81]

## Potassium

The epidemiological observation of low blood pressure in communities with a high average potassium intake (which is often combined with a low sodium intake) has been mentioned (page 18). While there is, therefore, evidence of a depressor effect of this dietary combination, it is not strong,[78] especially in comparison with the contrary influences of alcohol or body weight (see pages 33 and 26).

In contrast to the relationships found with body sodium, and discussed earlier (page 29), body potassium content is negatively correlated with arterial pressure in essential hypertension. The correlation with potassium is more marked in younger patients with mild hypertension.

Therapeutic trials of potassium supplementation have individually given variable but usually negative results; however, a meta-analysis of 19 such studies[45] did show a significant antihypertensive effect. The magnitude of the pressure drop has been considered by several workers to be too small, however, to be of great therapeutic value.[1,2,46] Moreover, there is concern about the side-effects, especially abdominal pain and diarrhoea, that such treatment may cause. Additionally, hyperkalaemia could result from potassium supplementation in subjects with renal impairment.

In this connection it should be emphasized that diuretic therapy for hypertension has often been accompanied by significant lowering of body potassium content in addition to hypokalaemia (Figure 7.6).[47] Such potassium depletion might well limit the effectiveness of antihypertensive therapy, and could be a reason additional to the risks of cardiac

arrhythmia for correction of potassium status in hypertensive patients being treated with diuretics.

## Magnesium

Despite suggestions that a high intake of magnesium could be accompanied by low blood pressure, this is not well-supported by epidemiological evidence.[1,2,4,78]

Moreover, intervention trials in which oral magnesium intake has been supplemented have usually,[2,48,49] but not always,[50] been negative. As with potassium, increasing the dietary content of magnesium salts could provoke diarrhoea.

However, magnesium sulphate given intravenously has been found in hypertensive crises to lower blood pressure acutely.[51]

## Calcium

Despite strong advocacy of calcium deficiency as an important cause of hypertension, and thus for calcium supplementation in treatment, the apparent importance of the role of dietary calcium has receded rather than advanced in recent years, although the interest in a parathyroid hypertensive factor, a substance with a slow pressor effect, occurring in a subset of patients with essential hypertension, and lowered by calcium supplementation, could lead to a revival.[84]

The theoretical and experimental studies underlying the concepts have been severely criticized,[1,2,4] and the results of several careful trials have failed to show an effect of calcium supplementation on blood pressure.[52–55]

It has been found that calcium supplementation does not limit the antihypertensive effect of calcium antagonist drugs.[56]

## Alcohol

There is clear evidence of a powerful association between alcohol consumption and hypertension

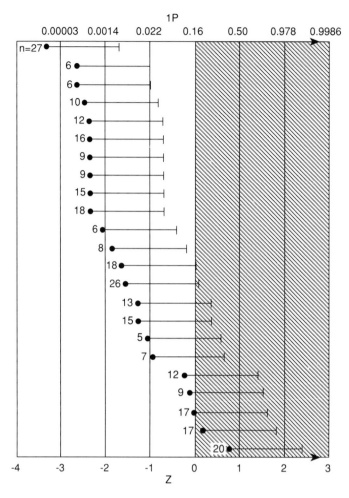

**Figure 7.6.** Omnibus test of the effects of therapy with potassium-wasting diuretics in 23 trials in hypertension on total body or total exchangeable potassium. The number of patients in each individual trial shown. Standard normal deviates (Z) and one-sided 95% confidence intervals also shown. Those individual studies in which 95% confidence intervals are clear of the shaded area are significant individually in demonstrating a fall in body potassium. Overall, diuretics lower body potassium content highly significantly ($P < 0.0001$). (Redrawn from Ref. 47, with permission.)

(Figure 7.7).[1,2,4,57] Although the relationship is seen most obviously with higher alcohol intake, it is also apparent with the consumption of as little as 30–40 g/day. The pressor effect of alcohol disappears within a few days of abstinence, an observation that indicates a causal relationship as well as providing encouragement therapeutically. Alcohol restriction effectively reduces blood pressure independently of falls in body weight. Limitation of alcohol intake could be important in other ways: heavy drinkers are less likely to be aware that they have hypertension, less likely to comply with treat-

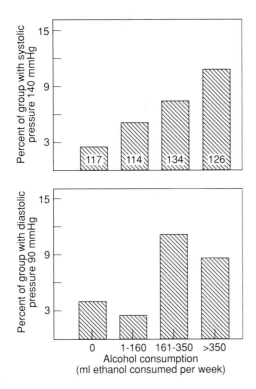

**Figure 7.7.** Percentage of subjects with systolic and diastolic hypertension according to alcohol consumption. Absolute numbers of subjects in each category given in upper set of columns. (Redrawn from Ref. 1, with permission.)

ment, and less likely to be adequately controlled with therapy.[1,2]

The aetiology of alcohol-induced hypertension remains obscure. The acute ingestion of alcohol does not alter plasma concentrations of renin, adrenaline, noradrenaline, aldosterone or cortisol; nor is there evidence of sympathetic activation.[58]

Some subjects who consume alcohol in excess resemble patients with Cushing's syndrome, and to them has been applied the term 'alcohol-induced pseudo-Cushing's syndrome'.[59] However, the reality of this as an entity has been questioned.[60] The issue is dealt with in more detail on page 207.

Other alcoholic subjects have been found to resemble patients with mineralocorticoid-induced hypertension, showing hypokalaemia and mild

hypernatraemia, albeit without excess of any mineralocorticoid substance being found.[61]

Hyponatraemia can occur with heavy drinking of beer in subjects who take little food.[62,63]

Magnesium supplementation has been shown to prevent experimental alcohol-induced hypertension in rats.[64]

Alcohol consumption has been associated with a small but significant fall in plasma calcium concentration. It has been suggested tentatively that alcohol may raise blood pressure acutely by a vasoconstrictor effect, possibly mediated by a shift in intracellular calcium.[65]

The partly contrary suggestions that modest alcohol consumption and that drinking wine, especially red wine, may confer protection against arterial morbidity,[66,67] are considered on page 93.

## Caffeine

The acute ingestion of caffeine, usually by drinking coffee, can cause a slight transient rise in blood pressure.[68-71] This is accompanied by clear increases in plasma renin, adrenaline and noradrenaline.[72] The pressor effect diminishes and often disappears with habitual caffeine administration.[68,73,74]

Salvaggio et al.[75] noted that those who drank coffee habitually had lower blood pressures than subjects who did not, and that blood pressures decreased with increasing coffee consumption. Elimination of caffeine from the diet has given conflicting results, variously being reported either to lower blood pressure slightly,[70,76] or to have no effect.[74]

The data suggest it is unlikely that habitual coffee consumption will raise arterial pressure long term. However the acute pressor effect, especially in persons unused to coffee, needs to be recognized, notably in short-term studies.

## Vegetarian Diets

Beilin and his colleagues have made spectacular progress in this difficult area.[1] The outcome of

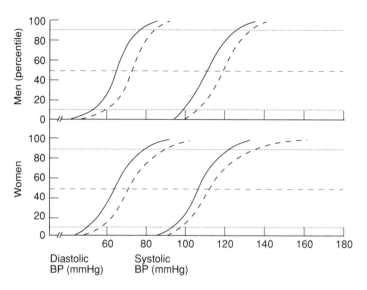

**Figure 7.8.** Cumulative frequency distributions of systolic and diastolic blood pressures in vegetarians (full curve) and omnivores (broken curve) aged 25–44 years. (Redrawn from Ref. 1, with permission.)

their studies has had, as a major consequence, recognition that 'essential' hypertension is not unavoidable. These workers[1] demonstrated that vegetarians (a term which encompasses a range of very different dietary habits) have lower blood pressures than do meat-eaters (Figure 7.8). There is suggestive but inconclusive evidence that lower blood pressures accompany increased dietary fibre intake. Changes in the ratio of polyunsaturated to saturated fat do not appear relevant. Neither the type nor the quality of ingested protein explain the differences in blood pressure between meat-eaters and vegetarians. Beilin concludes a review of the topic[1] by stating 'some combination of the dietary changes associated with but not dependent upon vegetarianism appears to be responsible'.

## Marine Oils

There are suggestive, but as yet inconclusive, reports that the consumption of diets rich in marine oils containing polyunsaturated fatty acids such as eicosapentanoic acid and docosahexanoic acid can result in lower blood pressures.[1] The potential effect of fish oils is believed to be mediated by relaxation of resistance arterial tone.

A powerful consideration limiting any therapeutic application of this approach is the pervasive unpleasant smell often accompanying these diets.

## Case study

See Case study 9, Appendix 2.

## References

1. Beilin LJ. Environmental and dietary aspects of primary hypertension. In *Handbook of Hypertension*, Vol. 15: *Clinical Hypertension* (ed. JIS Robertson). Amsterdam: Elsevier, 1992: 95–140.
2. Ramsay LE. Dietary aspects of prevention and treatment of hypertension. *Curr. Opinion Cardiol.* 1987; **2**: 758–63.
3. Swales JD. Non-pharmacological antihypertensive therapy. *Eur. Heart J.* 1988; **9** (suppl. G): 45–52.

4. Yeo WW, Ramsay LE. Non-pharmacological treatment of hypertension. In *Handbook of Hypertension*, Vol. 15: *Clinical Hypertension* (ed. JIS Robertson). Amsterdam: Elsevier, 1992: 709–46.

5. Reisin E. Obesity and hypertension: effect of weight reduction. In *Handbook of Hypertension*, Vol. 1: *Clinical Aspects of Essential Hypertension* (ed. JIS Robertson). Amsterdam: Elsevier, 1983: 30–43.

6. Andersson O, Sivertsson R, Sannerstedt R *et al.* Body fat and glucose tolerance in early blood pressure elevation: its relation to arteriolar hypertrophy. *Clin. Sci.* 1982; **63** (suppl.): 395–8.

7. Paul O. Epidemiology of hypertension. In *Arterial Hypertension* (eds FH Gross and JIS Robertson). London: Pitman Medical, 1979: 15–24.

8. Barker DJP, Osmond C, Golding J, Kuh D, Wadsworth MEJ. Growth in utero, blood pressure in childhood and adult life, and mortality from cardiovascular disease. *Br. Med. J.* 1989; **298**: 564–7.

9. Whincup PH, Cook DG, Shaper AG. Early influences on blood pressure: a study of children aged 5–7 years. *Br. Med. J.* 1989; **299**: 587–91.

10. Weinsier RL, Norris DJ, Birch R *et al.* The relative contribution of body fat and fat pattern to blood pressure level. *Hypertension* 1985; **7**: 578–85.

11. Shear CL, Freedman DS, Burke GL, Harsha DW, Berenson GS. Body fat patterning and blood pressure in children and young adults: the Bogalusa heart study. *Hypertension* 1987; **9**: 236–44.

12. Arkwright PD, Beilin LJ, Rouse I, Armstrong BK, Vandongen R. Effects of alcohol use and other aspects of life-style on blood pressure levels and prevalence of hypertension in a working population. *Circulation* 1982; **66**: 60–6.

13. Wallace RB, Barrett-Conner E, Crigui M *et al.* Alteration in blood pressure associated with combined alcohol and contraceptive use: the lipid research clinics prevalence study. *J. Chron. Dis.* 1982; **35**: 251–7.

14. Lavie CJ, Messerli FH. Cardiovascular adaptation of obesity and hypertension. *Chest* 1986; **90**: 275–9.

15. Raison J, Achimastos A, Asmar R, Simon A, Safar M. Extracellular and interstitial fluid volume in obesity with and without associated systemic hypertension. *Am. J. Cardiol.* 1986; **57**: 223–6.

16. Toto-Moukouo JJ, Achimastos A, Asmar RG, Hugues CJ, Safar ME. Pulse wave velocity in patients with obesity and hypertension. *Am. Heart J.* 1986; **112**: 136–42.

17. Langford HG, Stamler J, Wassertheil-Smoller S, Prineas RJ. All-cause mortality in the Hypertension Detection and Follow-up Program: Findings for the whole cohort and for persons with less severe hypertension, with and without other traits related to risk of mortality. *Prog. Cardiovasc. Dis.* 1986; **29** (suppl. 1): 29–54.

18. Reisin E, Abel R, Modan M *et al.* Effect of weight loss without salt restriction on the reduction of blood pressure in overweight hypertensive patients. *N. Engl. J. Med.* 1978; **298**: 1–6.

19. Ramsay LE, Ramsay MH, Hettiarachchi J *et al.* Weight reduction in a blood pressure clinic. *Br. Med. J.* 1978; **2**: 244–5.

20. MacMahon SW, Macdonald GJ, Bernstein L, Andrews G, Blacket RB. Comparison of weight reduction with metoprolol in treatment of hypertension in young overweight patients. *Lancet* 1985; **i**: 1233–6.

21. Simpson FO. Salt and hypertension: a sceptical review of the evidence. *Clin. Sci.* 1979; **57** (suppl.): 463–9.

22. Nicholls MG. Reduction of dietary sodium in Western society: benefit or risk? *Hypertension* 1984; **6**: 795–801.

23. Swales JD. Salt saga continued: salt has only small importance in hypertension. *Br. Med. J.* 1988; **297**: 307–8.

24. Swales JD. Studies of salt intake in hypertension: what can epidemiology teach us? *Am. J. Hypertens.* 1990; **3**: 645–9.

25. Muntzel M, Drüeke T. A comprehensive review of the salt and blood pressure relationship. *Am. J. Hypertens.* 1992; **5** (suppl.): 1–42.

26. Kurtz TW, Al-Bander HA, Morris RC. 'Salt-sensitive' hypertension in men: is the sodium ion alone important? *N. Engl. J. Med.* 1987; **317**: 1043–8.

27. Sharma AM, Shattenfroh S, Thiede HM, Oelkers W, Distler A. Effects of sodium salts on pressor reactivity in salt-sensitive men. *Hypertension* 1992; **19**: 541–8.

28. Lowder SC, Brown RD. Hypertension corrected by discontinuing chronic sodium bicarbonate ingestion. *Am. J. Med.* 1975; **58**: 272–9.

29. Swales JD. Dietary salt and hypertension. *Lancet* 1980; **i**: 1177–9.

30. Intersalt Cooperative Research Group. Intersalt: an international study of electrolyte excretion and blood pressure: results for 24 hour urinary sodium and potassium excretion. *Br. Med. J.* 1988; **297**: 319–28.

31. Khaw KT, Barrett-Connor E. Increasing sensitivity of blood pressure to dietary sodium and potassium with increasing age: a population study using casual urine specimens. *Am. J. Hypertens.* 1990; **3**: 505–11.

32. Alderman MH, Lamport B. Moderate sodium restriction: do the benefits justify the hazards? *Am. J. Hypertens.* 1990; **3**: 499–504.

33. Beretta-Piccoli C, Davies DL, Boddy K *et al.* Relation of arterial pressure with body sodium, body potassium, and plasma potassium in essential hypertension. *Clin. Sci.* 1982; **63**: 257–70.

34. Robertson JIS. The Franz Gross Memorial Lecture. The renin–aldosterone connection: past, present and future. *J. Hypertens.* 1984; **2** (suppl. 3): 1–14.

35. Overlack A., Ruppert M, Göbel B. *et al.* Characterization of hypertensive subjects responding to low salt intake with an increase in blood pressure. Abstracts, 6th European Meeting on Hypertension, Milan, 1993; no. 555.

36. Grobbee DE, Hofman A. Does sodium restriction lower blood pressure? *Br. Med. J.* 1986; **293**: 27–9.

37. MacGregor GA, Markandu ND, Sagnella GA, Singer DRJ, Cappuccio FP. Double-blind study of three sodium intakes and long-term effects of sodium restriction in essential hypertension. *Lancet* 1989; **ii**: 1244–7.

38. Law MR, Frost CD, Wald NJ. By how much does dietary salt reduction lower blood pressure? I: Analysis of observational data among populations. *Br. Med. J.* 1991; **302**: 811–5.

39. Frost CD, Law MR, Wald NJ. By how much does dietary salt reduction lower blood pressure? II: Analysis of observational data within populations. *Br. Med. J.* 1991; **302**: 815–8.

40. Law MR, Frost CD, Wald NJ. By how much does dietary salt reduction lower blood pressure? III: Analysis of data from trials of salt reduction. *Br. Med. J.* 1991; **302**: 819–24.

41. Law MR, Frost CD, Wald NJ. Dietary salt and blood pressure. *J. Hypertens.* 1991; **9** (suppl. 6): 37–41.

42. Swales JD. Dietary salt and blood pressure: the role of meta-analyses. *J. Hypertens.* 1991; **9** (suppl. 6): 42–6.

43. Collins R, Peto R, MacMahon S *et al.* Blood pressure, stroke and coronary heart disease: Part 2, short-term reductions in blood pressure: overview of randomised drug trials in their epidemiological context. *Lancet* 1990; **335**: 827–38.

44. Elliott P. Observational studies of salt and blood pressure. *Hypertension* 1991; **17** (suppl. 1): 3–8.

45. Cappuccio FP, MacGregor GA. Moderate potassium supplementation in hypertension: how useful? Abstracts, 5th European Meeting on Hypertension, Milan, 1991, no. 99.

46. Matlou SM, Isles CG, Higgs A *et al.* Potassium supplementation in blacks with mild to moderate essential hypertension. *J. Hypertens.* 1986; **4**: 61–5.

47. Singh BN, Hollenberg NK, Poole-Wilson PA, Robertson JIS. Diuretic-induced potassium and magnesium deficiency: relation to drug-induced QT prolongation, cardiac arrhythmias and sudden death. *J. Hypertens.* 1992; **10**: 301–16.

48. Cappuccio FP, Markandu ND, Beynon GW *et al.* Lack of effect of oral magnesium on high blood pressure: a double blind study. *Br. Med. J.* 1985; **291**: 235–8.

49. Henderson DG, Schierup J, Schödt T. Effect of magnesium supplementation on blood pressure and electrolyte concentrations in hypertensive patients receiving long term diuretic treatment. *Br. Med. J.* 1986; **293**: 664–5.

50. Widman L, Wester PO, Stegmayr BK, Wirell M. The dose-dependent reduction in blood pressure through administration of magnesium: a double blind placebo controlled cross-over study. *Am. J. Hypertens.* 1993; **6**: 41–5.

51. Winkler AW, Smith PK, Hoff HI. Intravenous magnesium sulfate in the treatment of nephritic convulsions in adults. *J. Clin. Invest.* 1942; **21**: 207–16.

52. Zoccali C, Mallami F, Delfino D *et al.* Long-term oral calcium supplementation in hypertension: a double-blind, randomized, cross-over study. *J. Hypertens.* 1986; **4** (suppl. 6): 676–8.

53. Kaplan NM, Meese RB. The calcium deficiency hypothesis of hypertension: a critique. *Ann. Intern. Med.* 1986; **105**: 947–55.

54. Bloomfield RL, Young LD, Zurek G *et al.* Effects of oral calcium carbonate in subjects with mildly elevated arterial pressure. *J. Hypertens.* 1986; **4** (suppl. 5): 351–4.

55. Cappuccio FP, Siani A, Strazullo P. Oral calcium supplementation and blood pressure: an overview of randomized controlled trials. *J. Hypertens.* 1989; **7**: 941–6.

56. Resnick LM, Nicholson JP, Gupta RK, Laragh JH. Interactive effects of oral calcium supplementation with calcium channel antagonist therapy in essential hypertension. Abstracts, 6th European Meeting on Hypertension, Milan, 1993, no. 612.

57. Saunders JB, Beevers DG, Paton A. Alcohol-induced hypertension. *Lancet* 1981; **ii**: 653–6.
58. Stott DJ, Ball SG, Inglis GC *et al.* Effects of a single moderate dose of alcohol on blood pressure, heart rate and associated metabolic and endocrine changes. *Clin. Sci.* 1987; **73**: 411–6.
59. Smals AG, Kloppenborg PW, Njo KT, Knoben JM, Ruland CM. Alcohol-induced Cushingoid syndrome. *Br. Med. J.* 1976; **iv**: 1298.
60. Jeffcoate W. Alcohol-induced pseudo-Cushing's syndrome. *Lancet* 1993; **341**: 676–7.
61. Dominiczak AF, Semple PF, Fraser R *et al.* Hypokalaemia in alcoholics. *Scot. Med. J.* 1989; **34**: 489–94.
62. Demanet JC, Bonnyns M, Bleiberg H, Stevens-Rocmans C. Coma due to water intoxication in beer drinkers. *Lancet* 1971; **ii**: 1115–7.
63. Hilden T, Svendson TL. Electrolyte disturbances in beer drinkers: a specific hypo-osmolality syndrome. *Lancet* 1975; **ii**: 245–6.
64. Hsieh ST, Sano H, Saito K *et al.* Magnesium supplementation prevents the development of alcohol-induced hypertension. *Hypertension* 1992; **19**: 175–82.
65. Potter JF, Watson RDS, Skan W, Beevers DG. The pressor and metabolic effects of alcohol in normotensive subjects. *Hypertension* 1986; **8**: 625–31.
66. St. Leger AS, Cochrane AL, Moore F. Factors associated with cardiac mortality in developed countries with particular reference to the consumption of wine. *Lancet*, **i**: 1017–20.
67. Sharp D. Coronary disease: when wine is red. *Lancet* 1993; **341**: 27–8.
68. Freestone S, Ramsay LE. Pressor effect of coffee and cigarette smoking in hypertensive patients. *Clin. Sci.* 1982; **63** (suppl.): 403–5.
69. Robertson D, Hollister AS, Kincaid D *et al.* Caffeine and hypertension. *Am. J. Med.* 1984; **77**: 54–60.
70. van Dusseldorp M, Smits P, Thien T, Katan MB. Effect of decaffeinated versus regular coffee on blood pressure: a 12-week, double-blind trial. *Hypertension* 1989; **14**: 563–9.
71. Myers MG, Reeves RA. The effect of caffeine on daytime ambulatory blood pressure. *Am. J. Hypertens.* 1991; **4**: 427–31.
72. Robertson D, Frölich JC, Carr RK *et al.* Effects of caffeine on plasma renin activity, catecholamines and blood pressure. *N. Engl. J. Med.* 1978; **298**: 181–6.
73. Casiglia E, Paleari CD, Petucco S *et al.* Haemodynamic effects of coffee and purified caffeine in normal volunteers: a placebo-controlled clinical study. *J. Human Hypertens.* 1992; **6**: 95–9.
74. MacDonald TM, Sharpe K, Fowler G *et al.* Caffeine restriction: effect on mild hypertension. *Br. Med. J.* 1991; **303**: 1235–8.
75. Salvaggio A, Periti M, Miano L, Zambelli C. Association between habitual coffee consumption and blood pressure levels. *J. Hypertens.* 1990, **8**: 585–90.
76. Bak AAA, Grobbee DE, A randomized study on coffee and blood pressure. *J. Human Hypertens.* 1990, **4**: 259–64.
77. Hall JE. Renal and cardiovascular mechanisms of hypertension in obesity. *Hypertension* 1994; **23**: 381–94.
78. Kesteloot H, Joossens J. Relationship of dietary sodium, potassium, calcium and magnesium with blood pressure. *Hypertension* 1988; **12**: 594–9.
79. Zhou C, Fan S, Zou L *et al.* Clinical observation of treatment of hypertension with calcium. *Am. J. Hypertens.* 1994; **7**: 363–7.
80. Moore TJ, Malarick C, Olmedo A, Klein RC. Salt restriction lowers resting blood pressure but not 24-hour ambulatory blood pressure. *Am. J. Hypertens.* 1991; **4**: 410–5.
81. Alderman MH, Cohen H, Madhaven S. Low urinary sodium and increased myocardial infarction and total cardiovascular disease among treated hypertensives. *J. Hypertens.* 1992; **10** (suppl. 4): 137.
82. Iwaoka T, Umeda T, Inoue J *et al.* Dietary NaCl restriction deteriorates oral glucose tolerance in hypertensive patients with impairment of glucose tolerance. *Am. J. Hyp.* 1994; **7**: 460–3.
83. Pan WH, Nanas N, Dyer A *et al.* The role of weight in the positive association between age and blood pressure. *Am. J. Epidemiol.* 1986; **124**: 612–23.
84. Hansson L, Hedner T, Jern S. The parathyroid hypertensive factor: facts and future. *Blood Pressure* 1994; **3**: 147.

# 8
# Cigarette smoking

The interrelations between cigarette smoking and arterial pressure are complex. Among the immediate effects of inhaling cigarette smoke are a rise in blood pressure and heart rate, almost certainly a result of an action of nicotine at various sites.[1-4] Gropelli et al.[3] showed that with the smoking of one cigarette every 15 min for 1 h, normotensive smokers showed an acute, marked and very variable rise in blood pressure. These authors speculated that such effects, which could elude clinic measurements made during temporary interruption of smoking, might account for some of the well-known cardiovascular complications of smoking.

However, many studies have reported lower blood pressures in persistent smokers than in non-smokers.[1-4] These associations are independent of gender, body mass, physical exertion and fitness, rural or urban habitat, caffeine consumption, and age. Indeed, St. George et al.[1] found lower blood pressures in 15-year-old cigarette smokers than in matched non-smokers.

The adverse effects of cigarette smoking are probably multifactorial. Smokers have lower levels of serum high density lipoprotein (HDL) cholesterol, and these increase after cessation of smoking.[5,6]

Blood fibrinogen levels are higher in smokers;[5,7] various biochemical markers of platelet aggregation are increased; white blood cell aggregation is enhanced;[8] and smoking appears to predispose to coronary artery spasm.[9]

Both in hypertensive and non-hypertensive subjects, smoking clearly increases the risk of a range of cardiovascular complications, including stroke, and coronary and peripheral arterial disease.[10-13]

Both fibromuscular dysplastic and atheromatous renal artery stenosis are more prevalent in smokers (pages 179 and 188–189). Several studies[14-18] have shown that the incidence of malignant phase hypertension is higher in smokers; moreover, its prognosis when treated is poorer in those who continue to smoke. Cessation of smoking decreases vascular risk.[19-21]

The capacity of antihypertensive drugs both to lower arterial pressure (especially notable with propranolol in black patients) and to limit the cardiovascular complications of hypertension, are poorer in persistent smokers.[22,23]

## Case studies

See Case studies 9, 10 and 13, Appendix 2.

## References

1. St. George IM, Williams S, Stanton WR, Silva PA. Smoking and blood pressure in 15 year olds in Dunedin, New Zealand. *Br. Med. J.* 1991; **302**: 89–90.
2. Benowitz NL. Pharmacologic aspects of cigarette smoking and nicotine addiction. *N. Engl. J. Med.* 1988; **319**: 1318–30.
3. Gropelli A, Giorgi DMA, Omboni S *et al*. Persistent blood pressure increases induced by heavy smoking. *J. Hypertens.* 1992; **10**: 495–9.
4. Simpson FO, Waal-Manning HJ, Bolli P, Spears GFS. A community study of risk factors for high blood pressure: possibilities for prevention. *Perspectives in Cardiovasc. Res.* 1979; **4**: 31–9.

5. Rangemark C, Wennmalm A. Cigarette smoking and urinary excretion of markers for platelet/vessel wall interaction in healthy women. *Clin. Sci.* 1991; **81**: 11–15.

6. Stubbe I, Eskilsson J, Nilsson-Ehle P. High-density lipoprotein concentrations increase after stopping smoking. *Br. Med. J.* 1982; **284**: 1511–13.

7. Meade TW, Imeson J, Stirling Y. Effects of changes in smoking and other characteristics on clotting factors and the risk of ischaemic heart disease. *Lancet* 1987; **ii**: 986–8.

8. Bridges AB, Hill A, Belch JJF. Cigarette smoking increases white blood cell aggregation in whole blood. *J. Roy. Soc. Med.* 1993; **86**: 139–40.

9. Sugiishi M, Takatsu F. Cigarette smoking is a major risk factor for coronary spasm. *Circulation* 1993; **87**: 76–9.

10. Doll R, Peto R. Mortality in relation to smoking: 20 years' observations on male British doctors. *Br. Med. J.* 1976; **2**: 1525–36.

11. Shinton R, Beevers DG. Meta-analysis of relation between cigarette smoking and stroke. *Br. Med. J.* 1989; **298**: 789–94.

12. Peto R, Lopez AD, Boreham J *et al*. Mortality from tobacco in developed countries: indirect estimation from national vital statistics. *Lancet* 1992; **339**: 1268–78.

13. West RA. Smoking: its influence on survival and cause of death. *J. Roy. Coll. Phys. Lond.* 1992; **26**: 357–66.

14. Isles CG. Excess smoking in malignant hypertension. *Am. Heart J.* 1980; **99**: 538–9.

15. Isles CG, Brown JJ, Cumming AMM *et al*. Excess smoking in malignant-phase hypertension. *Br. Med. J.* 1979; **1**: 579–81.

16. Bloxham CA, Beevers DG, Walker JM. Malignant hypertension and cigarette smoking. *Br. Med. J.* 1979; **1**: 581–3.

17. Elliot JM, Simpson FO. Cigarettes and accelerated hypertension. *N.Z. Med. J.* 1980; **91**: 447–9.

18. Tuomilehto J, Elo J, Nissinen A. Smoking among patients with malignant hypertension. *Br. Med. J.* 1982; **284**: 1086.

19. Rosenberg L, Kaufman DW, Helmrich SP, Shapiro S. The risk of myocardial infarction after quitting smoking in men under 55 years of age. *N. Engl. J. Med.* 1985; **313**: 1511–14.

20. Rosenberg L, Palmer JR, Shapiro S. Decline in the risk of myocardial infarction among women who stop smoking. *N. Engl. J. Med.* 1990; **322**: 213–17.

21. Kawachi I. *et al*. Smoking cessation and decreased risk of stroke in women. *J. Am. Med. Assoc.* 1993; **269**: 232–6.

22. Medical Research Council Working Party. MRC trial of treatment of mild hypertension: principal results. *Br. Med. J.* 1985; **291**: 97–104.

23. Materson BJ, Reda D, Freis ED, Henderson WG. Cigarette smoking interferes with treatment of hypertension. *Arch. Intern. Med.* 1988; **148**: 2116–19.

# 9
# Hormonal changes in essential hypertension

A variety of hormonal systems can influence arterial pressure both acutely and chronically. These systems are relevant to a consideration of essential hypertension, although several are more directly and obviously involved with a number of syndromes of secondary hypertension (see later).

The possibility that hormonal alterations might be concerned fundamentally with the pathogenesis of essential hypertension has attracted repeated attention, although so far no clear evidence of pathogenic involvement of any of the many hormones considered has emerged. Hitherto, most interest has been focused on the strictly endocrine aspects of these hormones, i.e. their actions as chemical messengers with the circulation. Although their local autocrine and paracrine functions have long been recognized, and have indeed been considered to be phylogenetically the oldest, they have been largely neglected until recent years (Figure 9.1). Increasing interest in autocrine and paracrine aspects has been re-awakened, especially in relation to the possible pathogenesis of essential hypertension.[2]

## Insulin, diabetes mellitus and hypertension

It is well-established epidemiologically that obesity, non-insulin-dependent diabetes mellitus, and essential hypertension frequently coexist.[3] The prevalence of all three conditions rises, moreover, with ageing. A pathogenic mechanism common to all three could be hyperinsulinaemia.[4,5] Whilst there are on presently available evidence alternative explanations, an attractive possibility is that insulin resistance and hyperinsulinaemia might be involved in blood pressure regulation. Young normotensive offspring of hypertensive parents, who are at increased risk of developing hypertension, are insulin-resistant.[6] Suggested mechanisms whereby these phenomena might lead to hypertension[5] include enhanced renal sodium and water reabsorption and/or increased pressor sensitivity to sodium (several authors have reported expansion of body sodium and of extracellular volume in diabetes mellitus);[7,84] heightened pressor and aldosterone responsiveness to angiotensin II; enhanced $\beta$-adrenergic responsiveness;[89] alterations in cellular transmembrane electrolyte transport (Chapter 11); increased intracellular calcium accumulation; and an enhanced influence of growth factors on resistance arterial structure. These possibilities are not mutually exclusive (Figure 9.2).

Epidemiological evidence has indicated that malnutrition in pregnancy, causing low fetal birth weight, can be associated with subsequent obesity, non-insulin-dependent diabetes and a predisposition to cardiovascular morbidity in the offspring[9,10] (page 26).

However, despite much current interest and investigation, the role of insulin resistance and/or hyperinsulinaemia in the pathogenesis of hypertension remains uncertain; for the present the frequent association of these phenomena cannot be affirmed as more than an association. Moreover, most untreated subjects with essential hypertension do not have raised plasma insulin values.

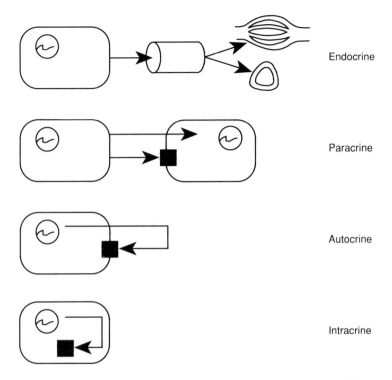

Endocrine

Paracrine

Autocrine

Intracrine

**Figure 9.1.** Distinction between endocrine, paracrine, autocrine, and intracrine hormonal actions. *Endocrine*: The hormone enters the circulation and produces its effects at target organs located at a distance. *Paracrine*: After secretion the hormone acts on receptors located on adjacent cells. *Autocrine*: After secretion the hormone acts on receptors located on the same cell. *Intracrine*: The substance acts within the cell of its own synthesis. (Redrawn from Ref. 1, with permission.)

The important, but quite separate, issues of the role of diabetes mellitus, whether insulin-sensitive or insulin-resistant, in compounding the vascular complications of hypertension, and of the interaction of some antihypertensive drugs with the stability of diabetic control, are discussed respectively on pages 92, 108, 140 and 273.

——— The renin–angiotensin system ———

Renin,[11] an enzyme formed in and released from the kidney, reacts with a circulating substrate, angiotensinogen, splitting off an inactive decapeptide, angiotensin I. In turn, angiotensin I is cleaved by angiotensin-converting enzyme (ACE), two amino acid residues are removed, and the principal active component of the system, the octapeptide angiotensin II, is formed (Figure 9.3).

Angiotensin II has a range of actions within the circulation. It raises arterial pressure via both an acute and a slower mechanism; it stimulates the sympathetic nervous system at various levels, while inhibiting vagal tone; it has several direct effects on the kidney; it can promote thirst and sodium appetite; and it stimulates the secretion of both antidiuretic hormone and aldosterone. In normal physiology, the renin–angiotensin system is reci-

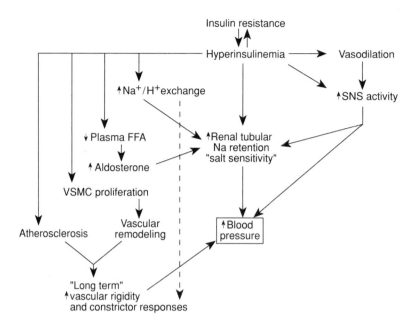

**Figure 9.2.** Schematic representation of some mechanisms by which hyperinsulinaemia could contribute to hypertension. SNS: sympathetic nervous system; FFA: free fatty acids; VSMC: vascular smooth muscle cell. (Redrawn from Ref. 8, with permission.)

procal with atrial natriuretic peptide. The neural effects of the renin–angiotensin system are also discussed on page 53.

All of these actions are directed to sustaining arterial pressure and the circulation, and the renin–angiotensin system can be seen as protecting the organism against salt and fluid loss or deprivation, haemorrhage or hypotension. For example, plasma renin is increased by sodium restriction and depressed by sodium loading.

Plasma renin values decline progressively with age, and this decline is more marked in essential hypertension. However, the sensitivity of the aldosterone response to angiotensin II is enhanced in essential hypertension, so that the concurrent fall in plasma aldosterone is relatively less marked.

Although some workers have proposed that in a proportion of young patients with essential hypertension, plasma renin and angiotensin II are raised, and thus that renin-mediated vasoconstriction could be an important pathogenic factor, the evi-

dence in favour is not strong. It seems unlikely that the circulating renin–angiotensin system makes much direct contribution to the blood pressure elevation of essential hypertension. Most patients with essential hypertension have low plasma renin and angiotensin II. The gene for angiotensinogen (renin-substrate) has been shown to be linked to essential hypertension, although the mechanisms of the raised blood pressure remain uncertain.[85]

Increased evidence suggests the presence of local tissue renin–angiotensin systems in the heart and in arterial walls. The full significance of these local systems remains to be explored, although it is an exciting possibility that such local renin could contribute severally in hypertension to thickening of the media of resistance arteries, to the reduced compliance of large arteries, and to left ventricular hypertrophy. The relevance of these changes in arterial and cardiac structure to the complications of hypertension, and to therapy, is discussed in Chapters 13, 17 and 19.

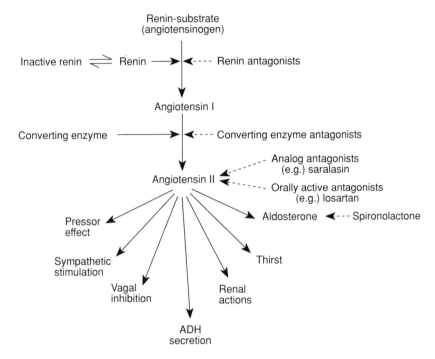

**Figure 9.3.** Outline of the renin–angiotensin system, showing some of the principal actions of angiotensin II. Also shown are sites of action of drugs antagonizing the system. (Modified from Ref. 79, with permission.)

Very high levels of plasma angiotensin II can cause myocardial necrotic lesions and acute renal tubular necrosis (Figure 9.4).[12]

A further and controversial proposal, that more modest elevation of plasma renin might be an independent risk factor for coronary artery disease and stroke, is discussed on pages 92–93.

Plasma renin may sometimes be high in malignant hypertension, although a raised plasma renin is not a requirement for the supervention of this complication. This topic is discussed in more detail on pages 65–66.

The notion that the level of circulating renin might be a useful guide to the class of antihypertensive drug to employ in essential hypertension, although advocated with enthusiasm, has so far been largely unrewarding. The marked changes in the renin system which occur in human pregnancy, and their modification with pregnancy hypertension, are described in Chapter 47.

——————— Catecholamines ———————

Plasma concentrations of noradrenaline and adrenaline are often taken as indicators respectively of sympathetic nerve activity and of adrenal medullary catecholamine secretion (see Chapter 10). The approximate nature of such estimations deserves emphasis. Values are influenced by discharge and secretion rates, uptake, metabolism and excretion, and via these by exercise, body posture, mental stress, sodium balance, smoking and age.[13–15]

Plasma noradrenaline has been shown in some but not all studies to rise with age, and this may

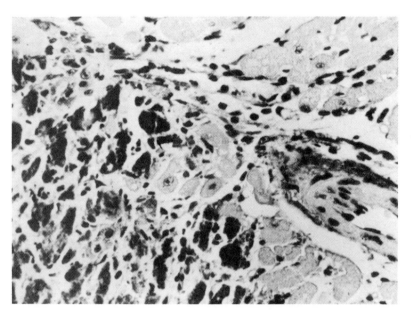

**Figure 9.4.** Myocardial necrotic lesion (dark area) induced in a rabbit by infusing angiotensin II at high dose. (Reproduced from Ref. 12, with permission.)

have suggested wrongly a causal relationship of noradrenaline with arterial pressure. This remains controversial. Plasma adrenaline does not seem to change with age, and thus reports of a correlation of plasma adrenaline with arterial pressure[16] may indicate a pathogenic connection, although interpretation is difficult.

A further attractive possibility is of repeated elevation of circulating adrenaline, released in a susceptible individual from the adrenal medulla, to be taken up in sympathetic nerve terminals, and later to stimulate neurotransmitter release, and to act also as a co-transmitter with noradrenaline. There have been speculations that such a mechanism may initiate essential hypertension.[17] Both in the rat and human, infused adrenaline can lead to neurotransmitter release and/or to elevation of arterial pressure.[15,19] However, in mildly hypertensive patients, many of whom were presumably in the early stages of the disorder, no evidence of excessive adrenaline or noradrenaline secretion was found in comparison with matched normotensive control subjects.[20]

High doses of catecholamines can cause multifocal myocardial necrotic lesions.[12]

Plasma noradrenaline can rise acutely after a stroke or subarachnoid haemorrhage, and be accompanied by transient hypertension, cardiac arrhythmias and myocardial necroses (page 71).[21]

The neurotransmitter role of catecholamines is discussed in Chapter 10.

## Atrial natriuretic peptide

Atrial natriuretic peptide (ANP; $\alpha$-ANP) is elaborated in and released from cardiac atria; higher amounts are found usually in the right than the left atrium.[11,22,23] It is cleared from the circulation by the liver and kidneys.[24] Atrial natriuretic peptide has potent diuretic and natriuretic effects, it relaxes vascular smooth muscle, it inhibits vasoconstriction caused by noradrenaline or angiotensin II, and it reduces the secretion of both renin and aldosterone. The inhibitory effect of ANP on renin release depends on normal perfusion of the kidney, and is

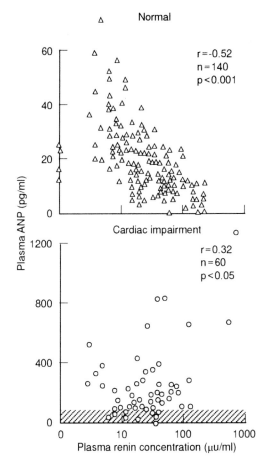

**Figure 9.5.** Plasma concentrations of active renin and atrial natriuretic peptide (ANP) in resting normal subjects with a wide range of dietary sodium intakes (upper panel); and with either treated or untreated cardiac failure (lower panel). In the lower panel, the normal range for ANP is indicated by the hatched area. (Redrawn from Ref. 25, with permission.)

lost with the impaired renal blood flow accompanying severe renal disease and in cardiac failure (Figure 9.5).[25] Atrial natriuretic peptide may also serve as a neurotransmitter (see Chapter 10).[23]

Atrial natriuretic peptide can be seen as normally counterpoised against the renin–angiotensin system and thus as protecting the organism against fluid overload. In cardiac impairment, peripheral plasma concentrations of ANP correlate with right

atrial pressure and pulmonary artery wedge pressure, findings consistent with the notion that increases in atrial pressure stimulate ANP secretion.[22,24]

Weak, but significant, correlations between plasma ANP and systemic arterial pressure have been found in patients with essential hypertension, notably in the presence of left ventricular hypertrophy.[26] This has been interpreted as showing impaired ventricular compliance in hypertension, leading to increased atrial work and a rise in mean atrial pressures.

Usually, as stated above, changes in circulating ANP and angiotensin II are inversely related.[11,25] However, both may be recruited in cardiac failure, a circumstance in which renal blood flow is depressed and thus the inhibitory action of ANP on renin release is lost.[25] In heart failure, ANP serves to promote water and electrolyte excretion, whilst the renin–angiotensin system assists renal function in the presence of a reduced renal blood flow.[11,25] Thus in this disease the normally antagonistic effects of the two systems are mutually reinforcing. Plasma ANP and renin are also both increased in pregnancy (page 240).

In addition to α-ANP discussed above, two related peptides, brain natriuretic peptide (BNP) and C-type natriuretic peptide (CNP) have been identified, and shown to possess vasorelaxant, natriuretic and diuretic properties.[23] BNP is found particularly in cardiac ventricles, where it predominates over α-ANP. BNP may be inolved in the response to left ventricular failure.[83,87]

─────────── Vasopressin ───────────

Vasopressin (posterior pituitary antidiuretic hormone) possesses both pressor and antidiuretic properties, and has been repeatedly considered as perhaps being involved in the pathogenesis of essential hypertension.[27] However, physiological variations in plasma vasopressin appear to take place at levels below the threshold concentrations required to affect arterial pressure directly.[27] Long-term exposure to elevated plasma levels of vaso-

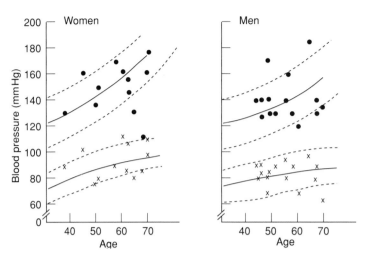

**Figure 9.6.** Relationships of systolic and diastolic blood pressure to age in 12 women and 16 men with inappropriately excessive secretion of vasopressin because of bronchial carcinoma. Also shown are mean values ±1 SD for a normal population. (Redrawn from Ref. 28, with permission.)

pressin does not lead to hypertension, as shown by the normal age-adjusted blood pressure values seen in a series of patients with bronchial carcinoma and chronic excess vasopressin secretion (Figure 9.6).[28]

However, very marked elevation of vasopressin, as following haemorrhagic hypotension, may help to sustain arterial pressure in these extreme circumstances.[27]

Plasma vasopressin values in patients with uncomplicated essential hypertension are in the same range as those in normotensive control subjects (Figure 9.7).[27,29] Plasma vasopressin may, however, be elevated in patients with malignant hypertension[29] and in cases of hypertension with severe renal artery stenosis;[30] in these circumstances, stimulation of vasopressin secretion is caused probably by very high plasma concentrations of angiotensin II.[31]

## – Serotonin (5-hydroxytryptamine, 5-HT) –

The possibility that circulating serotonin has a pressor role has long been controversial.[32–34] Little

or no serotonin circulates free in plasma, as the amine is avidly taken up by several mechanisms and especially by platelets. Thus, if it is to be invoked in the pathogenesis of hypertension by a peripheral action, it has to be released from platelets into plasma at the periphery. This could occur in the presence of peripheral vascular disease, with associated platelet aggregation and breakdown, or if the capacity of platelets to take up or retain serotonin were impaired. There is evidence that both of these mechanisms obtain in clinical hypertension, and are more marked with age. A further possibility is that endogenous ouabain may diminish the capacity of platelets to take up and retain serotonin (page 49).[35] Moreover, in the presence of endothelial damage, the vasoconstrictor effect of any free serotonin will be enhanced. It has been shown that the arterial contraction induced by serotonin is increased with age. Thus, serotonin could have a peripheral hormonal pressor effect, although this is inherently difficult to establish clinically.[33,34] The neurotransmitter[13,36] and vascular hypertrophic[37] roles of serotonin are discussed respectively on pages 54 and 83.

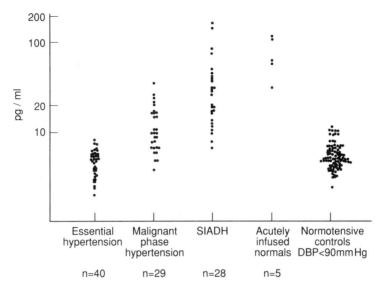

**Figure 9.7.** Plasma concentrations of vasopressin (pg/ml) in normal subjects and in various clinical states. DBP: fifth phase diastolic; SIADH: excessive secretion of vasopressin with bronchial carcinoma. (Redrawn from Ref. 27, with permission.)

## The kallikrein–kinin system

Kinins are peptides with a wide range of actions, including vasodilatation.[38-40] They are formed from precursor kininogen by the proteolytic action of kallikreins, which circulate in plasma and are, additionally, located in many solid tissues. Some kallikreins exist in these solid tissues in an active form, but most of such tissue kallikreins, and plasma kallikrein, are present as inactive precursors. The precursors are readily activated by various other enzymes, and, once active, can then release kinins. There are also endogenous kallikrein inhibitors which can bind to kallikreins.

Bradykinin is a nonapeptide which is released from kininogen by plasma kallikrein. Bradykinin is rapidly inactivated in the circulation by angiotensin-converting enzyme (ACE), which is also known as kininase II. Thus the administration of ACE inhibitors, whilst depressing the formation of the active peptide angiotensin II, could also theoretically enhance the persistence of bradykinin.[11,40] Kallidin (lysyl bradykinin) is a decapeptide formed from kininogen by tissue kallikrein. Bradykinin and kallidin show only minor differences in their pharmacological properties; they respond similarly moreover to many antagonists of kinins.

Kinins have a wide range of actions, causing arterial dilatation with consequent hypotension, cutaneous flushing, vascular permeability, pain, duodenal relaxation and bronchial constriction. Whilst the pharmacological properties of bradykinin and kallidin are such that they could well have a role in blood pressure regulation, this has been difficult to assess for two reasons: suitable assays have proved difficult to develop; and effective long-acting antagonists have also been wanting. The synthesis of potent long-acting antagonists has now been achieved.[38,41] The use of such agents possessing oral bioavailability should open up many hitherto obscure aspects. For example, the unproductive cough and occasional wheezing which can accompany the use of ACE inhibitors (page 125) has been suspected of being a result of accumulation of kinins in the tissues of the respiratory tract.[11] This hypothesis remains, however, unconfirmed. The issue may be resolved with the employment of suitable kinin antagonists.

## Reproductive hormones

Variations in blood pressure in the menstrual cycle are described on page 22.

## Endothelin

In 1988 a powerful vasoconstrictor peptide, endothelin, containing 21 amino acid residues, was identified in vascular endothelial cells, purified, sequenced and cloned.[42] Endothelin-1 is the naturally occurring isomer, and is produced in response to a range of stimuli.[43,44,58] Infused endothelin has been shown to elevate blood pressure in both animals and man. Endothelin augments the pressor response to infused angiotensin II in rats, whilst, also in rats, the ACE inhibitor captopril prevents chronic hypertension caused by endothelin infusion. In man, plasma endothelin concentration increases with orthostasis.

Whilst endothelin-1 acts mainly in paracrine fashion,[43] increased circulating plasma levels of endothelin have been reported in patients with essential hypertension;[45-47] in hypertensive diabetics, both insulin-sensitive and insulin-resistant;[48] and in hypertensive patients with chronic renal failure.[46] Plasma endothelin falls below the non-pregnant level in normal pregnant women, but is elevated to values higher than in essential hypertension in some women with pregnancy-induced hypertension[49] (see also page 244). In rats with severe experimental hypertension[50] and in patients with advanced atherosclerosis,[51] plasma endothelin concentrations have been reported to be increased in proportion rather to the extent of the arterial disease than to the severity of hypertension. Moreover, in the human studies, there was no correlation of plasma endothelin with age or cigarette smoking. Other experimental data in spontaneously hypertensive rats suggest that endothelin is likely to be involved in local vasoconstriction at sites of arterial injury rather than being integral with the development of hypertension.[52]

Yokokawa *et al.*[53] have provided evidence that human malignant haemangioendotheliomata may secrete excess endothelin and so contribute to clinical hypertension. More critical studies are needed, however, to confirm this[54] (see page 229).

These diverse observations suggest important involvement of endothelin in various aspects of hypertension, and especially with the associated arterial damage. The data are too fragmentary, however, at present for definitive presentation.

## Endothelium-derived relaxing factor (EDRF; nitric oxide)

Vascular endothelium synthesizes nitric oxide (endothelium-derived relaxing factor; EDRF) from L-arginine, a process which appears to be continuous in most arterial beds.[55-57,80,81] Nitric oxide has a vasodilator effect; it also inhibits platelet aggregation and adhesion.

Endothelium-derived nitric oxide is released in greater quantities, thus promoting arterial dilatation, with increased shear stress, as with a sudden rise in blood velocity; on stimulation by various circulating hormones, including serotonin, catecholamines, vasopressin, oxytocin, adenine nucleotides and thrombin; and in response to chemicals released in the vessel wall, including prostacyclin, arachidonic acid, histamine, bradykinin and substance P. Inhibition of nitric oxide synthesis raises blood pressure in normal men.[86]

The secretion of nitric oxide is impaired in the presence of lesions of the endothelium, and, as is mentioned later (page 63), these are more prevalent with ageing, in hypertension and with atherosclerotic disease. Such endothelial abnormalities will thus tend to promote and reinforce pressor and atherosclerotic processes, exacerbating both hypertension and the associated arterial disease.[59]

The possible involvement of disordered endothelial nitric oxide in pre-eclampsia is considered on page 244.

### Ouabain

Ouabain (earlier referred to as 'endogenous digitalis-like factor') and possibly but not certainly[88] of adrenal cortical origin, has been identified and queried,[88] in peripheral plasma.[60-63] Plasma ouabain concentrations have been reported as increased in essential hypertension in humans[64] and in spontaneous hypertension in the rat.[65]

It has been suggested that such endogenous ouabain may be pathogenetically linked to hypertension. One proposal is that a deficient renal capacity to excrete sodium in some way evokes an increase in plasma ouabain, which then, by inhibiting both renal tubular and arterial smooth muscle Na-K-ATPase, enhances sodium output directly by the renal action,[66] and also via pressure natriuresis[67] consequent upon the rise in arterial pressure. That such a mechanism could operate is supported by accounts that plasma ouabain is raised also in other syndromes in which there is sodium retention and hypertension, including aldosterone-secreting adenoma[68,69] (page 199), acromegaly[70] (page 220), and renal failure[71,82] (page 194). Plasma ouabain can be increased in clinical heart failure,[72] a condition likewise in which, despite therapy, body sodium content often remains elevated.[73]

This process could well operate in the older, and more severely affected patients with essential hypertension, in whom, as discussed earlier, body sodium content is often expanded.[74] However, it is difficult to reconcile the concept as an initiating mechanism in human essential hypertension with the observation that body sodium is significantly low in young subjects with mild blood pressure elevation[74,75] (see page 29 and Figure 7.4).

An alternative or additional pathogenetic possibility relates to the observation that endogenous ouabain can diminish the capacity of human platelets to take up and retain serotonin.[35] This could be a mechanism whereby free plasma serotonin is raised, then to have a vasoconstrictor and/or platelet aggregatory action[34,35] (see page 47).

Other possibly relevant observations are of facilitation by ouabain of adrenergic transmission;[76] of stimulation of release of atrial natriuretic peptide;[77]

and, via an increase in intracellular calcium, of inhibition of renin secretion.[66]

Increased plasma ouabain has further been reported in pregnancy-induced hypertension.[78]

These various aspects, now presenting as fragmentary observations, can confidently be expected to be considerably elucidated, and a more cohesive pattern discerned, in the near future.

An important aspect, which should not be neglected, is that the ingestion of dietary constituents containing ouabain-like substances can readily confound results.

### Case study

See also Case study 4, Appendix 2.

### References

1. Admiraal PJJ. *In vivo* production of angiotensins I and II. PhD thesis, Erasmus University, Rotterdam, 1993.
2. Dzau VJ, Pratt RE. Cardiac, vascular and intrarenal renin–angiotensin systems in normal physiology and disease. In *The Renin–Angiotensin System* (eds JIS Robertson and MG Nicholls). London/New York: Gower Medical, 1993: chapter 42.
3. Beretta-Piccoli C. Diabetes mellitus and hypertension. In *Handbook of Hypertension*, Vol. 15: *Clinical Hypertension* (ed. JIS Robertson). Amsterdam: Elsevier, 1992: 141–76.
4. Johnston CI, Cooper ME, Nicholls MG. Meeting report of the International Society of Hypertension Conference on hypertension and diabetes. *J. Hypertens.* 1992; **10**: 393–7.
5. Donnelly R, Connell JMC. Insulin resistance: possible role in the aetiology and clinical course of hypertension. *Clin. Sci.* 1992; **83**: 265–75.
6. Beatty OL, Harper R, Sheridan B *et al.* Insulin resistance in offspring of hypertensive parents. *Br. Med. J.* 1993; **307**: 92–6.
7. Weidmann P, Beretta-Piccoli C, Trost BN. Pressor factors and responsiveness in hypertension accompanying diabetes mellitus. *Hypertension* 1985; **7** (suppl. II): 33–42.

8. Epstein M, Sowers JR. Diabetes mellitus and hypertension. *Hypertension* 1992; **19**: 403–18.
9. Barker DJP. The fetal origins of adult hypertension. *J. Hypertens.* 1992; **10** (suppl. 7): 39–44.
10. Law CM, de Swiet M, Osmond C *et al.* Initiation of hypertension in utero and its amplification throughout life. *Br. Med. J.* 1993; **306**: 24–7.
11. Robertson JIS, Nicholls MG (eds). *The Renin–Angiotensin System.* London/New York: Gower Medical, 1993.
12. Gavras H, Kremer D, Brown JJ *et al.* Angiotensin- and norepinephrine-induced myocardial lesions: experimental and clinical studies in rabbits and man. *Am. Heart J.* 1975; **89**: 321–32.
13. Chalmers JP, West MJ. The nervous system in the pathogenesis of hypertension. In *Handbook of Hypertension*, Vol. 1: *Clinical Aspects of Essential Hypertension* (ed. JIS Robertson). Amsterdam: Elsevier, 1983: 64–96.
14. Goldstein DS, Kopin IJ. The autonomic nervous system and catecholamines in normal blood pressure control and hypertension. In *Hypertension: Pathophysiology, Diagnosis and Management*, Vol. 2 (eds JH Laragh and BM Brenner). New York: Raven Press, 1990: 711–48.
15. Ball SG. Catecholamines in hypertension. *Curr. Opinion Cardiol.* 1986; **1**: 622–7.
16. Franco-Morselli R, Elghozi SL, Joly E. *et al.* Increased plasma adrenaline concentrations in benign essential hypertension. *Br. Med. J.* 1977; **2**: 1251–4.
17. Majewski H, Rand MJ. Adrenaline-mediated hypertension: a clue to the antihypertensive effect of beta-adrenoceptor blocking drugs. *Trends Pharmacol. Sci.* 1981; **2**: 24–6.
18. Blankestijn PJ, Man in't Veld AJ, Tulen J *et al.* Support for the adrenaline-hypertension hypothesis: 18-hour pressor effect after 6 hours adrenaline infusion. *Lancet* 1988; **ii**: 1386–9.
19. Zabludowski J, Clark S, Ball SG *et al.* Pressor effects of brief and prolonged infusions of epinephrine in the conscious rat. *Am. J. Physiol.* 1984; **246**: H683–9.
20. Brown MJ, Causon RC, Barnes VF *et al.* Urinary catecholamines in essential hypertension: results of 24-hour urine catecholamine analyses from patients in the Medical Research Council trial for mild hypertension and from matched controls. *Q. J. Med.* 1985; **57**: 637–51.
21. Myers MG, Norris JW, Hachinski VC *et al.* Cardiac sequelae of acute stroke. *Stroke* 1982; **13**: 838–42.
22. Espiner EA, Richards AM. Atrial natriuretic peptide: an important factor in sodium and blood pressure regulation. *Lancet* 1989; **i**: 707–10.
23. Lang CC, Choy AMJ, Struthers AD. Atrial and brain natriuretic peptides: a dual natriuretic peptide system potentially involved in circulatory homeostasis. *Clin. Sci.* 1992; **83**: 519–27.
24. Richards AM, Cleland JGF, Tonolo G *et al.* Plasma α-natriuretic peptide in cardiac impairment. *Br. Med. J.* 1986; **293**: 409–12.
25. Richards AM, Tonolo G, Tree M *et al.* Atrial natriuretic peptides and renin release. *Am. J. Med.* 1988; **84** (3A): 112–18.
26. Montorsi P, Tonolo G, Polonia J *et al.* Correlates of plasma atrial natriuretic factor in health and hypertension. *Hypertension* 1987; **10**: 570–6.
27. Padfield PL, Morton JJ. Antidiuretic hormone and hypertension. In *Handbook of Hypertension*, Vol. 1: *Clinical Aspects of Essential Hypertension* (ed. JIS Robertson). Amsterdam: Elsevier, 1983: 348–64.
28. Padfield PL, Brown JJ, Lever AF *et al.* Blood pressure in acute and chronic vasopressin excess: studies of malignant hypertension and the syndrome of inappropriate antidiuretic hormone secretion. *N. Engl. J. Med.* 1981; **304**: 1067–70.
29. Padfield PL. Vasopressin in hypertension. *Am. Heart J.* 1977; **94**: 531–2.
30. Atkinson AB, Brown JJ, Davies DL *et al.* Hyponatraemic hypertensive syndrome with renal artery occlusion corrected by captopril. *Lancet* 1979; **ii**: 606–9.
31. Padfield PL, Morton JJ. Effects of angiotensin II on arginine vasopressin in physiological and pathological situations in man. *J. Endocrinol.* 1977; **74**: 251–9.
32. Vanhoutte P, Amery A, Birkenhäger W *et al.* Serotonergic mechanisms in hypertension: focus on the effects of ketanserin. *Hypertension* 1988; **11**: 111–33.
33. Robertson JIS. Serotonin, serotonin antagonists, hypertension, and vascular diseases. *Curr. Opinion Cardiol.* 1988; **3**: 702–14.
34. Robertson JIS. Serotonergic type-2 (5-HT$_2$) antagonists: a novel class of cardiovascular drugs. *J. Cardiovasc. Pharmacol* 1991; **17** (suppl. 5): 48–53.
35. Guicheney P, Devynck M.-A, Cloix J-F *et al.* Platelet 5-HT content and uptake in essential hypertension: role of endogenous digitalis-like factors and plasma cholesterol. *J. Hypertens.* 1988; **6**: 873–9.
36. Chalmers JP, Angus JA, Jennings GL, Minson JB. Serotonin and hypertension. In *Hypertension: Pathophysiology, Diagnosis, and Management* (eds JH Laragh

and BM Brenner). New York: Raven Press, 1990: 761–78.

37. Saxena PR, Wouters W. Interferences with 5-hydroxytryptamine. In *Pharmacology of Antihypertensive Therapeutics* (eds D Ganten and PJ Mulrow). Berlin: Springer-Verlag, 1990: 533–58.

38. Editorial. Kinins and their antagonists. *Lancet* 1991; **338**: 287–8.

39. Strick DM, Romero JC. Renin, the kidney, kallikrein, and prostaglandins. In *The Renin–Angiotensin System* (eds JIS Robertson and MG Nicholls). London: Gower Medical, 1993: chapter 38.

40. Campbell DJ, Kladis A, Duncan AM. Bradykinin peptides in kidney, blood, and other tissues of the rat. *Hypertension*, 1993; **21**: 155–65.

41. Lembeck F, Griesbacher T, Eckhardt M *et al.* New, long-acting, potent bradykinin antagonists. *Br. J. Pharmacol.* 1991; **102**: 297–304.

42. Yanagisawa M, Kurihara H, Kimura S *et al.* A novel potent vasoconstrictor peptide produced by vascular endothelial cells. *Nature* 1988; **332**: 411–15.

43. Webb DJ, Haynes WG. Endothelins come of age. *Lancet* 1993; **342**: 1439–40.

44. Hasegawa K, Fujiwara H, Doyama K *et al.* Endothelin-1-selective receptor in the arterial intima of patients with hypertension. *Hypertension* 1994; **23**: 288–93.

45. Saito Y, Nakao K, Mukoyama M, Imura H. Increased plasma endothelin level in patients with essential hypertension. *N. Engl. J. Med.* 1990; **322**: 205.

46. Schichiri M, Hirata Y, Ando K *et al.* Plasma endothelin levels in hypertension and chronic renal failure. *Hypertension* 1990; **15**: 493–6.

47. Schiffrin EL, Thibault G. Plasma endothelin in human essential hypertension. *Am. J. Hypertens.* 1991; **4**: 303–8.

48. Haak T, Jungmann E, Felber A *et al.* Increased plasma levels of endothelin in diabetic patients with hypertension. *Am. J. Hypertens.* 1992; **5**: 161–6.

49. Kamoi K, Sudo N, Ishibashi M, Yamaji T. Plasma endothelin-1 levels in patients with pregnancy-induced hypertension. *N. Engl. J. Med.* 1990; **323**: 1486–7.

50. Kohno M, Murakawa K, Horio T *et al.* Plasma immunoreactive endothelin-1 in experimental malignant hypertension. *Hypertension* 1991; **18**: 93–100.

51. Lerman A, Edwards BS, Hallett JW *et al.* Circulating and tissue endothelin immunoreactivity in advanced atherosclerosis. *N. Engl. J. Med.* 1991; **325**: 997–1001.

52. Takagi Y, Fukase M, Takata S *et al.* Role of endogenous endothelin in the development of hypertension in rats. *Am. J. Hypertens.* 1991; **4**: 389–91.

53. Yokokawa K, Tahara H, Kohno M *et al.* Hypertension associated with endothelin-secreting malignant hemangioendothelioma. *Ann. Intern Med.* 1991; **114**: 213–15.

54. Robertson JIS. Endothelin-secreting tumor. In *Handbook of Hypertension*, Vol. 15: *Clinical Hypertension* (ed. JIS Robertson). Amsterdam: Elsevier, 1992: 619–20.

55. Gryglewski RJ, Botting RM, Vane JR. Mediators produced by the endothelial cell. *Hypertension* 1988; **12**: 530–48.

56. Marshall JJ, Kontos HA. Endothelium-derived relaxing factors: a perspective from *in vivo* data. *Hypertension* 1990; **16**: 371–86.

57. Collier J, Vallance P. Physiological importance of nitric oxide: an endogenous nitrovasodilator. *Br. Med. J.* 1991; **302**: 1289–90.

58. Vanhoutte PM. Is endothelin involved in the pathogenesis of hypertension? *Hypertension* 1993; **21**: 747–51.

59. Lüscher TF. Imbalance of endothelium-derived relaxing and contracting factors: a new concept in hypertension? *Am. J. Hypertens.* 1990; **3**: 317–30.

60 Mathews WR, DuCharme DW, Hamlyn JM *et al.* Mass spectral characterization of an endogenous digitalislike factor from human plasma. *Hypertension* 1991; **17**: 930–5.

61. Ludens JH, Clark MA, DuCharme DW *et al.* Purification of an endogenous digitalis like factor from human plasma for structural analysis. *Hypertension* 1991; **17**: 923–9.

62. Ludens JH, Clark MA, Robinson FG, DuCharme DW. Rat adrenal cortex is a source of a circulating ouabainlike compound. *Hypertension* 1992; **19**: 721–4.

63. Hamlyn JM, Manunta P. Ouabain, digitalis-like factors and hypertension. *J. Hypertens.* 1992; **10** (suppl. 7): 99–111.

64. Devynck M-A, Pernollet M-G, Rosenfeld JB, Meyer P. Measurement of digitalis-like compound in plasma: application in studies of essential hypertension. *Br. Med. J.* 1983; **287**: 631–4.

65. Wauquier I, Pernollet M-G, Grichois M-L *et al.* Endogenous digitalis like circulating substances in spontaneously hypertensive rats. *Hypertension* 1988; **12**: 108–16.

66. Editorial. Welcome to ouabain: a new steroid hormone. *Lancet* 1991; **338**: 543–4.

67. Hall JE, Mizelle HL, Hildebrandt DA, Brands MW. Abnormal pressure natriuresis: a cause or a consequence of hypertension? *Hypertension* 1990; **15**: 547–59.

68. Masugi F, Ogihara T, Hasegawa T *et al.* Circulating factor with ouabain-like immunoreactivity in patients with primary aldosteronism. *Biochem. Biophys. Res. Commun.* 1986; **135**: 41–5.

69. Pedrinelli R, Clerico A, Panarace G *et al.* Does a digoxin-like substance participate in vascular and pressure control during dietary sodium changes in patients with primary aldosteronism? *J. Hypertens.* 1991; **9**: 457–63.

70. Deray G, Rieu MA, Devynck MG *et al.* Evidence of an endogenous digitalis-like factor in the plasma of patients with acromegaly. *N. Engl. J. Med.* 1987; **316**: 575–80.

71. Durakovic Z, Ivanovic D, Durakovic A. Digoxin-like substance in the serum of uremic patients before and after hemodialysis. *Cardiovasc. Drugs Ther.* 1989; **2**: 757–60.

72. Shilo L, Adawi A, Solomon G, Shenkman L. Endogenous digoxin-like immunoreactivity in congestive heart failure. *Br. Med. J.* 1987; **295**: 415–16.

73. Cleland JGF, Dargie HJ, Robertson JIS *et al.* Total body electrolyte composition in patients with heart failure: a comparison with normal subjects and patients with untreated hypertension. *Br. Heart J.* 1987; **58**: 230–8.

74. Beretta-Piccoli C, Davies DL, Boddy K *et al.* Relation of arterial pressure with body sodium, body potassium, and plasma potassium in essential hypertension. *Clin. Sci.* 1982; **63**: 257–70.

75. Robertson JIS. The Franz Gross Memorial Lecture. The renin–aldosterone connection: past, present and future. *J. Hypertens.* 1984; **2** (suppl. 3): 1–14.

76. Tsuda K, Tsuda S, Shima H, Masuyama Y. Facilitatory effects of ouabain and digitalis-like substance on adrenergic transmission in hypertension. *Am. J. Hypertens.* 1989; **2**: 465–7.

77. Morise T, Takeuchi Y, Okamoto S, Takeda R. Stimulation of atrial natriuretic peptide secretion and synthesis by Na-K-ATPase inhibitors. *Biochem. Biophys. Res. Commun.* 1991; **176**: 875–81.

78. Poston L, Morris JF, Wolfe CD, Hilton PJ. Serum digoxin-like substances in pregnancy-induced hypertension. *Clin. Sci.* 1989; **77**: 189–94.

79. Robertson JIS, Ball SG. Hypertension. In *Diseases of the Heart*, 1st edn (eds DG Julian, AJ Camm, KM Fox *et al.*). London: Baillière Tindall, 1989: 1227–92.

80. Moncada S, Higgs A. The l-arginine–nitric oxide pathway. *New Engl. J. Med.* 1993; **329**: 2002–12.

81. Anggard E. Nitric oxide: mediator, murderer and medicine. *Lancet* 1994; **343**: 1199–206.

82. Yamada K, Goto A, Nagoshi H *et al.* Participation of ouabain-like compound in reduced renal mass-saline hypertension. *Hypertension* 1994; **23** (suppl. 1): 110–13.

83. Davis M, Espiner E, Richards G *et al.* Brain natriuretic peptide in assessment of acute dyspnoea. *Lancet* 1994; **346**: 440–4.

84. Endre T, Mattiasson I, Berglund G *et al.* Insulin and renal sodium retention in hypertension-prone men. *Hypertension* 1994; **23**: 313–19.

85. Caulfield M, Lavender P, Farrall M *et al.* Linkage of the angiotensinogen gene to essential hypertension. *New Engl. J. Med.* 1994; **330**: 1629–33.

86. Haynes WG, Noon JP *et al.* Inhibition of nitric oxide synthesis raises blood pressure in healthy humans. *J. Hypertens.* 1993; **11**: 1375–80.

87. Lang CC, Motwani JG, Rahman AR *et al.* Effect of angiotensin-converting enzyme on plasma brain natriuretic peptide levels in patients with heart failure. *Clin. Sci.* 1992; **83**: 143–7.

88. Doris PA, Jenkins LA, Stocco DM. Is ouabain an authentic endogenous mammalian substance derived from the adrenal? *Hypertension* 1994; **23**: 632–6.

89. Gros R, Bonkowski KR, Feldman RD. Human insulin-mediated enhancement of vascular β-adrenergic responsiveness. *Hypertension* 1994; **23**: 551–5.

# 10
# The nervous system and blood pressure control

The central nervous system (CNS) plays a critical role in the regulation of the cardiovascular system.[1,2] However, evidence that an abnormality of central nervous function in any way accounts for essential hypertension is not forthcoming. Nevertheless, even if not directly implicated as a cause, the CNS fails in essential hypertension to correct the raised pressure, in spite of the ability of the CNS to affect profoundly cardiac output and peripheral resistance. Although certain structural nervous abnormalities, for example cerebral tumours (see Chapters 15, 44 and 45) may lead to raised blood pressure, these are rare causes of hypertension. No anatomical CNS abnormality is found in the majority of instances of raised blood pressure. The association between emotional stress and high pressure readings is dealt with elsewhere (Chapter 6).

There is a rapidly expanding growth in knowledge of central nervous cardiovascular regulation. Clearly the autonomic nervous system both centrally and peripherally plays a major role in circulatory control.[3,7] (See also page 43.) Whilst we continue to understand more of the complex relations between various areas of this system, we are left still with a bewildering array of complex pathways utilizing a multitude of transmitter substances.

## Role of the brainstem and hypothalamus

The nucleus of the tractus solitarius (NTS) lies in the dorsal medulla (Figure 10.1) and receives input from the peripheral baroreceptors and from numerous regulatory nuclei of the brain. Pathways from the NTS project on to the rostro-ventral lateral medulla (RVLM) which contains the $C_1$ adrenaline neurones linked to both the preganglionic sympathetic neurones in the intermediolateral columns and the AV3V ('antero ventral third ventricle region' of the anterior hypothalamus) region of the forebrain. Stimulation of the $C_1$ area raises blood pressure and heart rate through sympathetic activity. Lesions of the AV3V decrease pressure and prevent the expression of raised blood pressure in many animal models although not in the spontaneously hypertensive rat.

Some neurones in the AV3V region contain atrial natriuretic peptide (see Chapter 9) and lesions of this region have been associated with abnormalities of sodium and water excretion.

Caudal to the $C_1$ area are the $A_1$ noradrenaline-containing neurones. Stimulation of these lowers blood pressure by inhibiting sympathetic activity. This action is not direct but appears at least in part to go through the rostro-ventral lateral medulla. The dorsal motor nucleus of the vagus (DMVN) and the nucleus ambiguus (NA) are involved with cardiovascular parasympathetic activity but also have other complex interrelations with other nuclei.

The area postrema overlies the NTS and gives access to circulating substances because of the deficient blood–brain barrier, supporting the concept of circulating hormones (such as angiotensin II) influencing the central regulation of the circulation.

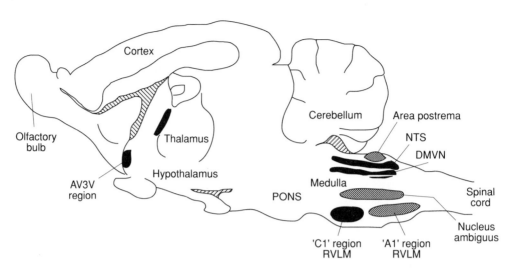

**Figure 10.1.** Diagram of a longitudinal section of a mammalian brain, showing some of the centres affecting blood pressure. See text for details..

## Neurotransmitters

The 'classic' neurotransmitters of the autonomic nervous system are acetylcholine and noradrenaline. However, other catecholamines such as adrenaline and dopamine may also act as transmitters.[4,5] Moreover, numerous non-adrenergic and non-cholinergic neurones exist within the central nervous system and at the level of the blood vessel. Transmitter substances include the amines such as serotonin (5-hydroxytryptamine), the excitatory amino acid glutamate and the inhibitory amino acid α-aminobutyric acid, atrial natriuretic peptide, and the purines. In addition, an extensive array of peptides containing up to 40 amino acid residues has been shown to be associated with various established or putative neurotransmitters (Table 10.1).

The classic concept of one neurotransmitter for each type of neurone no longer holds. Neurones can be defined by from 2 to 6 substances. Knowledge of the distribution of these proposed neurotransmitters far outweighs any understanding of their function and particularly of their relevance to blood pressure control. The proportions of putative transmitter substances in single nerve fibres appear to vary among different organs, species and physiological conditions. However, it is not clear to what extent such differences indicate lack of precision and sensitivity of techniques of identification, rather than reflecting truly physiologically relevant distinctions.

The expansion of knowledge of the diversity of neurotransmitters and hence of neurones possessing apparently distinct chemical coding has provided new impetus to long-continued studies which have concentrated on the topographical location of pressor and depressor pathways within the central nervous system and especially within the brainstem. The rapid development of this field offers the promise of antihypertensive drug design with the specific purpose of altering the actions of the heart, blood vessels and endocrine, paracrine or autocrine glands.

## Baroreflex Function

It is now increasingly accepted that the arterial and cardiac baroreceptors, whose efferent function is variously mediated by changes in autonomic nervous activity,[3] and possibly hormonal secretion, are concerned principally with short-term circulatory control, i.e. over seconds and minutes. The baroreceptors, however, have little influence on the long-term level of the prevailing tessitura of blood

**Table 10.1.** 'Classical' neurotransmitters and some associated peptides

| Transmitter | Associated peptides |
| --- | --- |
| Acetylcholine | Calcitonin gene-related peptide |
| | Vasoactive intestinal polypeptide |
| | Substance P |
| | Enkephalin |
| | Galanin |
| Noradrenaline | Neuropeptide Y |
| | Vasopressin |
| | Enkephalin |
| Adrenaline | Neuropeptide Y |
| | Substance P |
| | Neurotensin |
| Dopamine | Cholecystokinin |
| | Neurotensin |
| 5-Hydroxytryptamine (serotonin) | Substance P |
| | Thyrotrophin releasing hormone |
| | Cholecystokinin |
| | Enkephalin |
| α-Aminobutyric acid | Neuropeptide Y |
| | Cholecystokinin |
| | Vasoactive intestinal polypeptide |
| | Enkephalin |
| | Somatostatin |
| | Substance P |
| | Galanin |
| Glycine | Neurotensin |

**Table 10.2.** Neurogenic hypertension

Acute stroke
Intracranial tumour
Quadriplegia
Severe head injury
Guillain Barré syndrome
Encephalitis
'Autonomic' epilepsy
Sleep apnoea of central origin

of the thoraco-lumbar sympathetic outflow remove central nervous control and lead to systemic hypertension. Particularly in quadriplegic patients bladder distension can cause marked blood pressure elevation (autonomic hyperreflexia). Elevation of blood pressure through a central mechanism may be seen after carotid endarterectomy. A causative association between sleep apnoea and hypertension is accepted by some writers (page 24); this could also be regarded as a form of neurogenic hypertension.

pressure, i.e. that range in which pressure mostly lies, because their discharge threshold is adjusted to major shifts in resting blood pressure.[6]

## Various neurological disorders and blood pressure (Table 10.2)

Hypertension has been reported with Guillain–Barré syndrome (Chapter 44), encephalitis, and 'autonomic' epilepsy (page 219). There may be marked increases in blood pressure after a stroke for a period of hours to days (the 'Cushing reflex or effect'; pages 71, 150 and 231). With severely raised intracranial pressure, hypertension associated with bradycardia can occur. Intra-cranial tumours especially if in the posterior fossa may raise blood pressure and can cause confusion with phaeochromocytoma (see Chapter 45). Transverse lesions in the cervical spinal cord above the origins

─────────── References ───────────

1. Zanchetti A, Tarazi RC (eds). Neural mechanisms of cardiovascular regulation. *Handbook of Hypertension*, Vol. 8: *Pathophysiology of Hypertension: Regulatory Mechanisms*. Amsterdam: Elsevier, 1986: 1–277.
2. Wyss JM, Oparil S, Chen Y-F. The role of the central nervous system in hypertension. In *Hypertension: Pathophysiology, Diagnosis and Management* (eds JH Laragh, BM Brenner). New York: Raven, 1990: 679–701.
3. Julius S. Abnormalities of autonomic control in human hypertension. *Cardiovasc. Drugs Therap.* 1994; **8**: 11–20.
4. Hökfelt T, Millhorn K, Seroogy K *et al*. Coexistence of peptides with classical neurotransmitters. *Experientia* 1987; **43**: 768–70.
5. Robertson JIS, Ball SG. Hypertension. In *Diseases of the Heart*, 1st edn (eds DG Julian, AJ Camm, KM Fox *et al*.). London: Baillière Tindall, 1989: 1227–92.
6. Korner PI. Integrative neurohumoral control of the circulation. *Australian Soc. Exp. Biol. Proc.* 1988; **1**: 151–8.
7. Kjeldsen SE, Zweifler AJ, Petrin J *et al*. Sympathetic nervous involvement in essential hypertension: increased platelet noradrenaline coincides with decreased β-adrenoreceptor responsiveness. *Blood Pressure* 1994; **3**: 164–71.

# 11
# Abnormalities of cellular transmembrane electrolyte transport

Processes of ion transport across cell membranes, and especially of sodium, potassium and calcium, have been extensively studied in both clinical and experimental hypertension.[1-4] The principal aims of these endeavours have been to identify and elucidate distortions or abnormalities of the transmembrane transport systems, particularly in vascular smooth muscle and renal tubular epithelium, which could be involved in the pathogenesis of systemic hypertension. Because blood cells are those most readily available, erythrocytes, leucocytes and platelets have been more often examined, with the assumption, implicit or (less often) explicit, that a generalized membrane transport abnormality could be recognized in this haematological material, and would reflect, more or less faithfully, a more pathogenically relevant abnormality in cells of the kidney.[5,6] A further possible application of such studies could be to identify abnormalities with a particular genetic basis.[1] This latter approach has so far been most fruitful in the study of inherited hypertension in rat models.

One widely espoused hypothesis concerning the pathogenesis of essential hypertension, and which was mentioned in connection with endogenous ouabain (page 49), is that an abnormality of sodium/potassium transport at cell membranes could lead to cellular sodium overload, with consequent cellular calcium overload.[7] In vascular smooth muscle this would then enhance contractility and hence raise arterial pressure. An alternative hypothesis is that there might exist a primary abnormality leading more immediately to increased intracellular calcium.[6]

In human essential hypertension, the transmembrane ionic transport systems which have been most studied are the sodium/potassium pump, the frusemide-sensitive sodium/potassium co-transport system, sodium/lithium countertransport, and the sodium/hydrogen antiport (Figure 11.1). Amongst the extensive literature which has accumulated around these topics some brief comments can be entered here.

Examination of pooled data[8] indicates that, as a group, hypertensives exhibit enhanced sodium concentration in erythrocytes and, more consistently, in leucocytes. These observations might reflect decreased maximum sodium–potassium pump activity in these cells, possibly restricted to specific groups of patients.

There is extensive, but not wholly consistent, information showing that sodium/potassium co-transport differs in some groups of patients with essential hypertension from that in normal subjects.[6,9]

Extensive evidence[6] attests to the initial reaction velocity of the sodium/lithium countertransport being increased in many patients with essential hypertension.

There are several reports of increased activity of the sodium/hydrogen antiport when intracellular calcium concentration is raised.[6] It has also been reported that the platelets of patients with essential hypertension manifest hyperactivity of the sodium/hydrogen antiport.[10] However, the critical question of whether or not the platelets of patients with essential hypertension have a raised calcium content and a differential membrane stabilization

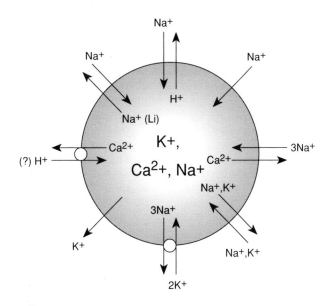

**Figure 11.1.** Sodium, potassium and calcium transport pathways across the cell membrane. (Redrawn from Ref. 6, with permission.)

by calcium as compared with controls is disputed.[11,12] Dean *et al.*[13] have found that plasma membrane $Ca^{2+}$-ATPase is decreased as a function of diastolic pressure, and that this could cause elevation of cytoplasmic calcium and enhancement of platelet sensitivity.

Despite the intense effort expended in studies of ion transport across cell membranes in hypertension, so far no unifying concepts in humans that should have reflected any widespread functional tissue disturbances perhaps responsible for increases in blood pressure in response to the relevant environmental stimuli have been attained. Although, as Bianchi especially has pointed out,[1] such studies were soundly based, they have not thus far been useful in the classification of patients or in providing the expected insight at the cellular level into the fundamental pathophysiology of essential hypertension. However, the employment of these approaches in animal models, in which the genetic background can be more easily controlled, has been valuable in identifying abnormalities linked with particular genotypes.[14]

Despite disappointments and reservations, these avenues continue to be pursued with enthusiasm, and still offer the possibility of enhanced understanding of pathophysiology in hypertension.

—————— References ——————

1. Bianchi G. Ion transport across blood cell membranes in essential hypertension. *Curr. Opinion Cardiol.* 1986; **1**: 634–9.
2. Bing RF, Heagerty AM, Thurston H, Swales JD. Ion transport in hypertension: are changes in the cell membrane responsible? *Clin. Sci.* 1986; **71**: 225–30.
3. Rosskopf D, Düsing R, Siffert W. Membrane sodium-proton exchanges and primary hypertension. *Hypertension* 1993; **21**: 607–17.
4. Postnov YV. An approach to the explanation of cell membrane alteration in primary hypertension. *Hypertension* 1990; **15**: 332–7.
5. Baudouin-Legros M, Cloix J-F, Crabos M *et al.* Membrane markers of arterial hypertension. In *Handbook of Hypertension*, Vol. 8: *Pathophysiology of Hypertension—Regulatory Mechanisms* (eds A Zanchetti and RC Tarazi). Amsterdam: Elsevier, 1986: 670–86.

6. Aviv A, Lasker N. Proposed defects in membrane transport and intracellular ions as pathogenic factors in essential hypertension. In *Hypertension: Pathophysiology, Diagnosis and Management* (eds JH Laragh and BM Brenner). New York: Raven Press, 1990: 923–37.

7. de Wardener HE. The primary role of the kidney and salt intake in the aetiology of essential hypertension: part II. *Clin. Sci.* 1990; **79**: 289–97.

8. Hilton PJ. Cellular sodium transport in essential hypertension. *N. Engl. J. Med.* 1986; **314**: 222–9.

9. Garay RP, Dagher G, Pernollet MG *et al.* Inherited defect in a $Na^+$-$K^+$ cotransport system in erythrocytes from essential hypertensive patients. *Nature* 1980; **284**: 281–3.

10. Livne A, Veitch R, Grinstein S *et al.* Increased platelet $Na^+$-$H^+$ exchange rates in essential hypertension: application of a novel test. *Lancet* 1987; **i**: 533–6.

11. Erne P, Bolli P, Burgisser E, Bühler FR. Correlation of platelet calcium with blood pressure: effect of antihypertensive therapy. *N. Engl. J. Med.* 1984; **310**: 1084–88.

12. Dominiczak AF, Semple PF, Bohr DF. Membrane stabilization of platelets by calcium in essential hypertension. Abstracts, 13th Scientific Meeting of the International Society of Hypertension, Montreal, 1990; S95.

13. Dean WL, Pope JE, Brier ME, Aronoff GR. Platelet calcium transport in hypertension. *Hypertension* 1994; **23**: 31–7.

14. Cusi D, Bianchi G. Genetic and molecular aspects of primary hypertension. In *Handbook of Hypertension*, Vol. 15: *Clinical Hypertension* (ed. JIS Robertson). Amsterdam: Elsevier, 1992: 63–94.

# 12
# Integrated control of the circulation

The various endocrine, paracrine, autocrine, neurological, structural, cellular and metabolic accompaniments of essential hypertension have, for ease of description, been described in Chapters 9–11, largely in isolation one from another. Although this is unavoidable for didactic purposes, it obscures to some extent the critical interactions between these fundamentally interdependent systems. The integrative approach has been especially emphasized by some authors, notably by Korner[1] and by Bianchi and his colleagues.[2] The latter have described the need to consider all levels of organization within the animal in studying the pathogenesis and evolution of hypertension: genetic, molecular, subcellular, cellular, tissue, organ and whole body. As already recognized, such an approach is more readily rewarding in sub-human animal models of hypertension, where genetic control can be strict. In humans, the inherited basis of hypertension, although undeniable, is genetically less pure, and abnormalities at the various organizational levels are less clear, although still discernible. However difficult it may be to achieve, the approach does offer the possibility of designing antihypertensive drugs that are directed at rectifying specifically relevant causative abnormalities (see also pages 20 and 126).

## References

1. Korner PI. Integrative neurohumoral control of the circulation. *Australian Soc. Exp. Biol. Proc.* 1988; **1**: 151–8.
2. Cusi D, Bianchi G. Genetic and molecular aspects of primary hypertension. In *Handbook of Hypertension*, Vol. 15: *Clinical Hypertension* (ed. JIS Robertson). Amsterdam: Elsevier, 1992: 63–94.

# 13
# Arterial changes in hypertension

Hypertension is associated with, and causes, progressively severe changes in the arteries, both large and small, from the aorta to the arterioles. The diverse modifications in arterial composition and geometry have long-term functional consequences in the various affected organs, whilst also predisposing to sudden catastrophes such as arterial thrombosis, embolism, dissection or rupture. We shall first describe the structural arterial changes which take place, and the haemodynamic accompaniments, and then proceed to a more detailed description of the way in which these arterial modifications affect those organs which are especially involved—the eyes, brain and kidneys (Chapters 14–16).

Additionally, major alterations in cardiac structure occur. The cardiac features of hypertension merit, and shall receive, separate exposition (Chapter 17).

The arterial and cardiac changes in hypertension derive from the interaction of several influences, including high arterial pressure as such, blood flow turbulence and shear, endothelial lesions with their consequent disordered biochemistry, and endocrine, paracrine and autocrine growth-promoting and growth-inhibiting substances.

## ───── Large arteries ─────

### Histological changes

In large and medium-sized arteries (>1 mm in diameter), with hypertension the internal elastic lamina is thickened and new layers are formed, especially towards the intima.[1,2] Smooth muscle becomes more prominent. In the later stages, elastic tissue can break up and be partly reabsorbed; there can be some replacement of the increased smooth muscle by fibrous tissue. The vessels become dilated, thickened, rigid, and often tortuous.

### Haemodynamic consequences of large arterial changes

Thickening and rigidity in larger arteries can render them resistant to compression by a sphygmomanometer cuff and hence lead to falsely high blood pressure readings ('pseudohypertension').[3] This is discussed further on page 134. Loss of distensibility and compliance in large arteries is associated with increased responses to constrictor stimuli, disproportionate elevation of systolic pressure, turbulent blood flow, endothelial lesions and atheroma formation.[4] Atheroma (or, as it is now more frequently termed, with insouciant disregard of etymological considerations,* atherosclerosis) is of especial relevance to the arterial pathology of hypertension, because its progressive worsening is accelerated by a raised arterial pressure. The pathology of atheroma is briefly summarized in the following section.

### Pathological consequences of large arterial changes: aneurysms and dissection

Hypertension-associated changes in large arteries can proceed also to the formation of saccular or fusiform aneurysms. Less commonly, but more

---

* 'Too many writers fail to understand that what they call "hardening through the agency of porridge" (atherosclerosis) is as ill-assorted a hotch-potch as its name implies.'[5]

seriously, large arterial or aortic dissection may occur in hypertension; it is not unusual with co-arctation of the aorta (Chapter 28). A tear in the intima, often transverse, permits blood to dissect through the media, with protean clinical manifestations, depending on the site and extent.

### Atheroma (atherosclerosis)

The development of atheromatous (atherosclerotic) lesions in large or medium-sized arteries has been described by Smith[6] as following initially either of two different paths, termed respectively fatty and proliferative. These two distinct varieties later converge as they evolve.

Fatty streaks consist microscopically of groups of macrophages containing large lipid droplets. These streaks may comprise from only a few cells immediately underlying the arterial endothelium, and with little accompanying intimal thickening, to moderately thickened patches containing several layers of fat-filled cells (Figure 13.1). Raised fatty lesions can form as focal proliferations of macrophages containing fat around a core of extracellular lipid, the latter derived from disintegrated cells.

Such lesions do not usually form large stenosing plaques, but the overlying endothelium can ulcerate, and platelets can then adhere, leading to the formation of mural thrombi.

Proliferative lesions are regarded as the main precursors of fibrous plaques.[6] Local accretions of exuberant subendothelial smooth muscle cells, initially devoid of fat-containing macrophages, progress with variable accumulation of fibrin to extensive fibrous plaques containing often substantial quantities of collagen together with the smooth muscle cells. About 50% of such atherosclerotic plaques contain a core of extracellular lipid.

It is considered that the fatty and the proliferative lesions at first develop independently, but that mixed fibro-fatty plaques can later form, with numerous fat-filled cells as well as extensive smooth muscular proliferation, presumably reflecting histological convergence of the two initially distinct types of lesion.

The importance of hypertension in the development of such atherosclerotic lesions requires emphasis. The responsible mechanisms include the following. In normal arteries, the fastest moving blood is in the centre of the lumen of the columnar

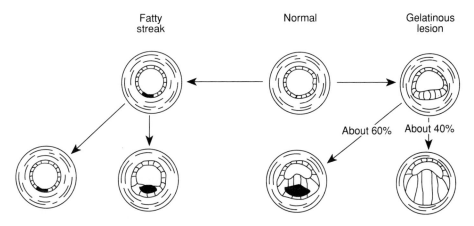

**Figure 13.1.** Diagram depicting two separate families of atherosclerotic lesions. On the left, fatty streaks consisting of small groups of cells (probably macrophages) filled with lipid droplets are found at all ages and may develop into small raised lesions containing masses of lipid, mainly intracellular. On the right, focal proliferations of smooth muscle cells, containing no fat-filled cells, are probable precursors of large stenosing fibrous plaques, of which about half accumulate a central core of extracellular lipid. (Redrawn from Ref. 6, with permission.)

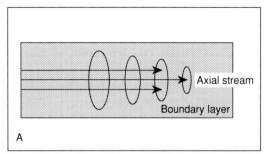
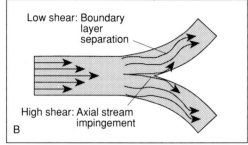
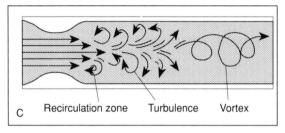
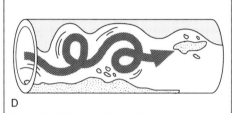

**Figure 13.2.** Blood flow patterns through an artery. (A) In normal circumstances, the fastest moving arterial blood is in the centre (the axial stream) and the blood closest to the endothelium (the boundary layer) is moving very slowly. Thus the endothelium is protected from the effects of kinetic energy in the blood. (B) When the haemodynamic circumstances in the parent artery are such that laminar flow cannot be maintained through a bifurcation, different parts of the bifurcation will be opposed to high shear (axial stream impingement) or low shear (boundary layer separation). Both types of flow disturbance will tend to occur under the same haemodynamic circumstances, but at different locations in the bifurcation. (C) Since blood has to accelerate to maintain volume flow through a stenosis, flow becomes non-laminar; vortex formation, recirculation zones and even turbulence will occur. (D) When there is non-laminar flow past a stenosis, platelets will be brought into contact with roughened surfaces and collagen in the base of ulcers, leading to the embolization of platelet thrombi; also, the swirling currents of blood will break off fragments of plaque, leading to embolization of atheromatous debris laden with cholesterol crystals. (Redrawn from Ref. 7, with permission.)

vessel, whilst the boundary layer closest to the endothelium moves slowly (Figure 13.2A). Thus the endothelium is relatively protected from the effects of kinetic energy in the blood.[4] Where an artery bifurcates, laminar flow cannot be maintained, and different parts of the artery will be subjected respectively to high shear, where there is axial stream impingement, and low shear, where there is boundary zone separation (Figure 13.2B)). Both types of flow disturbance will tend to occur under the same haemodynamic circumstances, but at different parts of the bifurcation. Zones of high shear will be subjected to the injurious effects of kinetic energy, which will be greater with hypertension. Endothelial damage is especially likely in

these high shear zones. Rapid, but limited, development of atherosclerotic plaques is prevalent at high shear sites of arterial bifurcations. Plaques also develop at places of low shear, more slowly, but eventually more extensively, than at loci of high shear.

With the formation of atherosclerotic arterial stenoses, because blood has to accelerate through the narrowing so as to maintain volume flow, the bloodstream becomes non-laminar. There can then appear vortices, recirculation zones and turbulence (Figure 13.2C). With non-laminar flow across a stenosis, platelets can be brought into contact with roughened surfaces and with collagen in ulcerated plaques. Consequences include embolization of platelet thrombi, or separation of plaque fragments, leading to emboli composed of atheromatous debris laden with cholesterol crystals (Figure 13.2D). Irrespective of embolization, atherosclerotic arterial stenoses can cause distal ischaemia and/ or infarction. Progression to occlusion of the affected artery is not unusual. The functional and pathological consequences of such atherosclerotic arterial lesions can be particularly serious in the renal, coronary, carotid and vertebral arteries.

──────────── Small arteries ────────────

### Medial and intimal thickening: endothelial lesions

The pattern of change in small arteries (of 1 mm diameter or less) differs substantially from that in large and medium-sized arteries. Medial thickening occurs, as in the larger arteries, but there is a more pronounced intimal expansion resulting from a concentric increase in the connective tissue. In these smaller arteries, there is progressive hyaline arteriosclerosis which eventually may involve the entire circumference apart from the endothelium. In contrast to the larger arteries, the lumen of the smaller arteries narrows, with important pathophysiological consequences. In the later stages of hypertensive disease, and with ageing, increasingly prevalent endothelial lesions also are found.

### Haemodynamic results of medial thickening

The structural change in smaller arteries, particularly the medial thickening and the luminal narrowing that occur in consequence, has been much studied, especially by Folkow and his colleagues (Figure 13.3).[8] Resistance to flow varies inversely with the fourth power of the luminal radius, and it has been emphasized that the hypertension-induced alterations will lead to narrowing of the lumen, even at maximal dilatation, and therefore to progressively increased vascular resistance which will thus reinforce the elevation of arterial pressure. It is likely that the upward re-setting of the limits of autoregulation of blood flow via various organs that occurs in hypertension results at least in part from such structural changes in small arteries, with the consequent narrowing of the lumen. This has been particularly well-studied in the brain[1,8,9] where it seems to hold true, even though small cerebral arteries are poorly muscled (Figure 13.4).[5] Obviously, such geometric

Increased wall / Lumen ratio

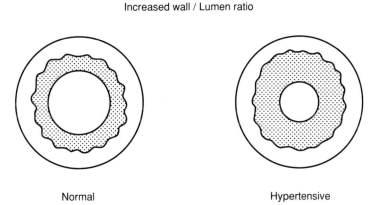

Normal                    Hypertensive

**Figure 13.3.** Diagrammatic representation of cross-section of a normal resistance artery and of a specimen in hypertension. The hypertensive artery shows thickening of the media with narrowing of the lumen.

Fig. 3.2.

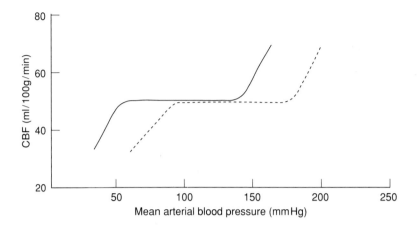

**Figure 13.4.** Diagram showing the limits of autoregulation of cerebral blood flow (CBF) in a normal person (continuous line) and patient with hypertension (dotted line). Cerebral blood flow is held constant over wide limits of systemic arterial pressure. If the systemic blood pressure exceeds the upper limit of autoregulation, the brain will be overperfused and become oedematous. If the pressure falls below the lower limit of autoregulation, cerebral ischaemia and possible infarction will result. (Redrawn from Ref. 1, with permission.)

changes will also limit the efficacy of those anti-hypertensive drugs which act mainly via arterial dilatation. Further, it is likely that the structural changes in resistance vessels contribute to persistence of hypertension in secondary hypertensive syndromes even after the causal lesion has been corrected.

Several lines of evidence have indicated that the medial thickening of resistance arteries is a main consequence neither of hypertrophy nor of hyperplasia of smooth muscle, but results principally from cellular rearrangement.[10,28] The proximate cause of the change is not solely the mechanical effect of raised blood pressure; biochemical and nervous influences, as will be discussed subsequently, appear also to be involved. These various factors are not mutually exclusive.

Reversal of medial thickening in resistance arteries, at least to a limited extent, has been demonstrated with antihypertensive drug treatment in essential hypertension.[11] An ACE inhibitor has been found superior to a $\beta$-blocker in this regard[26] (see also pages 79 and 108).

### Charcot–Bouchard aneurysms

These cerebral arterial aneurysms were described by Charcot and Bouchard in 1868,[12] then for long neglected, being rediscovered by Russell[13] nearly 100 years later. They are found on small arteries within the brain, and merit separate description because they are an important predisposing cause of cerebral haemorrhage in hypertension. Their structure is markedly different from that of smaller peripheral arteries in hypertension and as described in the preceding paragraph.

Charcot–Bouchard aneurysms are roughly spherical, and typically 0.2–1.0 mm in diameter (Figure 13.5). They are situated on small intracranial arteries of some 100–300 $\mu$m in cross-section, especially on lateral branches of the striate artery and on penetrating branches from the cortex. These lesions become increasingly prevalent with hypertension and with ageing. The muscular tissue of the parent artery usually terminates abruptly at the origin of the aneurysm, although remnants of elastica may extend for a short way into its wall.

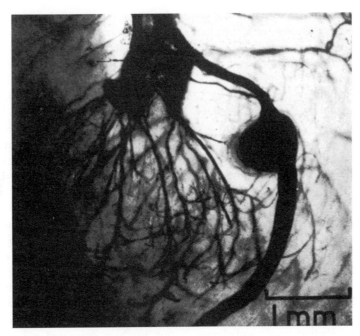

**Figure 13.5.** Charcot–Bouchard aneurysm on long penetrating artery from parietal cortex in man aged 71 who died from cerebral haemorrhage. Post-mortem injection specimen showing leakage from aneurysm. (Reproduced from Ref. 14, with permission.)

The aneurysm wall thus consists mainly only of connective tissue, with an inner hyaline layer derived from the intima fusing with an outer collagenous layer which is continuous with the adventitia of the parent vessel. The aneurysms not rarely show evidence variously of leakage or of thrombosis.

Charcot–Bouchard aneurysms appear to be peculiar to the cerebral circulation. Their characteristics have been attributed to the scanty musculature of cerebral arteries, which is possibly a consequence of the external support offered by the skull.[5] They are to be distinguished from the retinal microaneurysms of hypertension, which are of capillary origin[15] (see page 69), and from microaneurysms of the retinal venules found in diabetes mellitus.[16]

Cerebral Charcot–Bouchard aneurysms comprise a major reason for cerebral haemorrhage and for miliary brain infarcts in subjects with hypertension.

### Malignant phase

The most severe vascular lesions resulting from hypertension occur in the malignant phase, and this condition deserves detailed exposition.[1,2,17,18] Malignant ('accelerated') phase hypertension is the most severe of the arterial complications associated with a raised blood pressure. Untreated, it is inevitably fatal, usually within months. It is encountered most often at the highest levels of blood pressure, although it may supervene at rather lower values if the increase in blood pressure occurs rapidly.

Arterial lesions closely akin to those of the malignant phase are seen with the more advanced stages of pregnancy-induced hypertension (see page 249), a condition in which blood pressure rises very rapidly, although not necessarily to extremely high absolute values. While some authorities regard the arterial lesions of severe pregnancy-induced hypertension as examples of malignant hypertension,[2] other workers[25] consider these to be separate pathological conditions (page 249).

Similar arterial and retinal lesions to those of malignant phase (Figure 13.6) hypertension are found with collagen diseases such as polyarteritis nodosa and disseminated lupus erythematosus (page 180); these latter are almost certainly aetiologically distinct.[2,18] The ocular changes of malignant hypertension are described in more detail in Chapter 14.

The characteristic lesion of the malignant phase is necrosis ('fibrinoid necrosis' or 'plasmatic vasculosis') of small arteries and arterioles, which disrupt as a consequence of the very high blood pressure (Figure 13.6; Plate 16.1). Necrotic changes occur in already thickened and often hyaline arteriolar walls. The vascular endothelium breaks and plasma insudates into the media. Thrombotic occlusion of the lumen may occur, leading to infarction in the organ involved. At other sites, the vascular constriction and structural narrowing which are the early consequences of hypertension, are overcome and the vessels become overdistended and permeable. Thus, malignant hypertension leads in affected organs to a mixture of ischaemia in some areas and overperfusion in others.

The frequency with which different organs are involved in the malignant phase varies among species. In humans, the kidney, brain and retina are especially susceptible, with the pancreas, adrenal, heart, liver and gut also liable to involvement; skeletal muscle and skin are usually spared.

It requires emphasis that the malignant phase may supervene in hypertension of whatever aetiology—it is a consequence of very severe hypertension and the speed with which the pressure has risen. It is not a disease in its own right. Of all the known causes of hypertension, only aortic coarctation has been suggested as being immune to the complication of malignant hypertension, although

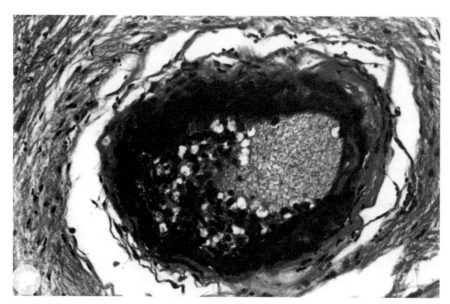

**Figure 13.6.** Malignant phase hypertension showing fibrinoid degeneration with invasion by macrophages in arterial wall ($\times$215). (Reproduced from Ref. 2 with permission.)

even in coarctation the malignant phase has occasionally been described.[19]

This concept of the malignant phase being simply a consequence of very severe hypertension[5] has important therapeutic consequences. Most, if not all, of the pathological accompaniments of the malignant phase can be arrested or corrected with appropriate antihypertensive treatment.

Untreated, the malignant phase of hypertension is invariably fatal, in humans within months at most. Progressive renal glomerular infarction, with renal failure, is an inevitable ultimate cause of death in this condition, although in many patients the course can be abruptly terminated by cardiac failure or cerebral haemorrhage before renal failure is sufficiently advanced to threaten life. Malignant phase hypertension remains common in the UK,[20-22] but has in recent years become rare in some countries such as Australia[23] and Sweden.[24] The reasons for this altered epidemiology are not agreed. It has been attributed by some writers to perhaps more efficient detection and control of hypertension in the latter countries.[23]

**Hypertensive encephalopathy**

A rarer complication, acute hypertensive encephalopathy, in which headache, confusion, coma and fits may occur, is, when it appears, almost always superimposed upon features of the malignant phase.[2] Hypertensive encephalopathy is a consequence of the systemic arterial pressure exceeding the upper limit of cerebral autoregulation, with consequent overperfusion and cerebral oedema.[1,2,27]

The ways in which raised blood pressure, and especially the arterial lesions which are its consequences, affect those organs, the eye, brain kidney and heart, that show particular susceptibility to such disease, and which manifest important clinical features as a result, will now be considered.

## Case studies

See Case studies 9, 10, 11 and 13, Appendix 2.

## References

1. Graham DI, Lee WR, Cumming AMM et al. Hypertension and the intracranial and ocular circulations: effect of antihypertensive treatment. In Handbook of Hypertension, Vol. 1: Clinical Aspects of Essential Hypertension (ed. JIS Robertson). Amsterdam: Elsevier, 1983: 174–201.
2. Spence JD, Arnold JMO, Gilbert JJ. Vascular consequences of hypertension and effects of antihypertensive therapy. In Handbook of Hypertension, Vol. 15: Clinical Hypertension (ed. JIS Robertson). Amsterdam: Elsevier, 1992: 621–54.
3. Spence JD, Sibbald WJ, Cape RD. Pseudohypertension in the elderly. Clin. Sci. 1978; 55 (suppl. 4): 399–402.
4. Robertson JIS. Left ventricular, large arterial, and resistance arterial changes, the J-curve, and antiplatelet agents. Curr. Opinion Cardiol. 1989; 4: 662–71.
5. Pickering GW. High Blood Pressure, 2nd edn. London: Churchill, 1968.
6. Smith EB. The pathogenesis of atherosclerosis. In: Diseases of the Heart, 1st edn. (eds DG Julian, AJ Camm, KM Fox et al.). London: Baillière Tindall, 1989: 1067–84.
7. Spence JD. In Hypertension and Coronary Atherosclerosis: Prevention and Intervention (eds Lie et al.). Amstelveen: Beecham Research Laboratories, 1988: 46–57.
8. Folkow B, Hansson L, Sivertsson R. Structural vascular factors in the pathogenesis of hypertension. In Handbook of Hypertension, Vol. 1: Clinical Aspects of Essential Hypertension (ed. JIS Robertson). Amsterdam: Elsevier, 1983: 133–50.
9. Strandgaard S, Paulson OB. Cerebral blood flow and its pathophysiology in hypertension. Am. J. Hypertens. 1989; 2: 486–92.
10. Heagerty AM, Aalkjaer C, Bund SJ et al. Small artery structure in hypertension: dual processes of remodelling and growth. Hypertension 1993; 21: 391–7.
11. Heagerty AM, Bund SJ, Aalkjaer C. Effects of drug treatment of human resistance arteriole morphology in essential hypertension: direct evidence for structural remodelling of resistance vessels. Lancet 1988; ii: 1209–12.
12. Charcot JM, Bouchard C. Nouvelles recherches sur la pathogénie de l'hémorrhagie cérébrale. Archs Physiol. 1868; 1: 110: 643, 725.
13. Russell RWR. Observations on intracerebral aneurysms. Brain 1963; 86: 425–40.

14. Pickering GW. *Hypertension: Causes, Consequences and Management*, 2nd edn. Edinburgh: Churchill Livingstone, 1974.

15. Ashton N, Harry J. The pathology of cotton wool spots and cytoid bodies in hypertensive retinopathy and other diseases. *Trans. Ophthal. Soc. UK* 1963; **83**: 91–114.

16. Ashton N. Arteriolar involvement in diabetic retinopathy. *Br. J. Ophthal.* 1953; **37**: 282–92.

17. Robertson JIS, Nicholls MG (eds). *The Renin–Angiotensin System*. London/New York: Gower Medical, 1993.

18. Robertson JIS. Renin and malignant hypertension. In *The Renin–Angiotensin System* (eds JIS Robertson and MG Nicholls). London: Gower Medical, 1993: chapter 60.

19. Cleland WP, Counihan TB, Goodwin JF, Steiner RE. Coarctation of the aorta. *Br. Med. J.* 1956; **2**: 379–90.

20. Isles CG, Brown JJ, Cumming AMM *et al.* Excess smoking in malignant-phase hypertension. *Br. Med. J.* 1979; **1**: 579–81.

21. Bloxham CA, Beevers DG, Walker JM. Malignant hypertension and cigarette smoking. *Br. Med. J.* 1979; **1**: 581–3.

22. Webster J, Petrie JC, Jeffers TA, Lovell HG. Accelerated hypertension: patterns of mortality and clinical factors affecting outcome in treated patients. *Q. J. Med.* 1993; **86**: 485–93.

23. Kincaid-Smith P. What has happened to malignant hypertension? In *Handbook of Hypertension*, Vol. 6: *Epidemiology of Hypertension* (ed. CJ Bulpitt). Amsterdam: Elsevier, 1985: 255–65.

24. Gudbrandsson T, Hansson L, Herlitz H, Andrén L. Malignant hypertension: improving prognosis in a rare disease. *Acta Med. Scand.* 1979; **206**: 495–9.

25. Redman C. Hypertension in pregnancy. In *The Circulation in the Female: From the Cradle to the Grave* (ed. J Ginsburg). New Jersey: Parthenon, 1989: 63–76.

26. Schiffrin EL, Deng LY, La rochelle P. Effects of a $\beta$-blocker or a converting enzyme inhibitor on resistance arteries in essential hypertension. *Hypertension* 1994; **23**: 83–91.

27. Dinsdale HB. Hypertensive encephalopathy. *Stroke* 1982; **13**: 717–19.

28. Mulvaney MJ. Mechanical and other factors involved in vascular injury related to hypertension. *Blood Pressure* 1994; **3** (suppl. 1): 11–17.

# 14
# The eye in hypertension

The fundus oculi provides the opportunity for the direct inspection of arteries by means of the ophthalmoscope or retinal camera. Detailed study of the eye allows the clinician to assess the evolution and severity of hypertension-associated arterial disease. In our opinion, the optic appearances in hypertension are best described objectively, rather than being arbitrarily 'graded'.

## Retinal lesions

In the early stages, the arterial consequences of hypertension are shown as thickening, irregularity and tortuosity of the retinal arteries. Occasionally, emboli may be seen traversing the retinal circulation. Central or sectorial retinal arterial or venous occlusions can accompany high blood pressure and may readily be diagnosed ophthalmoscopically.

The most striking retinal appearances accompany the malignant phase of hypertension (Chapter 13). The onset of the malignant phase can be recognized ophthalmoscopically by the appearance of usually bilateral retinal exudates, which may be circumscribed ('hard') or fluffy ('cottonwool'); haemorrhages; and, in the later stages, papilloedema and retinal oedema (Plate 14.1).

The pathology of the retinal lesions in malignant hypertension has been studied in detail.[1,2] Arteriolar leakage is demonstrable on fluorescein angiography. Focal microinfarction in the inner two-thirds of the retina gives rise to the 'cottonwool' exudates in the nerve fibre layer, and these exudates comprise the swollen bulbous ends of axons (cytoid bodies) containing both normal and degenerate organelles. 'Hard' exudates are caused by the accumulation of plasma and lipid in the outer plexiform layer of the retina in the 'watershed' zone between the retinal and choroidal circulations. In severe cases, they form a characteristic 'star' around the macula. Haemorrhages from pre-capillary arteries and from capillaries tend to be flame-shaped in the nerve fibre layer, and rounded ('blot' haemorrhages) in the outer plexiform layer. Microaneurysms appear as small evaginations in the capillary wall, and occur when the endothelial cells or pericytes are destroyed by ischaemia.[2] Papilloedema is the result of massive interference with axoplasmic flow at the disc. Elschnig's spots are small white areas in the fundus resulting from depigmentation in infarcted areas of the pigment epithelium.

## Effects of antihypertensive therapy

The various lesions of the malignant phase resolve with effective antihypertensive treatment. The ocular manifestations, which are often accompanied by marked visual disturbances, can clear completely in weeks or months (Plate 14.1).

Retinal infarction and/or optic nerve ischaemia and subsequent atrophy can result from sudden marked reduction of systemic arterial pressure.[1,3,4] These complications and their pathogenesis are described below in relation to changes in the autoregulation of cerebral blood flow (page 72).

## 'Malignant' versus 'accelerated' hypertension

For many years, several workers made a distinction between those patients in whom retinal haemorrhages and exudates were present, but in whom the optic disc was not swollen, and who were termed by them as having 'accelerated hypertension', and those in whom papilloedema was also apparent.[5] The term 'malignant hypertension' was reserved for the latter cases. There is now extensive evidence that renal arterial fibrinoid necroses are present even when retinal haemorrhages and exudates short of papilloedema have arisen, and the urgency of therapy is or should be as immediate. Thus, the terms 'accelerated' and 'malignant' hypertension are now regarded as synonymous, and are applied irrespective of the presence of optic disc swelling.[6–9]

## The Keith, Wagener and Barker terminology

A separate terminological approach, now largely discarded, is application of the classification of Keith, Wagener and Barker.[10] This was previously extensively employed, especially in North America. The classification, although much criticized,[8,9,11] does at least have the merit of emphasizing the importance of fundoscopy in assessing the arterial disease of hypertension. A major reason for the disparagement of this work, however, is that it embraces the now discredited concept of retinal artery spasm.[11]

In the Keith *et al.* classification,[10] group I patients, with the mildest disease, were those showing only minor narrowing or sclerosis of the retinal vessels; group II patients evinced more severe sclerotic changes; group III patients had retinal haemorrhages, exudates and oedema in addition to the arterial irregularities of group II; and in group IV swelling of the optic discs was also evident.

There can be little doubt that much of the attraction of this terminology, and hence of the relevance of the criticisms from its detractors, is the fascination which the use of clinical grades has for some doctors, and the pleasure they derive from employing, however inaccurately, sometimes misleadingly quantitative terms.

## Retinal photography

A renewed and highly appropriate interest in the evaluation of retinal vascular changes in hypertension is emerging with the advent of accurate photographic methods of assessment.[8,12] This approach promises well for the objective

quantitative interpretation of even minor ocular lesions.

## Case studies

See Case studies 9, 10,11 and 13, Appendix 2.

## References

1. Graham DI, Lee WR, Cumming AMM *et al.* Hypertension and the intracranial and ocular circulations: effect of antihypertensive treatment. In *Handbook of Hypertension*, Vol. 1: *Clinical Aspects of Essential Hypertension* (ed. JIS Robertson). Amsterdam: Elsevier, 1983: 174–201.
2. Ashton N, Harry J. The pathology of cotton wool spots and cytoid bodies in hypertensive retinopathy and other diseases. *Trans. Ophthal. Soc. UK* 1963; **83**: 91–114.
3. Cove DH, Seddon M, Fletcher RF, Dukes DC. Blindness after treatment for malignant hypertension. *Br.Med. J.* 1979; **3**: 245.
4. Hulse JA, Taylor DSI, Dillon MJ. Blindness and paraplegia in severe childhood hypertension. *Lancet* 1979; **ii**: 553–6.
5. Bulpitt CJ. Prognosis of treated hypertension 1951–1981. *Br. J. Clin. Pharmacol.* 1982; **13**: 73–9.
6. World Health Organization. *Arterial Hypertension. WHO Tech. Rep. Ser.* 1978; **628**: 57.
7. Brown JJ, Davies DL, Lever AF, Robertson JIS. Plasma renin concentration in human hypertension III: renin in relation to complications of hypertension. *Br. Med. J.* 1966; **1**: 505–508.
8. McGregor E, Isles CG, Jay JL *et al.* Retinal changes in malignant hypertension. *Br. Med. J.* 1986; **292**: 233–4.
9. Ahmed MEK, Walker JM, Beevers DG, Beevers M. Lack of difference between malignant and accelerated hypertension. *Br. Med. J.* 1986; **292**: 235–7.
10. Keith NM, Wagener HP, Barker NW. Some different types of essential hypertension: their course and prognosis. *Am. J. Med. Sci.* 1939; **196**: 332–43.
11. Pickering GW. *High Blood Pressure*, 2nd edn. London: Churchill, 1968.
12. Stanton AV, Mullaney PB, Mee K *et al.* Fundal blood vessel alterations are associated with mild to moderate hypertension. Abstracts, 5th European Meeting on Hypertension, Milan 1991; no. 699.

# 15
# Consequences of hypertensive disease in the brain

## Physiological changes: autoregulation of cerebral blood flow

Cerebral blood flow is held constant over wide limits of systemic arterial pressure. In a normal subject, cerebral blood flow increases only when mean arterial pressure rises above about 150 mmHg, and decreases only when mean arterial pressure drops below around 50 mmHg. Both the upper and lower limits of such autoregulation are shifted upwards in established hypertension[1-3] (Figure 13.4).

The arterial and arteriolar wall thickening in hypertension and described in Chapter 13, even though less pronounced in the cerebral circulation than in some other beds, is probably a major cause of the upward re-setting of the limits of systemic arterial pressure between which cerebral blood flow is kept constant.

The upward shift of the upper limit of autoregulation almost certainly has a protective effect, minimizing the likelihood of cerebral overperfusion and oedema, and thus of hypertensive encephalopathy (page 67), in the event of marked elevation of systemic arterial pressure. However, the upward shift also of the lower limit of cerebral autoregulation means that in hypertension, if the blood pressure is suddenly lowered, for example, by overzealous drug administration, cerebral and ocular underperfusion, ischaemia and possibly infarction can occur at higher absolute levels of blood pressure than would be the case in normal subjects.[4-7] This has important implications for antihypertensive therapy, especially in the elderly subject.[8,14]

## Pathological changes

### Stroke

Hypertension as such is a major cause of primary intracerebral haemorrhage, which accounts for some 20% of all strokes. About 80% of the bleeds occur in the cerebral hemispheres (Figure 15.1), 10% in the brainstem and 8% in the cerebellum.[1] Many of these events take place at the site of Charcot–Bouchard microaneurysms of the smaller arteries deep within the brain (page 65).[9]

Clinical stroke can more commonly result from cerebral infarction, for which hypertension is again an important predisposing factor. Lacunar brain infarcts are considered to be a consequence of hypertensive lesions in small deep-lying intracerebral arteries,[10,15] possibly a result of thrombosis originating in a Charcot–Bouchard aneurysm.[9] These complications are again in such cases direct consequences of elevated arterial pressure.

An often confounding issue is that blood pressure, particularly diastolic, can increase acutely and transiently after a stroke (page 55). This has been attributed to stroke-induced enhancement in sympathetic tone.[11] Cardiac arrhythmias or bradycardia can also be a feature. The therapeutic approach to this problem is considered on page 150.

Brain infarction can also frequently follow less directly from hypertension. Atherosclerotic plaques can lead to progressive occlusion of arteries or can act as a source of emboli, composed variously of atheromatous debris and cholesterol crystals, or mixtures of fibrin, leucocytes and platelets[12] (page 61).

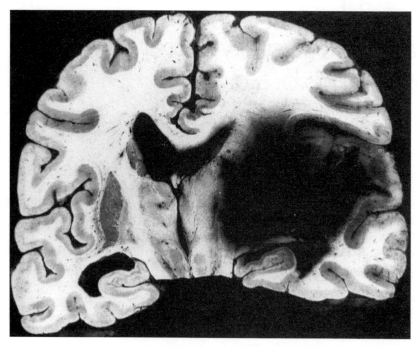

**Figure 15.1.** Large haematoma in basal ganglia of right cerebral hemisphere in a patient with chronic hypertension. Note displacement of lateral ventricle, midline shift and supracallosal hernia. (Reproduced from Ref. 1, with permission.)

The rarer cerebral and cerebellar infarcts that can result from sudden blood pressure reduction and consequent cerebral ischaemia have already been mentioned[1,6,7] (pages 64 and 71). They occur at the 'watershed' zones between the areas of distribution of major cerebral arteries, and are a consequence of the systemic arterial pressure falling suddenly—usually from overzealous antihypertensive drug therapy—below the lower limit of cerebral auto-regulation (Figure 15.2). They occur when the capacity of the underperfused ischaemic brain to extract oxygen from such blood as it does receive is exceeded.[13] The cerebral and cerebellar infarcts may be accompanied in these circumstances by retinal infarction and/or optic nerve ischaemia with subsequent optic atrophy; these ocular lesions have a similar pathophysiological basis[4,5] (page 69).

## Transient ischaemic attacks

Transient ischaemic attacks are defined as reversible disturbances of cerebral function lasting less than 24 h. They can result from temporary arterial occlusion by embolism, from external compression of an artery, especially if it is already the seat of disease, or from sudden hypotension, for example, that consequent upon cardiac dysrhythmia or aggressive antihypertensive therapy. It has been estimated that some 30% of transient ischaemic attacks evolve to a major stroke within 5 years.[1] It is further considered that hypertension is a potent factor predisposing to such an adverse sequel.

## Subarachnoid haemorrhage

The role of hypertension in the causation of subarachnoid haemorrhage is uncertain, although

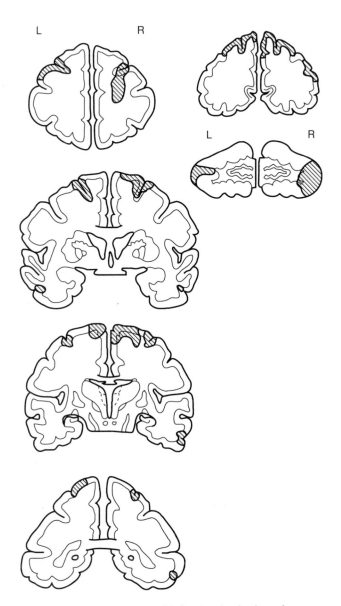

**Figure 15.2.** Distribution of infarction in the boundary zones between the major arterial territories of the cerebral and cerebellar hemispheres (hatched) in a previously hypertensive patient who died following sudden lowering of arterial pressure. (Reproduced from Ref. 6, with permission.)

associations have been reported between subarachnoid haemorrhage and coarctation of the aorta, polycystic kidneys or fibromuscular dysplasia of the renal arteries.[1] However, in these conditions, the link may be a widespread disorder of mesodermal development rather than one of raised blood pressure. Nevertheless, prognosis following subarachnoid rupture of a saccular aneurysm of a superficial artery to the brain is worse in a hypertensive patient, and appropriate antihypertensive therapy is needed.

Blood pressure can rise acutely after subarachnoid haemorrhage, as with stroke, considered above (pages 55 and 71). This has, likewise, been thought to be due to transiently enhanced sympathetic discharge; again, cardiac arrhythmias or catecholamine-induced myocardial necrosis (page 44) can be associated.[11]

## Dementia

The association between dementia and hypertension is often obscure.[1,10] However, so-called multi-infarct dementia, in which progressive deterioration of mental function is accompanied by focal neurological signs, is usually associated with hypertension, and such patients could benefit from antihypertensive therapy.

Binswanger's encephalopathy is sometimes distinguished as a separate entity;[1] in this condition, again associated with hypertension, dementia is accompanied by pseudobulbar palsy and periventricular white matter lucency.[14]

## Hypertensive encephalopathy

This was described on page 67.

--------- References ---------

1. Graham DI, Lee WR, Cumming AMM *et al.* Hypertension and the intracranial and ocular circulations: effect of antihypertensive treatment. In *Handbook of Hypertension*, Vol. 1: *Clinical Aspects of Essential Hypertension* (ed. JIS Robertson). Amsterdam: Elsevier, 1983: 174–201.

2. Folkow B, Hansson L, Sivertsson R. Structural vascular factors in the pathogenesis of hypertension. In *Handbook of Hypertension*, Vol. 1: *Clinical Aspects of Essential Hypertension* (ed. JIS Robertson). Amsterdam: Elsevier, 1983: 133–50.

3. Strandgaard S, Paulson OB. Cerebral blow flow and its pathophysiology in hypertension. *Am. J. Hypertens.* 1989; **2**: 486–92.

4. Cove DH, Seddon M, Fletcher RF, Dukes DC. Blindness after treatment for malignant hypertension. *Br.Med.J.* 1979; **3**: 245.

5. Hulse JA, Taylor DSI, Dillon MJ. Blindness and paraplegia in severe childhood hypertension. *Lancet* 1979; **ii**: 553–6.

6. Graham DI. Ischaemic brain damage of cerebral perfusion type following treatment of severe hypertension: a report of two cases. *Br. Med. J.* 1975; **4**: 739.

7. Ledingham JGG, Rajagopalan B. Cerebral complications in the treatment of accelerated hypertension. *Q. J. Med.* 1979; **48**: 25–41.

8. Robertson JIS. The nature of hypertension. In *Handbook of Hypertension*, Vol. 15: *Clinical Hypertension* (ed. JIS Robertson). Amsterdam: Elsevier, 1992: 1–13.

9. Russell RWR. Observations in intracerebral aneurysms. *Brain* 1963; **86**: 425–40.

10. Spence JD, Arnold JMO, Gilbert JJ. Vascular consequences of hypertension and effects of antihypertensive therapy. In *Handbook of Hypertension*, Vol. 15: *Clinical Hypertension* (ed. JIS Robertson). Amsterdam: Elsevier, 1992: 621–54.

11. Myers MG, Norris JW, Hachinski VC. *et al.* Cardiac sequelae of acute stroke. *Stroke* 1982; **13**: 838–42.

12. Robertson JIS. Left ventricular, large arterial, and resistance arterial changes, the J-curve, and antiplatelet agents. *Curr. Opinion Cardiol.* 1989; **4**: 662–71.

13. Strandgaard S., Haunsø S. Why does antihypertensive treatment prevent stroke but not myocardial infarction? *Lancet* 1987; **ii**: 548–661.

14. Matsushita K, Kuriyama Y, Nagatsuka K *et al.* Periventricular white matter lucency and cerebral blood flow autoregulation in hypertensive patients. *Hypertension* 1994; **23**: 565–8.

15. Hankey GJ, Warlow CP. Lacunar transient ischaemic attacks: a clinically useful concept? *Lancet* 1991; **337**: 335–8.

# 16
# Consequences of hypertensive disease in the kidney

## Physiological changes

In the kidney, arterial and arteriolar narrowing in hypertension has been invoked as the cause of the upward re-setting of the levels of systemic arterial pressure that can induce natriuresis ('pressure natriuresis').[1,2] Guyton and his colleagues[3] have emphasized the importance of the consequent tendency for salt and water retention to occur unless the kidney is perfused at higher arterial pressure. Thus, the 'renal barostat' has been regarded by some workers as representing an extension of the concept of arterial and arteriolar wall thickening in hypertension which could be especially relevant to the pathogenesis of the raised arterial pressure. Mulvany has speculated,[4] for example, that the renal arteriolar changes could be more important than those in the periphery in the pathogenesis of hypertension. A prospective study[13] has shown serum creatinine to be an independent predictor of hypertension.

## Pathological changes

### Malignant hypertension

Renal lesions occurring in the malignant phase of hypertension (page 65) are serious. In a majority of such patients, the kidney sustains most of the consequences of the malignant phase, with extensive and progressive fibrinoid necrosis of afferent glomerular arterioles, glomerular infarction and consequent renal impairment (Plate 16.1).[5-8] Thus, as has been mentioned earlier, in malignant hypertension, provided the course is not terminated abruptly by a catastrophic cerebral lesion or by cardiac failure, left untreated the patient will eventually succumb to renal failure.

Renal arterial lesions in the malignant phase can stimulate excessive release of renin which can compound the pathology.

The urinary accompaniments of renal lesions of the malignant phase are proteinuria, haematuria and granular casts.

### Renal parenchymal lesions

Short of the malignant phase, the clinical effects of hypertension on the kidney are not prominent. However, the decline in renal function with age is faster in the presence of a raised arterial pressure,[9,12] and end-stage renal disease attributed to hypertension is said to have increased in the past decade,[14] although the diagnostic criteria are not unassailable (see page 194). It is possible that effective antihypertensive therapy could slow down this progressive renal impairment, although this has been difficult to demonstrate in antihypertensive treatment trials, which have probably been too brief for this benefit to be apparent.[10] Elevation of plasma renin could arise from hypertension-induced intrarenal arterial lesions,[5,10,11] short of the malignant phase discussed above. A related, albeit controversial concept, which is dealt with in more detail on page 92, is that such elevated plasma renin and hence angiotensin II could constitute an independent risk factor for myocardial infarction.

## Main renal artery stenosis

Atheroma and fibromuscular dysplasia of the renal artery are the commonest causes of renal artery stenosis (page 178).

———————— Case studies ————————

See Case studies 11 and 13, Appendix 2.

———————— References ————————

1. Hall JE, Mizelle HL, Hildebrandt DA, Brands MW. Abnormal pressure natriuresis: a cause or a consequence of hypertension? *Hypertension* 1990; **15**: 547–59.

2. Folkow B, Hansson L, Sivertsson R. Structural vascular factors in the pathogenesis of hypertension. In *Handbook of Hypertension*, Vol. 1: *Clinical Aspects of Essential Hypertension* (ed. JIS Robertson). Amsterdam: Elsevier, 1983: 133–50.

3. Guyton AC, Hall JE, Lohmeier TE *et al*. Role of the kidney and volume control in the pathogenesis of hypertension. In *Handbook of Hypertension*, Vol. 1: *Clinical Aspects of Essential Hypertension* (ed. JIS Robertson). Amsterdam: Elsevier, 1983: 216–38.

4. Mulvany MJ. Are vascular abnormalities a primary cause or a secondary consequence of hypertension? *Hypertension* 1991; **18** (suppl. 1): 52–7.

5. Robertson JIS, Nicholls MG (eds). *The Renin–Angiotensin System*. London/New York: Gower Medical, 1993.

6. Spence JD, Arnold JMO, Gilbert JJ. Vascular consequences of hypertension and effects of antihypertensive therapy. In *Handbook of Hypertension*, Vol. 15: *Clinical Hypertension* (ed. JIS Robertson). Amsterdam: Elsevier, 1992: 621–54.

7. Robertson JIS. Renin and malignant hypertension. In *The Renin–Angiotensin System* (eds JIS Robertson and MG Nicholls). London: Gower Medical, 1993: chapter 60.

8. Brown JJ, Davies DL, Lever AF, Robertson JIS. Plasma renin concentration in human hypertension III: renin in relation to complications of hypertension. *Br. Med. J.* 1966; **1**: 505–508.

9. Whelton PK, Perneger TV, Brancati FL, Klag MJ. Epidemiology and prevention of blood pressure-related renal disease. *J. Hypertens.* 1992; **10** (suppl. 7): 77–84.

10. Ruilope LM, Alcazar JM, Rodicio JL. Renal consequences of arterial hypertension. *J. Hypertens.* 1992; **10** (suppl. 7): 85–90.

11. Brown JJ, Owen K, Peart WS *et al*. The diagnosis and treatment of renal artery stenosis. *Br. Med. J.* 1960; **2**: 327–38.

12. Schmieder RE, Schädinger H, Messerli FH. Accelerated decline in renal perfusion with aging in essential hypertension. *Hypertension* 1994; **23**: 351–7.

13. Miura K, Nakagawa H, Nakamura H *et al*. Serum creatinine level in predicting the development of hypertension: ten year follow-up of Japanese adults in a rural community. *Am. J. Hypertens.* 1994; **7**: 390–5.

14. Epstein M. Hypertension as a risk factor for progression of chronic renal disease. *Blood Pressure* 1994; **3** (suppl. 1): 23–8.

# ─────17─────
# The heart in hypertension

## ─────Left ventricular hypertrophy─────

### Structural changes

An early and consistent feature of hypertension is left ventricular hypertrophy (Figure 17.1). This appears to be closely akin both in its genesis and rate of development to the medial thickening of small arteries and arterioles already described. There may also be similarities between the heart and small blood vessels in regression of the changes with treatment of hypertension.[2-4] Nevertheless, the cardiac and arterial processes also show distinct differences both in their development and in their

response to therapy.[5-7] The increase in left ventricular mass in hypertension is associated with enlargement of cardiac myocytes but does not involve an increase in their numbers.

The mechanical effect of blood pressure elevation in the genesis of hypertensive left ventricular hypertrophy, although important, is only one of several factors involved. Numerous studies have failed to show a close correlation between the arterial pressure and the extent of cardiac hypertrophy,[3,5] although the relationship becomes closer if blood pressure measurements made over 24 h (page 12) rather than single readings are

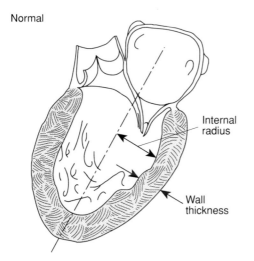
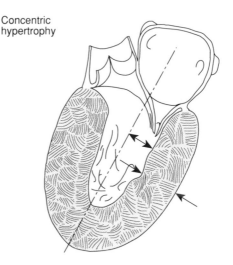

**Figure 17.1.**    Diagram contrasting normal left ventricle with that in concentric hypertrophy. The ventricle in the latter empties well but fills poorly; cavity size is reduced, there is raised end-diastolic pressure and elevation of plasma atrial natriuretic peptide; myocardial ischaemia (especially subendocardial) and ventricular dysrhythmias are prevalent. (Redrawn from Ref. 1, with permission.)

utilized.[8-10] There are numerous possible neural and humoral influences,[3] which are discussed in Chapters 9 and 10. Male gender and early increased left ventricular hypertrophy are independent predictors of left ventricular hypertrophy in adolescents.[28]

Greater wall thickness without enlargement of the ventricular cavity is called concentric hypertrophy.[3] End-diastolic left ventricular volume is normal with concentric left ventricular hypertrophy.

Enlargement of the ventricular cavity without increase in the ratio of wall thickness to chamber size despite an increase in left ventricular mass is called eccentric hypertrophy, in which left ventricular end-diastolic volume is increased. With elevation of end-diastolic pressure plasma atrial natriuretic peptide (ANP) becomes raised.[11]

A third variety of left ventricular hypertrophy ('irregular left ventricular hypertrophy') characterized by asymmetrical hypertrophic zones has been recognized.

It has been speculated that, although left ventricular hypertrophy may initially be adaptive and hence beneficial, later increased collagen deposition will reduce ventricular compliance and hinder left ventricular relaxation and filling, even when systolic function remains good. Because coronary filling is mainly during diastole, and may be impaired with left ventricular hypertrophy, subendocardial ischaemia and fibrosis, even in the absence of main coronary artery stenosis, is frequent in these circumstances.[1,3,4,12] Irregular left ventricular hypertrophy has been particularly associated with coronary microarterial disease.[13,14]

Frank atherosclerotic change in coronary arteries is also especially prevalent in hypertension. Cardiac functional impairment in hypertension may further be a partial consequence of thickening of the media (page 63), of coronary arterioles, or of coronary arteriolar fibrinoid necrosis in the malignant phase (page 66). Another possible contributory factor is multifocal ventricular myocardial necrosis, which can be caused by high circulating concentrations either of angiotensin II or of catecholamines.[15]

In some patients with mild hypertension and little evidence of left ventricular hypertrophy, it appears that the pressure load is supported by increased myocardial contractility rather than by ventricular hypertrophy.[5]

Left ventricular hypertrophy in hypertension has, however, been found to be accompanied by a reduction in adrenoceptor numbers, and in these circumstances there may be a greater dependence on the Frank–Starling mechanism than on neurohumoral factors to maintain cardiac function.[5] Herein, it is supposed, lies a major reason for progression to cardiac failure in hypertension.

### Accompanying morbidity

It has long been known that left ventricular hypertrophy in hypertension, assessed electrocardiographically (see pages 142 and 143), is associated with increased morbidity and mortality. More recent and more accurate methods of measuring left ventricular dimensions, for example, echocardiography, have reinforced these findings.[3,16] Ventricular ectopic rhythms and sudden death are more frequent in the presence of hypertensive left ventricular hypertrophy; these events cannot be attributed solely to coexistent main coronary artery disease or to left ventricular dysfunction, but are related to the extent of cardiac hypertrophy and subendocardial fibrosis.[17,18] It has been further proposed that left ventricular hypertrophy sensitizes the heart to the arrhythmogenic effects of hypokalaemia as can frequently result from diuretic therapy.[19]

--------- Cardiac failure ---------

The subtle and pervasive effects of hypertension on left ventricular morphology and function, the increased workload imposed directly by the raised arterial pressure, the decline in ventricular adrenoceptor numbers, the diminution in coronary reserve, myocardial ischaemia, and possible myocardial necrotic lesions, provide substantial reasons for the supervention of cardiac failure in this condition. Four decades ago, before the widespread availability of effective antihypertensive drug treatment, overt cardiac failure was one of the most common complications of hypertension, and one of the most frequent causes of death in that condition.[3,27] It is now much rarer. It is especially likely to appear nevertheless in the malignant phase, where the occasional occurrence of fibrinoid necroses in the coronary arterial tree may also contribute; however, the major cause of heart failure in malignant hypertension is almost certainly the extremely high systemic arterial pressure imposed on a heart given little time to adapt functionally.

Even so, although overt cardiac failure is now uncommon in patients with hypertension, coronary artery disease accompanying high blood pressure is one of the commonest causes of more subtle long-term impairment of cardiac function (see below).

## Coronary artery atheromatous disease

Coronary artery atheroma is one of the most frequent accompaniments of raised arterial pressure (Plate 17.1).[3,20] It has come into increasing prominence in recent years with greater attention being paid to mild elevation of blood pressure, and with therapeutic attention to long-term cardiac impairment. With hypertension, and in the lower ranges of hypertension especially, coronary disease predominates over both stroke and cardiac failure in frequency.[21] Although some workers have questioned whether the relationship is causal,[22,23] it is likely that, as with atheromatous changes in other arteries, the flow disturbances which are a feature of hypertension (see earlier and below) are largely responsible.[4,24] The presence of coronary artery atherosclerosis in hypertension has implications, moreover, for the concept of the so-called 'J-curved' relationship between the level of diastolic pressure during antihypertensive treatment and the risk of myocardial infarction[4,25] (page 81).

Remodelling of coronary arteries with anti-

hypertensive treatment is distinctly limited, and this may explain the only partial success of such therapy in reducing this complication.[26]

## Case study

See Case study 12, Appendix 2.

## References

1. Katz AM. A physiological approach to the treatment of heart failure. *Hosp. Pract.* 1987; **22**: 117–48.
2. Messerli F, Sclant RC (eds). Left ventricular function in hypertension: mechanisms and therapy. *Am. J. Med.* 1983; (suppl.): 1–120.
3. Frohlich ED, Apstein C, Chobanian AV *et al*. The heart in hypertension. *N. Engl. J. Med.* 1992; **327**: 998–1008.
4. Robertson JIS. Left ventricular, large arterial, and resistance arterial changes, the J-curve, and antiplatelet agents. *Curr. Opinion Cardiol.* 1989; **4**: 662–71.
5. Fouad-Tarazi FM. Structural cardiac and vascular changes in hypertension: response to treatment. *Curr. Opinion Cardiol.* 1987; **2**: 782–5.
6. Novo S, Abrignani MG, Corda M, Strano A. Cardiovascular structural changes in hypertension: possible regression during long-term antihypertensive treatment. *Eur. Heart J.* 1991; **12** (suppl. G): 47–53.
7. Lucarini AR, Spessot M, Picano E *et al*. Lack of correlation between cardiac mass and arteriolar structural changes in mild-to-moderate hypertension. *J. Hypertens.* 1991; **9**: 1187–91.
8. Drayer JL, Weber MA, De Young JL. Blood pressure as a determinant of left ventricular mass. *Arch. Intern. Med.* 1983; **143**: 90–2.
9. Devereux RB, Pickering TG, Harschfield GA *et al*. Left ventricular hypertrophy in patients with hypertension: importance of blood pressure response to regularly recurring stress. *Circulation* 1983; **68**: 470–6.
10. Devereux RB. Does increased blood pressure cause left ventricular hypertrophy or vice versa? *Ann. Intern. Med.* 1990; **112**: 157–9.

11. Montorsi P, Tonolo G, Polonia J. *et al.* Correlates of plasma atrial natriuretic factor in health and hypertension. *Hypertension* 1987; **10**: 570–6.

12. O'Gorman DJ, Sheridan DJ. Abnormalities of the coronary circulation associated with left ventricular hypertrophy. *Clin. Sci.* 1991; **81**: 703–13.

13. Strauer BE. *Das Hochdruckherz*, 3rd edn. Berlin: Springer-Verlag, 1991.

14. Vogt M, Motz W, Strauer BE. Coronary haemodynamics in hypertensive heart disease. *Eur. Heart J.* 1992; **13** (suppl. D): 44–9.

15. Gavras H, Kremer D, Brown JJ. *et al.* Angiotensin- and norepinephrine-induced myocardial lesions: experimental and clinical studies in rabbits and man. *Am. Heart J.* 1975; **89**: 321–32.

16. Kannel WB. Left ventricular hypertrophy as a risk factor in arterial hypertension. *Eur. Heart J.* 1992; **13** (suppl. D): 82–8.

17. McLenechan JM, Dargie HJ. Left ventricular hypertrophy as a factor in arrhythmias and sudden death. *Am. J. Hypertens.* 1989; **2**: 128–31.

18. McLenechan JM, Dargie HJ. Ventricular arrhythmias in hypertensive left ventricular hypertrophy; relationship to coronary artery disease, left ventricular dysfunction, and myocardial fibrosis. *Am. J. Hypertens.* 1990; **3**: 735–40.

19. James MA, Jones JV. An interaction between LVH and potassium in hypertension? *J. Human Hypertens.* 1991; **5**: 475–8.

20. Doyle AE. Vascular complications of hypertension. In *Handbook of Hypertension*, Vol. 1: *Clinical Aspects of Essential Hypertension* (ed. JIS Robertson). Amsterdam: Elsevier, 1983: 365–77.

21. MacMahon S, Peto R, Cutler J *et al.* Blood pressure, stroke, and coronary artery disease. Part 1: prolonged differences in blood pressure: prospective observational studies corrected for the regression dilution bias. *Lancet* 1990; **335**: 765–74.

22. Doyle AE. Future directions in mild hypertension research. In *Mild Hypertension: Recent Advances* (eds F Gross and T Strasser). New York: Raven Press, 1983: 389–92.

23. Robertson JIS. Concluding remarks: cum grano salis. In *Mild Hypertension: Recent Advances* (eds F Gross and T Strasser). New York: Raven Press, 1983: 413–18.

24. Spence JD, Arnold JMO, Gilbert JJ. Vascular consequences of hypertension and effects of antihypertensive therapy. In *Handbook of Hypertension*, Vol. 15: *Clinical Hypertension* (ed. JIS Robertson). Amsterdam: Elsevier, 1992: 621–54.

25. Cruickshank JM. Coronary flow reserve and the J curve relation between diastolic blood pressure and myocardial infarction. *Br. Med. J.* 1988; **297**: 1227–30.

26. Cooper A, Heagarty A. Small arteries and hypertension. *J. Hypertens.* 1994; **12** (suppl. 1): 33–5.

27. Doyle AE. Hypertension and vascular disease. *Am. J. Hypertens.* 1991; **4** (suppl.): 103–6.

28. Himmelmann A, Svensson A, Sigström L, Hansson L. Predictors of blood pressure and left ventricular mass in the young: the hypertension in pregnancy offspring study. *Am. J. Hypertens.* 1994; **7**: 381–9.

# 18
# Haemodynamic characteristics of hypertension

## — Evolution of haemodynamic features —

The haemodynamic accompaniments of hypertension are in conformity with the structural and functional changes which have already been described in both large and small arteries and in the heart (Chapters 13 and 17).[1,2]

In young subjects with borderline and often very labile hypertension, interindividual variations in haemodynamics may be considerable.

More consistent findings are apparent in young adults with established hypertension (more than 140/90 mmHg) that remains uncomplicated. In these subjects, the characteristic pattern is a high cardiac index with an elevated heart rate, and a numerically normal calculated total peripheral resistance.

With progression of the disease, the dominant haemodynamic disturbance is an increase in total peripheral resistance. At this later stage, cardiac index is lower than that in normotensive control subjects and lower than in the usually younger milder hypertensives. Heart rate may still be slightly elevated.

With increasing severity of hypertension and the onset of organ damage, there is a markedly increased total peripheral resistance, a decreased cardiac index and a reduced stroke volume.[1,2] Disproportionate elevation of systolic pressure is a feature of ageing,[3] and can be exaggerated in hypertension.

Regional measurements have shown that in established hypertension there is an increased vascular resistance across the kidneys, liver and skeletal muscle.[1,2] As previously mentioned (Chapter 17), the coronary vascular reserve is characteristically reduced,[4,5] particularly with supervention of atheromatous coronary artery stenosis.

A continuing problem in the assessment of haemodynamic aspects of hypertension is the difficulty of measuring cardiac output non-invasively.[12]

## Possible dangers of overzealous reduction of diastolic pressure: ——— the 'J- curve' ———

It has been proposed that in hypertensive patients with coronary artery disease, the optimum range of fifth-phase diastolic pressure during treatment should be around 85–90 mmHg.[6,7] (see also pages 12, 79 and 108). Higher pressures than this are not desirable, while conversely, too marked a reduction of diastolic pressure will be associated, it is suggested, with an increased risk of myocardial infarction (Figure 18.1). Thus, it is claimed, the relationship between the achieved diastolic pressure and myocardial infarction is 'J-shaped'. Since diastolic pressure may fall by a further 25% during sleep, the hypothetical risk may be enhanced nocturnally.[8,9]

Coronary artery filling is dependent on diastolic pressure, and it has been pointed out that the coronary circulation has less capacity for blood flow autoregulation than has the cerebral circulation. Further, while the brain has some capacity to extract more oxygen from blood when its perfusion pressure has fallen below the lower autoregulatory limit, the myocardium lacks this property.[10,11]

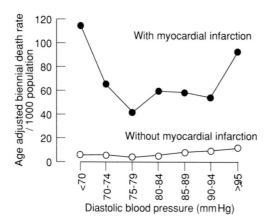

**Figure 18.1.** Coronary heart disease deaths relative to diastolic pressure in men and women with or without previous myocardial infarction. (Data from the Framingham study, Ref. 9.)

Considerable evidence has been provided both from epidemiological and therapeutic studies in support of the concept,[6,7] while it has also been vehemently denied by others.[7] A 'J-curve' as described must indeed exist; the main controversy surrounds the critical diastolic range below which therapy enhances, rather than diminishes, risk.

While there is no doubt of the pathophysiological and therapeutic interest in this important topic, most physicians might accept that their main difficulty is to achieve adequate blood pressure reduction. Excessive falls in diastolic are less often encountered in clinical practice.

## References

1. Lund-Johansen P. The hemodynamics of essential hypertension. In *Handbook of Hypertension*, Vol. 1:

*Clinical Aspects of Essential Hypertension* (ed. JIS Robertson). Amsterdam: Elsevier, 1983: 151–73.

2. Lund-Johansen P, Omvik P. Hemodynamic patterns of untreated hypertensive disease. In *Hypertension: Pathophysiology, Diagnosis, and Management* (eds JH Laragh and BM Brenner). New York: Raven Press, 1990: 305–27.

3. Staessen J, Fagard R, Lijnen P, Amery A. The effects of aging on blood pressure. In *Mild Hypertension: Recent Advances* (eds F Gross and T Strasser). New York: Raven Press, 1983: 315–27.

4. Frohlich ED, Apstein C, Chobanian AV *et al.* The heart in hypertension. *N. Engl. J. Med.* 1992; **327**: 998–1008.

5. Strauer BE. *Das Hochdruckherz,* 3rd edn. Berlin: Springer-Verlag, 1991.

6. Cruickshank JM. Coronary flow reserve and the J curve relation between diastolic blood pressure and myocardial infarction. *Br. Med. J.* 1988; **297**: 1227.

7. Zanchetti A, Amery A, Berglund G *et al.* How much should blood pressure be lowered? The problem of the J-shaped curve. *J. Hypertens.* 1989; **7** (suppl. 6): 338–48.

8. Floras JS. Antihypertensive treatment, myocardial infarction, and nocturnal myocardial ischaemia. *Lancet* 1988; **ii**: 994.

9. D'Agostino RB, Belanger AJ, Kannel WB, Cruickshank JM. Relation of low diastolic pressure to coronary heart disease death in presence of myocardial infarction: the Framingham study. *Br. Med. J.* 1991; **303**: 385–9.

10. Strandgaard S., Haunsø S. Why does antihypertensive treatment prevent stroke but not myocardial infarction? *Lancet* 1987; **ii**: 548–661.

11. Strandgaard S, Paulson OB. Hypertensive disease and the cerebral circulation. In *Hypertension: Pathophysiology, Diagnosis and Management* (eds JH Laragh and BM Brenner). New York: Raven Press, 1990: 399–416.

12. Robertson JIS, Birkenhäger WH (eds). Cardiac Output Measurement. London/Philadelphia: W. B. Saunders, 1991.

# 19
## Causes of cardiac and vascular changes in hypertension: therapeutic correction

The importance of the progressive cardiac structural and functional changes in the evolution of hypertension and its complications should be clear from the foregoing account. The loss of distensibility and compliance in large arteries leads to disproportionate elevation of systolic pressure and to end-systolic stress, thus contributing to the development of left ventricular hypertrophy.[1-4] Concurrently, there is greater turbulence of blood flow, promoting both endothelial damage and atheroma formation. The progressive thickening of the media of resistance arteries is similarly crucial to the increasing severity of the hypertension and its circulatory pattern, as well as to the sequential changes in renal function with the advance of the disease.

## Causes

Although the mechanical effect of elevation of arterial pressure as such provides a stimulus to cardiac and arterial changes, and thus to further progression of the hypertension, reasons have been advanced for its inadequacy as a sole explanation.[1,3,4,28] Extensive efforts have been devoted to the elucidation of additional stimuli. In this connection, most workers have regarded such influences as probably affecting the heart and resistance vessels alike, although conceding that there could be some differences in both the pattern and speed of the changes.[4-6]

The raised haematocrit which is a consistent feature of hypertension, with the accompanying increase in blood viscosity, could be one physical stimulus.[7-10]

Additionally, there are numerous vascular growth factors, demonstrable or speculative, around which an extensive literature has accumulated.[3,4,11-15,25] These include enhanced sympathetic activity, with consequent elevation of adrenaline and/or noradrenaline locally or within the circulation; corticosteroids; serotonin (5-hydroxytryptamine); angiotensin II, either in peripheral blood or generated locally within the muscle of heart or blood vessels; growth hormone; insulin; somatomedin C; platelet-derived growth factor; endothelial-derived growth factor; epidermal-derived growth factor; monocyte-derived growth factor; β-transforming growth factor; heparin; bradykinin; prostaglandins; vasopressin; thyroid hormone; and substance P.

## Therapeutic correction of left ventricular, large arterial and resistance arterial changes in hypertension

Numerous attempts have been made in recent years to identify and to utilize drugs in the treatment of hypertension that would be useful not only in simply lowering blood pressure but also in arresting and more particularly reversing left ventricular hypertrophy and medial thickening in resistance arteries, whilst improving compliance in large arteries.

Concerning the first two of these requirements, animal studies have indicated that the centrally acting agents methyldopa and reserpine, calcium antagonists of classes I and II, angiotensin-converting enzyme (ACE) inhibitors, and serotonin antagonists could be particularly useful. By contrast, vasodilators such as hydralazine, α-adrenergic blockers such as prazosin, and diuretics have appeared less efficacious.[16] These experiments have also shown that although hypertensive left ventricular hypertrophy and the medial thickening of smaller arteries share corrective responses to several drugs, therapeutic effects also can diverge between these tissues, indicating differences, despite some common influences, in causation.[6] Moreover, the clinical data are not always in full accord with the results of animal studies.

### Reversal of clinical left ventricular hypertrophy

Several reviewers have attempted comparisons of different classes of antihypertensive agents in affecting left ventricular hypertrophy. Their conclusions do not fully agree.

Hachamovitch et al.,[17] in an extensive review of the literature up to 1988, found that centrally acting sympatholytic agents, β-blockers, α-blockers, calcium antagonists and ACE inhibitors reduced left ventricular mass, while diuretics had a variable effect, and non-specific vasodilators were adverse.

Cruickshank et al.,[18] in a review of 104 studies, observed that left ventricular hypertrophy was most effectively corrected by ACE inhibitors, followed by methyldopa, α-blockers, non-dihydropyridine calcium antagonists, diuretics, β-blockers and dihydropyridine calcium antagonists, in that order. Non-specific vasodilators were ineffective, but on average, not adverse.

Dahlöf et al.,[19] surveying 109 trials, concurred that ACE inhibitors were the most effective, followed by diuretics, with β-blockers and calcium antagonists (which latter they did not subdivide) roughly equipotent. In their evaluation, which did not include non-specific vasodilators, α-blockers were least effective. Other forms of drug treatment, including methyldopa, clonidine, ketanserin and urapidil, were also shown to reduce left ventricular mass. There was a clear relationship overall between the therapeutic reduction of arterial pressure and of left ventricular mass.

Reassuringly, neither Cruickshank et al.,[18] nor Dahlöf et al.,[19] found placebo to be associated with any effect.

The differing results and emphases emerging from these three major reviews indicate the limitations of retrospective analyses of diverse trials initially designed for other purposes. Reliable comparisons could more readily be made prospectively, and within the same study.

### Improvement in large arterial compliance

Amongst the limited number of clinical studies so far reported, ACE inhibitors, various types of calcium antagonists, and several cardioselective and/or vasodilating β-blockers, as well as the β-blocker pindolol, which possesses marked intrinsic sympathomimetic activity, have shown their capacity to improve large arterial compliance. By contrast, the β-blockers propranolol and metoprolol, both potassium-wasting and potassium-conserving diuretics, and the direct-acting vasodilator dihydralazine, have been ineffective. Ketanserin improves arterial compliance, although urapidil does not.[20-22]

### Correction of medial thickening in resistance arteries

Heagerty et al.,[23] observed that hypertensive patients treated for a mean of 13 months showed, in subcutaneous resistance arteries, a substantial, but still incomplete, regression of media thickness. In this study, an assortment of drugs, in various combinations, was employed, so that no information was provided on any possible differential efficacy of antihypertensive agents. However, an ACE inhibitor has been found superior to atenolol in this regard.[26] This important field merits extensive future study.[24,27]

## References

1. Spence JD, Arnold JMO, Gilbert JJ. Vascular consequences of hypertension and effects of antihypertensive therapy. In *Handbook of Hypertension*, Vol. 15: *Clinical Hypertension* (ed. JIS Robertson). Amsterdam: Elsevier, 1992: 621–54.

2. Robertson JIS. Left ventricular, large arterial, and resistance arterial changes, the J-curve, and antiplatelet agents. *Curr. Opinion Cardiol.* 1989; **4**: 662–71.

3. Frohlich ED, Apstein C, Chobanian AV *et al.* The heart in hypertension. *N. Engl. J. Med.* 1992; **327**: 998–1008.

4. Strauer BE. *Das Hochdruckherz*, 3rd edn. Berlin: Springer-Verlag, 1991.

5. Lucarini AR, Spessot M, Picano E *et al.* Lack of correlation between cardiac mass and arteriolar structural changes in mild-to-moderate hypertension. *J. Hypertens.* 1991; **9**: 1187–91.

6. Agabiti-Rosei E, Muiesan ML, Geri A *et al.* Long-term antihypertensive treatment may induce normalization of left ventricular mass before complete regression of vascular structural changes: consequences for cardiac function at rest and during stress. *J. Hypertens.* 1988; **6** (suppl. 4): 94–6.

7. Göbel BO, Schülte-Göbel A, Weisser B *et al.* Arterial blood pressure: correlation with erythrocyte count, hematocrit, and hemoglobin concentration. *Am. J. Hypertens.* 1991; **4**: 14–19.

8. Koenig W, Sund M, Ernst E *et al.* Association between plasma viscosity and blood pressure. *Am. J. Hypertens.* 1991; **4**: 529–36.

9. Cirillo M, Laurenzi M, Trevisan M, Stamler J. Hematocrit, blood pressure and hypertension. *Hypertension* 1992; **20**: 319–26.

10. Fowkes FGR, Lowe GDO, Rumley A *et al.* The relationship between blood viscosity and blood pressure in a random sample of the population aged 55 to 74 years. *Eur. Heart J.* 1993; **14**: 597–601.

11. Frohlich ED. The mosaic of hypertension: past, present and future. *J. Hypertens.* 1988; **6** (suppl. 4): 2–11.

12. Schelling P, Fisher H, Ganten D. Angiotensin and cell growth: a link to cardiovascular hypertrophy? *J. Hypertens.* 1991; **9**: 3–15.

13. Janssen H, Rooman R, Robertson JIS (eds). *Wound Healing.* Petersfield/Chicago: Wrightson Biomedical, 1991.

14. Lever AF, Harrap SB. Essential hypertension: a disorder of growth with origins in childhood? *J. Hypertens.* 1992; **10**: 101–20.

15. Dustan HP. Growth factors and racial differences in severity of hypertension and renal diseases. *Lancet* 1992; **339**: 1339–40.

16. Fouad-Tarazi FM. Structural cardiac and vascular changes in hypertension: response to treatment. *Curr. Opinion Cardiol.* 1987; **2**: 782–5.

17. Hachamovitch R, Strom JA, Sonnenblick EH, Frishman WH. Left ventricular hypertrophy in hypertension and the effects of antihypertensive drug therapy. *Curr. Problems Cardiol.* 1988; **13**: 369–422.

18. Cruickshank JM, Lewis J, Moore V, Dodd C. Reversibility of left ventricular hypertrophy by differing types of antihypertensive therapy. *J. Human Hypertens.* 1992; **6**: 85–90.

19. Dahlöf B, Pennert K, Hansson L. Reversal of left ventricular hypertrophy in hypertensive patients: a metaanalysis of 109 studies. *Am. J. Hypertens.* 1992; **5**: 95–110.

20. Safar ME. Pulse pressure in essential hypertension: clinical and therapeutic implications. *J. Hypertens.* 1989; **7**: 769–76.

21. Arcaro G, Laurent S, Jondeau G *et al.* Stiffness of the common carotid artery in treated hypertensive patients. *J. Hypertens.* 1991; **9**: 947–54.

22. Van Bortel L, Hoeks APG, Kool MJF, Struijker-Boudier HA. Introduction to large artery properties as a target for risk reduction by antihypertensive therapy. *J. Hypertens.* 1992; **10** (suppl. 6): 123–6.

23. Heagerty AM, Bund SJ, Aalkjaer C. Effects of drug treatment of human resistance arteriole morphology in essential hypertension: direct evidence for structural remodelling of resistance vessels. *Lancet* 1988; **ii**: 1209–12.

24. Heagerty AM. Changes in vascular morphology in essential hypertension. *J. Human Hypertens.* 1991; **5** (suppl. 1): 3–8.

25. Gibbons GH, Dzau VJ. The emerging concept of vascular remodelling. *N. Engl. J. Med.* 1994; **330**: 1431–8.

26. Schiffrin EL, Deng LY, La rochelle P. Effects of a β-blocker or a converting enzyme inhibitor on resistance arteries in essential hypertension. *Hypertension* 1994; **23**: 83–91.

27. Cooper A, Heagerty A. Small arteries and hypertension. *J. Hypertens.* 1994; **12** (suppl. 1): 33–5.

28. Mulvaney MJ. Mechanical and other factors involved in vascular injury related to hypertension. *Blood Pressure* 1994; **3** (suppl. 1): 11–17.

# 20
# Factors influencing the complications of hypertension

Although raised blood pressure *per se* plus the accompanying disturbances of blood flow have been considered herein as principal causes of the complications associated with hypertension, these are affected by various additional factors. Some have already been mentioned in relation to cardiac hypertrophy and arterial modifications. There are several other important influences, as follows.

## Age

Advancing age predisposes to stroke, cardiac failure, coronary heart disease and progressive renal failure.[1] Ageing is accompanied by more prevalent Charcot–Bouchard aneurysms in intra-cerebral arteries, and more extensive arterial endothelial lesions. Concomitant hypertension, probably independently, compounds all of these tendencies.

Alone among the complications of hypertension, the malignant phase is less likely to occur after the age of 60 years than before.[1,2]

## Gender

For any given blood pressure value, the complication attack rate is higher in men than in women both before and during treatment (Figure 20.1).[3] The differential is more marked for coronary artery disease than for stroke. Most workers concur that the male to female differential risk is less marked, but still distinct, particularly for coronary morbid-ity, after the menopause. Colditz *et al.*,[4] however, in a prospective study conducted over 6 years in 121 700 American women, could find no evidence of an increased risk of coronary disease in those with a natural menopause, although there was an increased risk of coronary heart disease among women who had undergone bilateral oopho-rectomy and who did not take oestrogen supple-ments.

These concepts do not imply that women are immune to the consequences of high blood pressure. Hypertensive women are at risk when compared with their sisters who have lower blood pressure values, but in absolute terms much less so than are men with comparable blood pressure.

A number of reasons have been advocated for the lesser susceptibility of women to the cardio-vascular hazards of hypertension. One possibility is that women smoke less than men. This cannot, however, provide a full explanation, since the differential remains when comparing non-smoking men and women.[3] Serum total cholesterol concen-tration, which has unfavourable cardiovascular connotations, is lower in young women than in men of similar age; after the menopause, when the incidence of cardiovascular disease increases in women, total cholesterol values increase, and beyond the age of 50 may be even higher in women than in men.[3] However, as discussed in more detail on page 90, in hypertensive men and women over 60, the adverse influence of serum cholesterol on coronary artery disease is slight, and a higher serum cholesterol is then associated with a longer survival.[5,6]

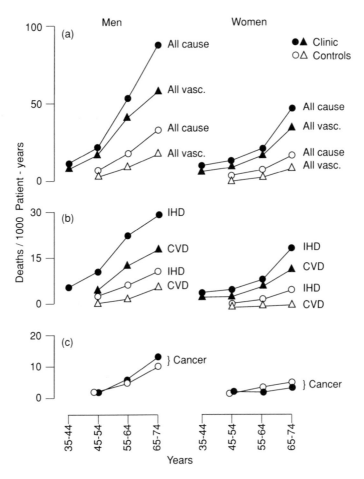

**Figure 20.1.** Age-, sex- and cause-specific mortality rates in the Glasgow Blood Pressure Clinic (closed symbols) and in the Renfrew–Paisley control population (open symbols). IHD = ischaemic heart disease; CVD = cerebrovascular disease; Vasc. = vascular. The vascular attack rate is higher in men than in women both in the treated hypertensives and in the control population. (Redrawn from Ref. 16, with permission.)

The pattern of low density lipoproteins (LDL), which are similarly believed to be adverse, at least in those under 60, tends to parallel that of total cholesterol. By contrast, high density lipoproteins (HDL), which carry a favourable cardiovascular prognosis, are higher in women than in men at all ages.[7]

After the menopause, plasma levels of factor VIIc and fibrinogen increase; these could heighten vascular risk.[8] Reduced insulin sensitivity might also contribute.[91]

Sarrell[9] has put forward a strong case for the loss of 17-$\beta$-oestradiol at the menopause as the critical factor in the subsequent enhanced risk of vascular disease in women. He has pointed out that this hormone can raise high density lipoprotein, lower low density lipoprotein, reduce platelet adhesiveness, regulate arteriolar tone and improve the phagocytic function of the reticulo-endothelial system. An additional hypothesis is that 17-$\beta$-oestradiol has a calcium antagonist effect.[10]

The vexed and inadequately studied problem[9,11-13] of the cardiovascular effects of long-term post-menopausal oestrogen replacement therapy is discussed on page 160.

## Social class

Social class, and also some behavioural accompaniments of social differentiation, such as smoking, markedly affect not only the prevalence (page 21) but also the consequences of high blood pressure.[14] Ménard and his colleagues[15] have testified, for example, to the more ready access of members of the higher social classes to the medical care of hypertension and thus presumably to a more satisfactory response to treatment. By contrast, social class was, surprisingly, not found to be related to risk among treated hypertensive patients in the Glasgow Blood Pressure Clinic.[16]

In the American HDFP study,[17] those hypertensive patients allocated to 'Stepped Care' received substantial financial support, with the costs of travel to the clinic, of laboratory tests and drugs being reimbursed (Table 21.3, page 104). The 'Referred Care' patients were simply returned to the care of their regular physician. The lower mortality of the Stepped Care patients at the end of the study was most marked in black women, followed by black men and white men. It seems likely that in large part these differences in outcome reflect more thorough provision of health care facilities overall for the Stepped Care group, the differential, and hence the benefits, being most striking, as would be expected, in those persons least privileged socially.

## Race and geography

Racial differences, which often tend to be associated with social privilege, demonstrate variations in the pattern of hypertension-related compli-

cations.[89] In an English study, it was shown that, when correction was made for differences in social class, there remained distinctions in the pattern of hypertension-related complications in whites, blacks (mainly of West Indian origin) and Asians (mainly from the Indian subcontinent). The West Indians had proportionately more strokes and fewer heart attacks than did the whites or Asians. Both non-white groups had a higher prevalence of diabetes mellitus.[18]

The population of Japan was, in the first half of the twentieth century, relatively immune to myocardial infarction, whilst being prone to stroke. However, residents of the west coast of the USA who were of Japanese extraction had lost this immunity to coronary artery disease, evincing a pattern of cardiovascular morbidity similar to that of other US citizens in that region. Genetic Japanese living in Hawaii showed a distribution of cardiovascular disease intermediate between that of Japan and the US west coast. Moreover, the pattern of disease within Japan has changed in recent decades, with coronary artery disease becoming progressively more prevalent. The reasons for this shift are not elucidated, but many epidemiologists attribute them to alterations in dietary preferences.[89] The traditional Japanese food was high in fish but low in other animal meat; this pattern has been modified considerably under American influence since 1945.

In China, likewise, coronary artery disease, whilst uncommon, is increasing in prevalence. Changing dietary habits have similarly been suspected as being largely responsible. Even so, it is remarkable that the increase in coronary disease in Chinese people has been observed in cities as far apart as Beijing, Taipei and Hong Kong, with their notable differences in lifestyle, culture, politics and diet.[19]

Amongst occidental nations, the prevalence of coronary artery disease is rising sharply in Hungary, a country in which a recent high dietary intake of fat has been blamed.[92] In contrast, some ethnic groups show remarkable immunity to the arterial complications of hypertension. Lindholm *et al.*,[20] reported on a community in the island of

(A)

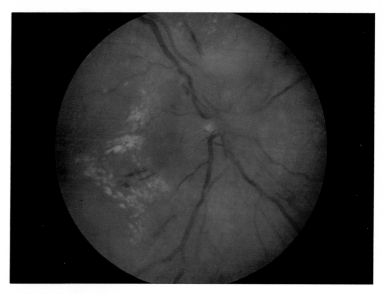

**Plate 14.1** Optic fundus of 35-year-old man presenting with malignant hypertension (blood pressure about 230/130 mmHg). (A) Papilloedema, haemorrhages and exudates can be seen. (B) Two years later, after effective antihypertensive drug treatment (blood pressure about 135/80 mmHg), the papilloedema and retinal lesions have resolved. (Reproduced from Ref. 1, with permission.)

(B)

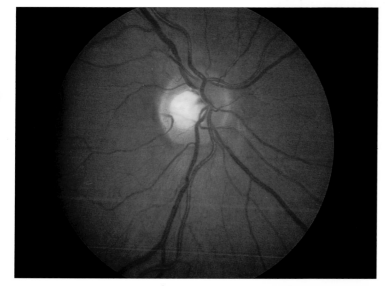

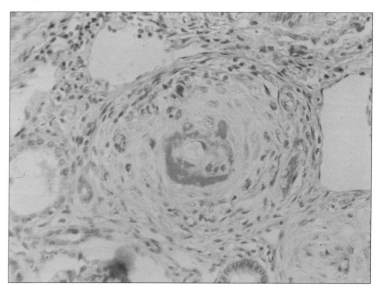

**Plate 16.1** Malignant hypertension, showing fibrinoid arterial necrosis in an intrarenal artery.

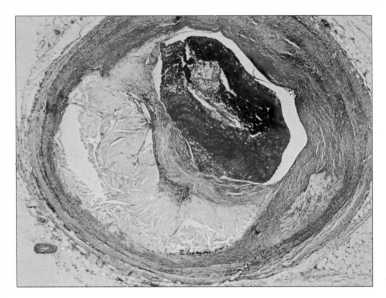

**Plate 17.1** Coronary thrombosis on a pre-existing atheromatous lesion in a patient with hypertension.

**Plate 25.1** Collection of uneaten antihypertensive drugs recovered from the locker of a 16-year-old girl with apparent drug-resistant hypertension (diastolic pressures 120–150 mmHg). She was observed to be taking tablets into her mouth, then surreptitiously spitting them out. Following further discussions, blood pressure was controlled at around 120/90 mmHg on atenolol 100 mg plus bendrofluazide 10 mg daily. (Reproduced from Ref. 31, with permission.)

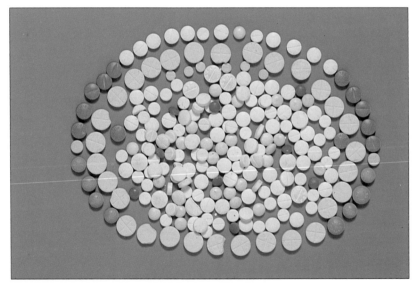

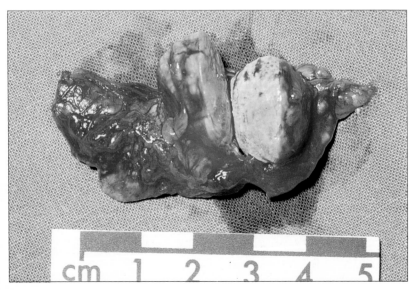

**Plate 35.1** Aldosterone-secreting adenoma of the adrenal cortex after removal. (Reproduced from Ref. 9, with permission.)

Crete, Greece, where coronary artery disease was almost absent, despite the usual Western prevalence of hypertension, diabetes mellitus, hypercholesterolaemia and cigarette smoking.

Remarkable differences in the pattern of cardiovascular morbidity can be seen even when the racial composition appears to be broadly uniform. Thus within the UK, coronary artery disease is especially prevalent in Northern Ireland and western Scotland, and much effort has been expended in attempts to elucidate the cultural, genetic and dietary factors underlying the problem. Coronary disease is especially prevalent also in eastern Finland, the former Soviet Union, and amongst the white races of South Africa.[21,89,90]

In Sweden and in Australia, there has been an apparent decline in the incidence of the malignant phase of hypertension in the past decade or so.[22,23] The reasons for this change are not understood, but one possibility is more effective screening, prevention and therapy (page 67). No such decline is evident in the UK; although figures are difficult to obtain, there is no obvious dearth of patients who have malignant hypertension in cities such as Birmingham and Glasgow.[24,25]

Much remains to be learned of the reasons for these often strikingly different patterns of cardiovascular disease, and hence of the complications of hypertension, between different races and cultures. The variations should serve to warn against extrapolating widely from epidemiological and therapeutic studies performed in a particular geographical area or circumscribed population group. The observations made in the small towns of Framingham[26] and Tecumseh[27] in the USA, for example, have been of substantial value, but the conclusions should not be translated incautiously to other places.

## Ambient temperature

As discussed on page 22, blood pressure values are consistently higher in cold weather, both in untreated and treated hypertensive men and women.[28,29] A seasonal variation in coronary morbidity and mortality has been seen in several countries, with higher rates in the cold periods of the year. Detailed Swedish studies have shown that the strong association between cold exposure and coronary mortality is not affected by regional variations in fat consumption, tobacco use, or hypertension (Figure 20.2).[30] In part the reason may be corresponding seasonal changes in the risk factors plasma fibrinogen and factor VII.[88]

## Body weight

Body weight, as has been discussed on page 26, is positively correlated with arterial pressure. The relation of weight to the complications of hypertension is more complex, these being more frequent in persons both with the highest and also the lowest body mass indices; subjects intermediate in body weight appear to do best.[17,31]

## Smoking

Of all the factors influencing the frequency and pattern of hypertension-related disease, cigarette smoking is pre-eminent. Smoking is such a powerful independent risk factor for cardiovascular disease that it may overwhelm a raised blood pressure in importance, and will severely restrict the benefits obtained from antihypertensive therapy. Several of these aspects are discussed in more detail in Chapter 8.

Smoking, predictably, greatly compounds the effects of high blood pressure *per se*. For example, the incidence of the malignant phase is more frequent, and its prognosis, even when treated, is distinctly poorer, in smokers than in non-smokers.[24] Hypertension-related stroke and coronary disease are also much more frequent in smokers, both in untreated and in treated subjects. Renal artery stenosis is more prevalent in hypertensive patients who smoke;[32,33] this holds true both for atherosclerotic and for fibromuscular dysplastic renovascular disease. The risks become less with cessation of smoking.[34,35]

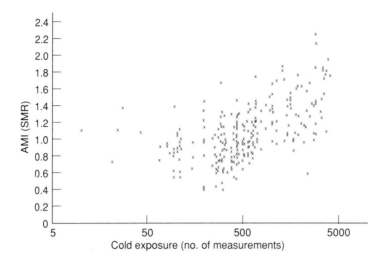

**Figure 20.2.** Standardized mortality rates (SMR) from acute myocardial infarction (AMI) 1975–84 for men aged 40–64 and cold exposure expressed as the number of measurements below −10°C during five measurements per day over the same period in 284 Swedish municipalities. (Redrawn from Ref. 30, with permission.)

## Serum cholesterol

Serum total cholesterol, LDL cholesterol and triglyceride are independent risk factors for cardiovascular morbidity. Thus the complications of hypertension, at any rate below the age of 60, increase in proportion to these values, of which the most often recorded is serum cholesterol.[26] By contrast, there is a negative correlation between coronary heart disease and HDL cholesterol (see also Appendix 3). These observations have given rise to diverse concerns and controversies. Some physicians have proposed that antihypertensive agents that *inter alia* elevate serum cholesterol or distort the serum lipid pattern in a potentially adverse way, such as many of the thiazide diuretics and some $\beta$-blockers, should, consequently, be used with caution.[36,37] According to these views, the employment of such drugs has been one reason why antihypertensive therapy has been less successful than had been hoped in limiting hypertension-related coronary artery morbidity.[38] Consequently, it has been suggested that the greater use of agents which have a potentially beneficial effect on the

serum lipid pattern, such as $\alpha$-blockers, hydralazine or serotonergic type 2 antagonists, or which are neutral in this respect, such as ACE inhibitors, are to be preferred. Other writers have derided these notions.[39]

Any worsening cardiovascular morbidity incurred by a high serum cholesterol seems, as mentioned above, to be restricted to those under about the age of 60. In an important survey, Staessen *et al.*[5] found that in hypertensive men and women over the age of 60, a high serum cholesterol was associated with longer survival (Figure 20.3). Possible confounding by cholesterol reduction in patients with cancer was avoided. Their results demonstrated a lower non-cardiovascular mortality with high serum cholesterol, and an absence, in this elderly population, of a positive relationship between serum cholesterol and cardiovascular mortality. The MRC trial in hypertensive subjects over 65 provided similar evidence[6] of a beneficial association with higher serum cholesterol.

A further intricacy has been introduced with observations, made in both Western and Oriental patients, that dietary sodium restriction can, at least

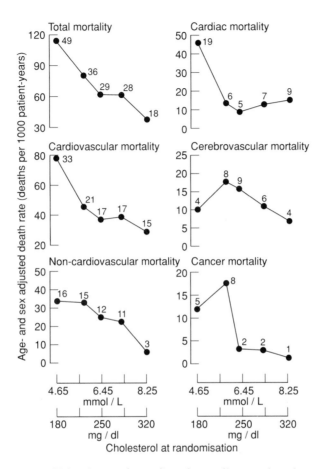

**Figure 20.3.**   Age- and sex-adjusted mortality rates in quin-
tiles of the distribution of serum total cholesterol at randomiza-
tion in hypertensive men and women over 60. Number of
deaths also given. Those with the higher cholesterol values had
better prognosis. (Redrawn from Ref. 5, with permission.)

short term, elevate serum cholesterol.[40–42] Not all
reports have confirmed this.[43] Studies of longer
duration are needed on this potentially important
topic.

The issue has become even more complex with
the increasing recognition that, while lowering
serum cholesterol may diminish the danger of
coronary artery disease, the risks of cancer and of
death from violence (including suicide) can, even in
those under the age of 60, be enhanced.[44,45]

Further concerns are introduced by claims that
selective analyses have misrepresented both the
dangers and benefits of cholesterol reduction;[46]
and that dietary measures intended to lower serum
cholesterol are in any event largely ineffective.[47,48]

The therapeutic implications, not surprisingly,
have generated fierce controversy, first concerning
whether serum cholesterol should or should not be
lowered, and second whether this has, or should
have, any bearing on the choice of antihypertensive
drug or on dietary attempts to lower blood pressure. If serum cholesterol is to be lowered, more
thorough measures than the dietary advice usually
offered currently are required.[47,48] Again, it should

be emphasized that elderly hypertensive men and women survive longer if their serum cholesterol is high.[5,6]

────────── Uric acid ──────────

There is no conclusive evidence that either spontaneous or diuretic-induced elevation of serum uric acid in hypertension worsens vascular risk.[49] However, as discussed on page 248, relative elevation of uric acid in pregnancy can indicate the onset of pre-eclampsia.

────────── Diabetes mellitus ──────────

The possible relationship of diabetes mellitus to the pathogenesis of hypertension is discussed on page 40. Additionally, there are important prognostic and therapeutic implications. Diabetes mellitus is associated with more prevalent vascular lesions, and thus the coexistence of diabetes with hypertension increases the risk of vascular disease.[26,50] Diabetes also introduces problems into the management of hypertension, because certain classes of drugs, notably thiazide diuretics and $\beta$-adrenoceptor blocking agents, can impair glucose tolerance and destabilize diabetic control.[50]

────────── Renin and angiotensin II ──────────

There is substantial experimental evidence, with some clinical support, that very high circulating levels of renin, and hence of its vasoactive product, angiotensin II, can, especially but not necessarily when combined with raised arterial pressure, cause arterial damage, renal tubular necrosis and multifocal myocardial necrosis.[51] The myocardial lesions, when extensive, can coalesce and come to resemble closely myocardial infarction from other causes. Moreover, while elevation of plasma renin and angiotensin II is not necessary for the supervention of malignant phase hypertension, there is much to suggest that if plasma angiotensin II is raised in hypertension, progression to the malignant phase is facilitated.[52]

The wider and potentially important issue of whether more modest long-term elevation of plasma renin constitutes an independent risk factor for some of the complications of hypertension remains controversial. Brunner et al.,[53] in a retrospective analysis, proposed that a raised plasma renin could predispose hypertensive patients to both stroke and myocardial infarction. A bigger retrospective survey from the same group appeared to confirm the relationship with heart attack, but not with stroke.[54] Epidemiological flaws in these studies were criticized by several writers.[51,55]

A later and larger retrospective analysis by Meade et al.,[56] which was also not above reproach, suggested contrarily that low, rather than high, plasma renin levels were likely to be associated with an increased risk of organ damage in hypertension.

Brown and Brown,[57] interpreting therapeutic data, proposed that a high plasma renin level might help prevent, rather than precipitate, stroke.

Alderman et al.,[58] in a prospective study, found evidence that a raised plasma renin level was associated with an increased risk of myocardial infarction; there was no association with stroke. The absolute numbers of myocardial infarctions in this trial were remarkably few; 7 with high renin, 15 with normal renin, and 5 with low renin. Although initial therapy was with a $\beta$-blocker (which would tend to lower renin) in 33% of patients, and with a diuretic (which should elevate renin) in 52%, no evidence was obtained that the outcome was affected by the class of antihypertensive drug used. Moreover, the results were insufficient to deter the principal author from recommending a diuretic as initial therapy in hypertension.[59] (See also page 303.)

In a very large prospective study of a predominantly normotensive male population, Meade et al.[60] could find no association between plasma renin activity and myocardial infarction or sudden coronary death.

A tangential demonstration is that a variant gene controlling the formation of angiotensin-converting enzyme (ACE) has been found to be strongly associated epidemiologically with myocardial infarction.[61] The relevance of these findings to the foregoing controversy is unclear; neither plasma renin activity nor angiotensin II were measured.[61] It is unlikely that variations in plasma ACE in the range observed[61] would be rate-limiting for angiotensin II generation. It remains uncertain for the present, therefore, whether the biochemical links are pathogenically related to the causation of myocardial infarction.

Thus, despite the possible importance of whether or not modest, as contrasted with marked, elevation of renin and angiotensin II is an independent risk factor for any of the complications of hypertension, this remains obscure. Most elusive still is the critical practical aspect of whether antihypertensive treatment should best be undertaken with a drug which raises or lowers plasma renin and hence angiotensin II.[51]

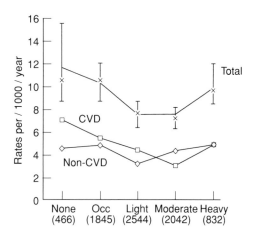

**Figure 20.4.** Total, cardiovascular (CVD) and non-cardiovascular mortality rates in five groups arranged by alcohol intake. Absolute numbers in each group shown. Vertical bars = 95% confidence intervals for total mortality. X = adjusted for age, social class and cigarette smoking. (Redrawn from Ref. 69, with permission.)

―――――――― Alcohol ――――――――

### Alcohol and adverse effects on morbidity

The pressor action of alcohol, and the additional adverse influences of heavy drinking on the compliance with, and the effectiveness of, antihypertensive therapy, have been described on pages 31–33.

Alcohol ingestion can further worsen prognosis by predisposing to stroke,[62] cardiac myopathy[63] and/or arrhythmias.[64,65]

Moreover, an alcoholic binge has been reported often to be followed by a stroke,[66,67] although this is disputed.[68]

### Modest alcohol consumption, wine drinking and arterial protection

Notwithstanding the undoubted baneful cardiovascular influences of heavy consumption of alcohol, there have been repeated epidemiological observations of a 'J-shaped' or 'U-shaped' relationship between alcohol intake and the prevalence of cardiovascular disease (Figure 20.4). These studies have shown that subjects with a modest consumption of

alcohol fare better than those who are total abstainers;[70-74] this benefit seems to extend to the elderly[75] and to women.[76,77] Possible mechanisms whereby any such protection might be conferred are via elevation of HDL cholesterol; reduction of plasma fibrinogen concentration; and reduced platelet activity.[72]

Not all epidemiologists have accepted that modest alcohol consumption is, in cardiovascular terms, superior to total abstention.[69,78] The issue has aroused fierce controversy,[79-83] perhaps not surprisingly, given the undoubted hazards of excessive alcohol intake, and the emotive accompanying propaganda.

A related topic is the apparent protective effect of wine, and especially of red wine, against myocardial infarction. St. Leger et al.[84] reported in 1979 that data from 18 developed countries showed a strong and specific negative association between deaths from coronary artery disease and alcohol consumption; this was attributable to wine intake (Figure 20.5). The beneficial properties are apparently associated with red rather than

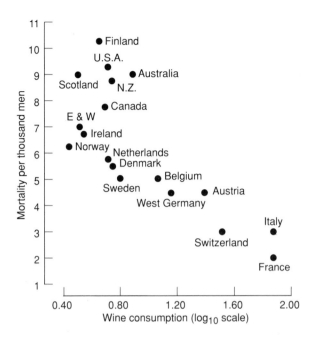

**Figure 20.5.** Relationship between coronary artery disease mortality rate and wine consumption in men aged 55–56. (Reproduced from Ref. 84, with permission.)

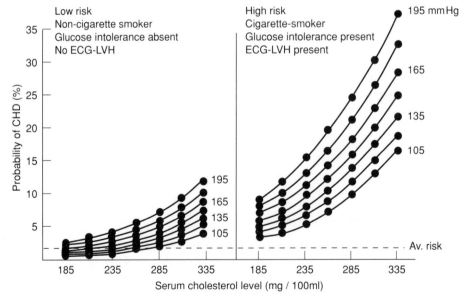

**Figure 20.6.** The interaction of several risk factors with systolic arterial pressure in relation to the development of coronary heart disease. The information is taken from a 16-year follow-up in 40-year-old men, and indicates the risk of developing coronary disease in 6 years. 185 mg/100 ml (4.8 mmol/litre); 335 mg/100 ml (8.7 mmol/litre) serum cholesterol. (Redrawn from Ref. 87, with permission.)

white wine,[85] although not all studies have shown this.

Features associated with red wine which might confer benefit are a capacity to inhibit platelet activity, and alterations in serum lipoprotein patterns. Frankel *et al.*[86] have reported that the non-alcoholic components of red wine have potent antioxidant effects on human LDL cholesterol, properties likely to limit thrombosis and ameliorate atheroma.

──────── Compounding of risk ────────

The manner in which some of the recognized additional factors can compound the cardiovascular dangers of hypertension is shown in Figure 20.6 (opposite).

──────────── Case study ────────────

See Case study 5, Appendix 2.

──────────── References ────────────

1. Pickering GW. *Hypertension: Causes, Consequences and Management*, 2nd edn. Edinburgh: Churchill Livingstone, 1974.
2. Pickering GW. *High Blood Pressure*, 2nd edn. London: Churchill, 1968.
3. Robertson JIS. Hypertension in the female. In *The Circulation in the Female: From the Cradle to the Grave* (ed. J Ginsburg). New Jersey: Parthenon, 1989: 51–9.
4. Colditz GA, Willett WC, Stampfer M *et al.* Menopause and the risk of coronary heart disease in women. *N. Engl. J. Med.* 1987; **316**: 1105–10.
5. Staessen J, Amery A, Birkenhäger W. Is a high serum cholesterol level associated with a longer survival in elderly hypertensives? *J. Hypertens.* 1990; **8**: 755–61.
6. MRC Working Party. Medical Research Council trial of treatment of hypertension in older adults: principal results. *Br. Med. J.* 1992; **304**: 405–12.
7. Gordon T. Coronary heart disease in young women: incidence and epidemiology. In *Coronary Heart Disease in Young Women* (ed. MF Oliver). Edinburgh: Churchill Livingstone, 1978: 12–23.
8. Meade TW. Epidemiology of atheroma, thrombosis and ischaemic heart disease. In *Haemostasis and Thrombosis* (eds AL Bloom and DP Thomas). Edinburgh: Churchill Livingstone, 1987: 697–720.
9. Sarrell P. The effects of ovarian steroids on the cardiovascular system. In *The Circulation in the Female: From the Cradle to the Grave* (ed. J Ginsburg). New Jersey: Parthenon, 1989: 117–40.
10. Collins P, Rosano GMC, Jiang C *et al.* Cardiovascular protection by oestrogen: a calcium antagonist effect? *Lancet* 1993; **341**: 1264–5.
11. Pfeffer RI, van den Noort S. Estrogen use and stroke risk in postmenopausal women. *Am. J. Epidemiol.* 1976; **103**: 445–56.
12. Wren BG, Routledge DA. Blood pressure changes: oestrogens in climacteric women. *Med. J. Aust.* 1981; **2**: 528–31.
13. Wilson PWF, Garrison RJ, Castelli WP. Postmenopausal estrogen use, cigarette smoking, and cardiovascular morbidity in women over 50. *N. Engl. J. Med.* 1985; **313**: 1038–43.
14. Angell M. Privilege and health: what is the connection? *N. Engl. J. Med.* 1993; **329**: 126–7.
15. Ménard J, Degoulet P, Chatellier G *et al.* Influence of educational and sociocultural factors on hypertension care. *J. Hypertens.* 1985; **3** (suppl. 2): 45–9.
16. Isles CG, Walker L, Beevers DG *et al.* Mortality in patients of the Glasgow Blood Pressure Clinic. *J. Hypertens.* 1986; **4**: 141–56.
17. Hypertension Detection and Follow-up Program Cooperative Group. Five-year findings of the hypertension detection and follow-up program: I. Reduction in mortality of persons with high blood pressure, including mild hypertension. *J. Am. Med. Assoc.* 1979; **242**: 2562–71.
18. Cruickshank JK, Beevers DG, Osbourne VL *et al.* Heart attack, stroke, diabetes and hypertension in West Indians, Asians and Whites in Birmingham, England. *Br. Med. J.* 1980; **281**: 1108.
19. Woo KS, Donnan SPB. Epidemiology of coronary arterial disease in Chinese. *Int. J. Cardiol.* 1989; **24**: 83–93.
20. Lindholm L, Koutis A, Leonis C *et al.* Risk factors for IHD in a Greek population: a cross-sectional study of men and women living in the village of Spili in Crete. *Eur. Heart J.* 1992; **13**: 291–8.

21. Wyndham CH. Trends with time of cardiovascular mortality rates in the populations of the RSA for the period 1968–1977. *South African Med. J.* 1982; **61**: 987–93.

22. Kincaid-Smith P. What has happened to malignant hypertension? In *Handbook of Hypertension*, Vol. 6: *Epidemiology of Hypertension* (ed. CJ Bulpitt). Amsterdam: Elsevier, 1985: 255–65.

23. Gudbrandsson T, Hansson L, Herlitz H, Andrén L. Malignant hypertension: improving prognosis in a rare disease. *Acta Med. Scand.* 1979; **206**: 495–9.

24. Isles CG, Brown JJ, Cumming AMM *et al.* Excess smoking in malignant-phase hypertension. *Br. Med. J.* 1979; **1**: 579–81.

25. Ahmed MEK, Walker JM, Beevers DG, Beevers M. Lack of difference between malignant and accelerated hypertension. *Br. Med. J.* 1986; **292**: 235–7.

26. Kannel WB. Hypertension and the risk of cardiovascular disease. In *Hypertension: Pathophysiology and Management* (eds JH Laragh and BM Brenner). New York: Raven, 1990: 101–17.

27. Higgins MW, Killer JB, Metzner HL *et al.* Studies of high blood pressure in Tecumseh, Michigan. II: antecedents in childhood of high blood pressure in young adults. *Hypertension* 1980; **2** (suppl. 1): 117–23.

28. Brennan PJ, Greenberg G, Miall WE, Thompson SG. Seasonal variation in blood pressure. *Br. Med. J.* 1982; **285**: 919–23.

29. Kunes J, Tremblay J, Bellevance F, Hamet P. Influence of environmental temperature on the blood pressure of hypertensive patients in Montreal. *Am. J. Hypertens* 1991; **4**: 422–6.

30. Gyllerup S. Cold as a risk factor for coronary mortality: a study of aggregated data from different regions in Sweden. M.D. thesis, University of Lund, Dalby, Sweden, 1992.

31. Langford HG, Stamler J, Wassertheil-Smoller S, Prineas RJ. All-cause mortality in the Hypertension Detection and Follow-up Program: Findings for the whole cohort and for persons with less severe hypertension, with and without other traits related to risk of mortality. *Prog. Cardiovasc. Dis.* 1986; **29** (suppl. 1): 29–54.

32. MacKay A, Brown JJ, Cumming AMM *et al.* Smoking and renal artery stenosis. *Br. Med. J.* 1972; **2**: 770–2.

33. Nicholson JP, Teichman SL, Alderman MH *et al.* Cigarette smoking and renovascular hypertension. *Lancet* 1983; **ii**: 765–6.

34. Rosenberg L, Kaufman DW, Helmrich SP, Shapiro S. The risk of myocardial infarction after quitting smoking in men under 55 years of age. *N. Engl. J. Med.* 1985; **313**: 1511–4.

35. Kawachi I. *et al.* Smoking cessation and decreased risk of stroke in women. *J. Am. Med. Assoc.* 1993; **269**: 232–6.

36. Ames RP. the effects of antihypertensive drugs on serum lipids and lipoproteins. I. Diuretics. *Drugs* 1986; **32**: 260–78.

37. Ames RP. The effects of antihypertensive drugs on serum lipids and lipoproteins. II. Non-diuretic drugs. *Drugs* 1986; **32**: 335–7.

38. Poulter N, Sever P, Thom S. Antihypertensive and adverse biochemical effects of bendrofluazide. *Br. Med. J.* 1990; **300**: 1465.

39. Ramsay LE, Yeo WW. Antihypertensive and adverse biochemical effects of bendrofluazide. *Br. Med. J.* 1990; **301**: 240–41.

40. Masugi F, Ogihara T, Hashizume K *et al.* Changes in plasma lipids and uric acid with sodium loading and sodium depletion in patients with hypertension. *J. Human Hypertens.* 1988; **1**: 293–8.

41. Egan BM, Weder AB, Petrin J *et al.* Neurohumoral and metabolic effects of short-term dietary NaCl restriction in men: relationship to salt-sensitivity status. *Am. J. Hypertens.* 1991; **4**: 416–21.

42. Ruppert M, Diehl J, Kolloch R *et al.* Short-term dietary sodium restriction increases serum lipids and insulin in salt-sensitive and salt-resistant normotensive adults. *Klin. Wschr.* 1991; **69** (suppl. 25): 51–7.

43. Kjeldsen SE, Taylor I, Westheim I *et al.* Severe sodium restriction alone and with potassium supplementation does not alter blood lipoproteins in essential hypertension. *Eur. J. Clin. Invest.* 1987; **17**: 182–6.

44. Muldoon MF, Manuck SB, Matthews KA. Lowering cholesterol concentrations and mortality: a quantitative review of primary prevention trials. *Br. Med. J.* 1990; **301**: 309–14.

45. Oliver MF. National cholesterol policies. *Eur. Heart J.* 1993; **14**: 581–3.

46. Ravnskov U. Cholesterol lowering trials in coronary heart disease: frequency of citation and outcome. *Br. Med. J;* 1992; **305**: 15–19.

47. Ramsay LE, Yeo WW, Jackson PR. Dietary reduction of serum cholesterol concentration: time to think again. *Br. Med. J.* 1991; **303**: 953–7.

48. Hunninghake DB, Stein EA, Dujovne CA *et al.* The efficacy of intensive dietary therapy alone or combined with lovastatin in outpatients with hyper-

cholesterolemia. *N. Engl. J. Med.* 1993; **328**: 1213–19.

49. Editorial. Uric acid in hypertension. *Lancet* 1987; **i**: 1124–5.

50. Beretta-Piccoli C. Diabetes mellitus and hypertension. In *Handbook of Hypertension*, Vol. 15: *Clinical Hypertension* (ed. JIS Robertson). Amsterdam: Elsevier, 1992: 141–76.

51. Gavras I, Gavras H. Angiotensin II-possible adverse effects on arteries, heart, brain and kidney: experimental, clinical and epidemiological evidence. In *The Renin–Angiotensin System* (eds JIS Robertson and MG Nicholls). London: Gower Medical, 1993: chapter 40.

52. Robertson JIS. Renin and malignant hypertension. In *The Renin–Angiotensin System* (eds JIS Robertson and MG Nicholls). London: Gower Medical, 1993: chapter 60.

53. Brunner HR, Laragh JH, Baer L *et al.* Renin and aldosterone, heart attack and stroke. *N. Engl. J. Med.* 1972; **286**: 441–9.

54. Brunner HR, Gavras H, Laragh JH *et al.* The risk of low renin hypertension: an updated analysis. *Eur. Soc. Clin. Invest. 9th Annual Meeting.* Rotterdam 1975; Abstract No. 53.

55. Kirkendall WM, Hammond JJ, Overturf ML. Renin as a predictor of hypertensive complications. *Ann. NY Acad. Sci.* 1978; **304**: 161–4.

56. Meade TW, Imeson TD, Gordon D *et al.* The epidemiology of plasma renin. *Clin. Sci.* 1983; **64**: 273–80.

57. Brown MJ, Brown J. Does angiotensin II protect against strokes? *Lancet* 1986; **i**: 427–9.

58. Alderman MH, Madhavan S, Ooi WL *et al.* Association of the renin-sodium profile with the risk of myocardial infarction in patients with hypertension. *N. Engl. J. Med.* 1991; **324**: 1098–104.

59. Alderman MH. Which antihypertensive drugs first—and why. *J. Am. Med. Assoc.* 1992; **267**: 2786–7.

60. Meade TW, Cooper JA, Peart WS. Plasma renin activity and ischemic heart disease. *N. Engl. J. Med.* 1993; **329**: 616–19.

61. Cambien F, Poirier O, Lecerf L *et al.* Deletion polymorphism in the gene for angiotensin-converting enzyme is a potent risk factor for myocardial infarction. *Nature* 1992; **359**: 641–4.

62. Gill JS, Zezulka AV, Shipley MJ *et al.* Stroke and alcohol consumption. *N. Engl. J. Med.* 1986; **315**: 1041–6..

63. Diamond I. Alcoholic myopathy and cardiomyopathy. *N. Engl. J. Med.* 1989; **320**: 458–60.

64. Thornton JR. Atrial fibrillation in healthy non-alcoholic people after an alcoholic binge. *Lancet* 1984; **ii**: 1013–15.

65. Koskinen P, Kupari M. Alcohol and cardiac arrhythmias. *Br. Med. J.* 1992; **304**: 1394–5.

66. Wilkins MR, Kendall MJ. Stroke affecting young men after alcoholic binges. *Br. Med. J.* 1985; **291**: 1342.

67. Gorelick PB, Kelly MA. Alcohol as a risk factor for stroke. *Heart Dis. Stroke* 1992; **1**: 255–8.

68. Gill JS, Zezulka AV. Beevers DG. Stroke affecting young men after alcoholic binges. *Br. Med. J.* 1985; **291**: 1645.

69. Shaper AG, Wannamethee G, Walker M. Alcohol and mortality in British men: explaining the U-shaped curve. *Lancet* 1988; **ii**: 1267–73.

70. Marmot MG, Rose GA, Shipley MJ *et al.* Alcohol and mortality: a U-shaped curve. *Lancet* 1981; **i**: 580–3.

71. Kreitman N. The perils of abstention? *Br. Med. J.* 1982; **284**: 444–5.

72. Marmot M, Brunner E. Alcohol and cardiovascular disease: the status of the U-shaped curve. *Br. Med. J.* 1991; **303**: 565–8.

73. Rimm EB, Giovannucci EL, Willet WC *et al.* Prospective study of alcohol consumption and risk of coronary disease in men. *Lancet* 1991; **338**: 464–8.

74. Jackson R, Scragg R, Beaglehole R. Alcohol consumption and the risk of coronary heart disease. *Br. Med. J.* 1991; **303**: 211–16.

75. Scherr PA *et al.* Light to moderate alcohol consumption and mortality in the elderly. *J. Am. Geriat. Soc.* 1992; **40**: 651–7.

76. Stampfer MJ, Colditz G, Willett WC *et al.* A prospective study of moderate alcohol consumption and the risk of coronary disease and stroke in women. *N. Engl. J. Med.* 1988; **319**: 267–73.

77. Razay G, Heaton KW, Bolton CH *et al.* Alcohol consumption and its relation to cardiovascular risk factors in British women. *Br. Med. J.* 1992; **304**: 80–3.

78. Editorial. Alcohol and mortality: the myth of the U-shaped curve. *Lancet* 1988; **i**: 1292–3.

79. Skrabanek P. Alcohol and the U-shaped curve. *Lancet* 1989; **i**: 105.

80. Burton JG. Alcohol and the U-shaped curve. *Lancet* 1989; **i**: 105.

81. Al-Bachari M, Acharya P. Alcohol and the U-shaped curve. *Lancet* 1989; **i**: 105.

82. Unwin N. Alcohol and the U-shaped curve. *Lancet* 1989; **i**: 105.

83. Cullen K. Alcohol and mortality. *Lancet* 1989; **i**: 363–4.

84. St. Leger AS, Cochrane AL, Moore F. Factors associated with cardiac mortality in developed countries with particular reference to the consumption of wine. *Lancet*, **i**: 1017–20.

85. Sharp D. Coronary disease: when wine is red. *Lancet* 1993; **341**: 27–28.

86. Frankel EN, Kanner J, German JB *et al*. Inhibition of human low-density lipoprotein by phenolic substances in red wine. *Lancet* 1993; **341**: 454–7.

87. Kannel WB, Stokes JS. Hypertension as a cardiovascular risk factor. In *Handbook of Hypertension*, Vol. 6: *Epidemiology of Hypertension* (ed. CJ Bulpitt). Amsterdam: Elsevier, 1985: 15–34.

88. Woodhouse PR, Khaw KT, Plummer M *et al*. Seasonal variations in plasma fibrinogen and factor VII activity in the elderly: winter infections and death from cardiovascular disease. *Lancet* 1994; **343**: 435–9.

89. Oliver MF. Diet and coronary heart disease. *Br. Med. Bull.* 1981; **37**: 49–58.

90. Cooper R. Rising death rates in the Soviet Union: the impact of coronary heart disease. *N. Engl. J. Med.* 1981; **304**: 1259–65.

91. Razay G, Heaton KW, Bolton CH. Coronary heart disease risk factors in relation to the menopause. *Quart J. Med.* 1992; **85**: 889–96.

92. Kesteloot H, Sasaki S *et al*. Secular trends in cerebrovascular mortality. *J. Hum. Hypertens.* 1994; **8**: 401–7.

# Section 3
## Treating essential hypertension

Section 3

# 21
# Benefits from treating hypertension

## Rationale of antihypertensive therapy

The various cardiovascular complications associated with raised systemic arterial pressure are described in detail in Chapters 13–17. Specifically, they comprise the malignant phase, hypertensive encephalopathy, cardiac failure, stroke, coronary heart disease and its consequences, and progressive impairment of renal function (Table 21.1). Antihypertensive therapy is directed to the prevention or correction of these disorders.

## Pharmacological and non-pharmacological therapy

The effectiveness of treatment has been evaluated in a succession of trials since the introduction of drugs capable of lowering arterial pressure in the 1950s. From that time, virtually all of the progress in this respect has been derived from pharmacological therapy.[1] Although there has been steady and increasing interest in non-pharmacological means of blood pressure reduction (pages 129 and 303), such approaches have so far had limited application, and any effects they may have in obviating complications have not been assessed.[2]

## Benefits ancillary to blood pressure reduction

For many years it was assumed, with good reason, that the complications were the result of high blood pressure as such, and that treatment should therefore be directed at lowering the raised pressure by whatever means available. Recently, there has been increasing interest in possible ancillary benefits of certain drug classes beyond their ability to lower blood pressure.[3] Several such potential effects are listed in Table 21.2. These aspects are discussed later (page 108).

Nevertheless, there has been some caution in assigning potential benefit to newly introduced types of agent, for example, ACE inhibitors or calcium antagonists, because these have not yet been employed in trials evaluating benefit with blood pressure reduction. The uncertainty surrounding these topics is illustrated in the quite differing positions taken by authors of various guidelines for initiating antihypertensive therapy.

**Table 21.1.**   Principal complications of hypertension

Malignant ('accelerated') phase
Hypertensive encephalopathy
Hypertensive heart failure
Stroke
Coronary artery disease
Renal function impairment

**Table 21.2.**   Possible additional benefits of some antihypertensive drugs

Neutral or potentially beneficial effects on plasma lipids
Preservation of total body potassium and of plasma potassium level
Facilitation of regression of left ventricular hypertrophy
Improvement of large arterial compliance
Facilitation of correction of medial thickening in resistance arteries
Antiplatelet action

The WHO/ISH recommendations are that first treatment may be with any of diuretic, $\beta$-blocker, calcium antagonist or ACE inhibitor.[4] The US Joint National committee restricts 'first-line' drugs to diuretic or $\beta$-blocker.[5] The British Hypertension Society was unable to reach a consensus position on this issue.[6] These matters are discussed further in Appendix 3.

### —— Diastolic versus systolic pressure ——

Many of the earlier intervention studies focused on diastolic rather than systolic blood pressure in assessing benefit. It is now clear that systolic blood pressure is important in indicating cardiovascular risk, although the relative weight of diastolic and systolic pressure as risk indicators is controversial.[49,50,51,52]

### —— Gender and treatment benefit ——

As the incidence of complications is, for any level of blood pressure at any age, and especially before the menopause, lower in women than in men (see also page 86), evidence of benefit is less clear in women. Moreover, some trials have included only men.

### Trials of antihypertensive treatment: —— an evaluation ——

#### Uncontrolled studies

Very soon after the availability of antihypertensive drugs, it became evident that these could correct

the malignant phase (provided that this had not progressed to severe renal failure), hypertensive encephalopathy and overt clinical hypertensive heart failure.[1,45] These benefits were sufficiently clear to preclude the need for formal controlled studies; indeed, these would have been doubtful to justify ethically.

#### Controlled trials focused on diastolic pressure

The demonstration of benefit from the prophylactic treatment of hypertension did, by contrast, require controlled clinical trials (Figure 21.1), which have been conducted in adults and with progressive refinement, since the pioneering papers of Hamilton *et al.*, in 1964,[1,7] and Wolff and Lindemann in 1966.[8] The various studies have demonstrated, despite their several and sometimes major faults (see below), a progressive lowering of the threshold of presenting diastolic pressure (fifth phase), above which a protective effect against hypertension-related cardiovascular morbidity may be discerned, to 90 mmHg. With such a low threshold at which, at least statistically, benefit can be seen, the advantages at the more modest levels of raised pressure are numerically slight, despite the increasingly large numbers of subjects qualifying potentially for therapy. Protection is apparent in middle-aged men, but less clear in middle-aged women.

#### Trials in subjects aged over 60

In hypertensive subjects over 60 years of age, and indeed up to the age of 80 and possibly higher, more distinct advantages of therapy in lessening the frequency of complications of hypertension are evident.[9-13] One study in the elderly has shown,

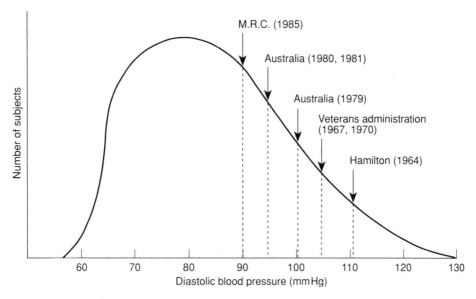

**Figure 21.1.** Schematic representation of the distribution of diastolic pressures within an adult Westernized population. Also shown are the thresholds of presenting diastolic pressure above which a protective effect of antihypertensive drug therapy has been seen in various controlled trials. For further details see Refs 7, 19 and 40. (Redrawn from Ref. 1, with permission.)

individually, a significant reduction in all cause mortality with active antihypertensive therapy.[13] Over the age of 60, the benefits of treatment are found in women as well as men. In the elderly, so defined, evidence of limitation of coronary artery disease and its consequences can be discerned, in contrast to the situation in younger hypertensive patients; these aspects are discussed in more detail below.

### Isolated systolic hypertension

Moreover in two trials,[9,12] but not in a third,[11] conducted in patients over 60, benefit has been found with the treatment of 'isolated systolic' hypertension, that is, with the systolic pressure above 159, but the diastolic below 90 mmHg. A curiosity of one of these, SHEP,[12] is that there was a progressive diminution of the treatment benefit for stroke as the baseline systolic pressure was higher.[42]

## —— Critique of some individual trials ——

Some individual trials and their interpretation require more detailed discussion.

### HDFP and the Collins meta-analysis

These two ventures require separate attention in the present context. The failings of the first[14] are directly responsible for the misconceptions of the second.[15] Regrettably, both have to be judged as unacceptable in several respects.

The American Hypertension Detection and Follow-up Program (HDFP)[14] was not, despite claims by its proponents, a trial of antihypertensive drug treatment, but rather a comparison of two different systems of health care as provided for patients with hypertension (see also pages 27 and 30). The special intervention group of HDFP (Stepped Care; SC) comprised patients assigned at random to a systematic programme of therapy, usually provided in a special centre. Antihypertensive treatment was prescribed according to a predetermined regimen. In addition, other factors, including overweight, hypercholesterolaemia and cigarette smoking, were addressed by counselling. SC participants were advised further to avoid a high salt intake.[14] The reference group (Referred Care; RC) consisted of patients referred to their local practitioner, there to receive whatever care he or she might consider appropriate. The SC patients were seen more frequently and in usually more favourable circumstances than those of the RC group; economic barriers to adherence were removed as far as possible; drugs, laboratory tests and if necessary, transportation were provided at no cost to the participant; waiting times were minimized; appointments were made at convenient hours; and a Program physician was on call at all times.[14]

Thus the services offered to the SC and RC groups were widely disparate; moreover, the disparity was likely to be greater for those patients less socially privileged (Table 21.3) (see also pages 21 and 88). The SC patients were certainly likely to receive more effective antihypertensive drug treatment, although the circumstances of blood pressure measurement were so different in the SC and RC groups that probably no valid comparison of the treated blood pressures can be made. Moreover, multiple cardiovascular risk factors were addressed in the SC patients. Last, the SC patients had usually more ready access to diagnostic and

therapeutic facilities, for whatever reason, cardiovascular or otherwise.

Not surprisingly, lower blood pressure values were recorded overall in the SC group, in which patients showed also a lower cardiovascular morbidity, including a lower death rate from coronary artery disease. However, also not surprisingly, deaths from a range of non-cardiovascular cases were fewer in the SC patients.[14] The superior outcome in the SC group was more marked in black than in white subjects, probably reflecting the economic advantages offered to the SC patients; these predictably would be most evident in the least financially privileged classes.

It is impossible, therefore, to discern how much of the advantage enjoyed by the SC over the RC patients was due to antihypertensive drugs, how much to other cardiovascular risk factor interventions, and how much to the more readily available medical facilities.

As was pointed out by one[16] of many critics,[1,10] HDFP 'which has had much influence on practice in the USA, was not really a trial of hypertension at all'.[16]

In 1990, Collins *et al.* surprisingly published a meta-analysis[15] of the outcome of what they described as the '14 unconfounded randomized trials of antihypertensive drugs'. However, the two subgroups of the VA study[43,44] were regarded by them separately; thus only 13 distinct trials were included in their evaluation. They assessed HDFP

**Table 21.3.** Potential confounding factors in the HDFP study: interventions and facilities offered to Stepped Care (SC) participants

Anti-smoking counselling given
Correction of overweight attempted
Dietary reduction of hypercholesterlaemia attempted
Dietary reduction sodium intake advised
Drugs, laboratory tests and transportation available free
Appointments at convenient hours
Waiting times minimized
More frequent visits than for referred care participants
HDFP physician available at all times
More ready availability of diagnostic and therapeutic facilities for any reason

*Source:* From Ref. 14.

amongst these 13, an important inclusion, because this was a very big study, with therefore weighty statistical implications. Collins *et al.* stated in detail in their paper[15] what they intended by 'unconfounded'—'Trials of multiple risk factor interventions, including not only blood pressure reduction but also separate interventions to alter some other risk factor(s), were ... not included ... the only confounding that remains is that due to any direct or indirect side-effects of the drugs tested in these trials.'[15] HDFP does not in our view, for the reasons given above, meet these criteria.

With HDFP contributing to their meta-analysis, Collins *et al.* concluded[15] that antihypertensive treatment caused a highly significant average 42% reduction in stroke. Whilst a prevention of stroke with antihypertensive drug treatment was to be expected, the magnitude was perhaps surprising, since it eliminated virtually completely the risk predicted epidemiologically. Apparent therapeutic success of this order should have made the authors wary of confounding influences in their calculations. There was also a marginal, but nevertheless nominally significant, average 14% reduction in coronary events. The latter, however, was entirely dependent on the dubiously appropriate inclusion of HDFP. When HDFP was excluded, as we and others consider it should have been,[17] the number of coronary events was almost identical in treated and control subjects (277 versus 282 events).

In a separate critique, Kaplan[18] has advanced arguments for omitting certain others of the trials than HDFP included by Collins and his colleagues in their review.[15]

For these various reasons, we consider it is advisable to omit both HDFP[14] and the meta-analysis of Collins *et al.*[15] when evaluating the benefits of antihypertensive drug therapy.

## The first MRC trial

One of the principal declared aims of the first Medical Research Council (MRC) trial, conducted in middle-aged hypertensive men and women, was to examine any possible differential benefit between a thiazide diuretic or a $\beta$-blocker given as initial

therapy.[19] However, little was made of this in the first report on the trial. Two later accounts did, however, show some interestingly relevant aspects.

In 1988 the trialists reported in detail on coronary heart disease in the MRC study.[20] This revealed that sudden death rates (defined as death within 1 h of the onset of new symptoms) were very different in those patients allocated at random to placebo, propranolol and bendrofluazide. The figures are most remarkable for men, in whom the great majority of these events occurred. The absolute numbers of such deaths in men were for bendrofluazide 29, propranolol 12 and placebo 41 (the number of patients allocated to placebo was equivalent to those allocated to the thiazide and $\beta$-blocker groups combined). These figures provide sudden death rates per 1000 patient-years on bendrofluazide as 2.6, on propranolol 1.1 and on placebo 1.8. The differences between the rates for bendrofluazide and propranolol were highly significant ($P < 0.01$). While the sudden death rate on thiazide was higher, and on $\beta$-blocker lower, than on placebo, in neither case was the comparison against placebo nominally significant.

In 1991 Green, who had originally been a member of the steering committee of the MRC trial, published his own independent analysis[21] of coronary events, both overt and symptomless, the latter assessed by ECG Minnesota coding at follow-up. Green emphasized[21] that his analysis of the MRC trial was independent of the official account. He found that coronary events were very much more frequent in those allocated to bendrofluazide rather than to propranolol, the age-adjusted rates per 1000 patient-years being respectively 27.4 and 20.4 ($P < 0.001$). Moreover, the rates on propranolol were significantly lower ($P < 0.05$) than on placebo (rate 23.9).

Why the official MRC trial reports[19,20] are so reticent about these potentially important findings remains obscure.

## The second MRC trial

The later MRC trial of hypertension in old patients[9] was single-blind, with initial random allocation to atenolol, or hydrochlorothiazide in a fixed combination with amiloride, or placebo. During the course of the trial there was substantial cross-contamination between these initial groups, with diuretic and $\beta$-blocker frequently being given together, and other drugs often being added. Moreover, active treatment was initiated in 11% of those allocated to placebo. Despite this contamination of the treatment groups as allocated, the authors presented an analysis on an 'intention to treat' basis. This showed that those subjects randomized to diuretic had a 31% less risk of stroke, a 44% less risk of a coronary event, and a 35% less risk of any cardiovascular event, all statistically significant as compared with placebo. Those patients randomized to $\beta$-blocker showed no significant reduction in these endpoints.

The eagerness of the MRC authors to present the analysis from the second trial[9] comparing the allocated treatment groups contrasts with their coyness on several such aspects of the earlier MRC study.[19,20] The wisdom and value of their later enthusiasm are questionable, given the seemingly greater shortcomings of the study in old patients.

Even so, the very big differences in the outcome when diuretics and $\beta$-blockers are compared in the two trials could be genuine. It is noteworthy that the $\beta$-blocker was propranolol in the earlier trial and atenolol in the later study; Kendall has suggested[22] that this difference of drug might be relevant. Another aspect is that the dose of thiazide was less, whilst the potassium-conserving agent amiloride was also prescribed, in the second trial. These differences could well have moderated hypokalaemia, with consequent cardiac advantages, although no information on this aspect was provided in the report on the second MRC trial.[9]

### The HAPPHY and MAPHY trials

Neither of these trials included a placebo group and hence both have limited application. However, they concern the later analyses of the two MRC trials,[20,21] hence deserve mention.

The HAPPHY trial (Heart Attack Primary Prevention in Hypertension)[23] was conducted in hypertensive men who were allocated at random to an open study of the effects of initial antihypertensive treatment with either of the $\beta$-blockers atenolol or metoprolol versus either of the thiazide diuretics hydrochlorothiazide or bendrofluazide. The results were inconclusive, with 101 deaths in those treated with diuretic versus 96 on $\beta$-blocker. The coronary event rates were respectively 9.48 and 10.62 per 1000 patient-years.

The MAPHY trial (Metoprolol Atherosclerosis Prevention in Hypertension) involved a later and separate analysis of the data from only those centres participating in the above-mentioned HAPPHY study where metoprolol was prescribed. These centres using metoprolol began the trial earlier and finished later than was the case with those prescribing atenolol, the mean duration of follow-up being 5 years on metoprolol versus 3 years on atenolol. Substantially more adverse cardiovascular events occurred at those centres studying metoprolol rather than atenolol. Deaths from all causes were fewer in the hypertensive men allocated to metoprolol than to thiazide diuretic (65 versus 83, $P = 0.028$); there were fewer sudden deaths (32 versus 45, $P = 0.017$); and fewer total coronary events, both overt and latent (111 versus 144, $P = 0.001$).[24-26]

Thus the MAPHY data with metoprolol,[24-26] but not the combined HAPPHY results,[23] which were derived employing either atenolol or metoprolol, are in broad accord with the data from the first MRC study,[20,21] and indicate an advantage of $\beta$-blocker over thiazide diuretic as initial therapy for hypertension in men.

### The IPPPSH trial

The International Primary Prospective Prevention Study in Hypertension (IPPPSH)[27] was an attempt to discern whether antihypertensive therapy based on the $\beta$-blocker oxprenolol conferred especial benefit. No such benefit was seen. However, so many patients in both the oxprenolol-treated and the comparison groups also received a diuretic, whilst additionally many patients had been exposed to a wide range of drugs before the trial started, that confident conclusions are, in our opinion, unwise.

## Complications corrected or prevented — by antihypertensive drug treatment —

Antihypertensive drug therapy can, as mentioned earlier, clearly correct hypertensive encephalopathy, the malignant phase and overt hypertensive heart failure.[1] Moreover, the controlled intervention trials have demonstrated, unequivocally, substantial prevention of stroke[1] (Table 21.4). The malignant phase apart, treatment has not, however, shown slowing of the rate of decline of renal function, almost certainly because such decline is very gradual, and the trials have been too brief for any benefit in this regard to be manifest.[28] Whilst, as already discussed, a reduction in both fatal and non-fatal myocardial infarction has been found in some, but not all,[12,29] trials in hypertensive subjects over the age of 60, this has not been so apparent, despite some unsuitably euphoric claims discussed above, in younger patients. Because coronary artery disease is now by far the most frequent cause of clinical cardiac failure, this unmet therapeutic need implies that the early success of antihypertensive treatment in correcting overt hypertensive heart failure has not been accompanied by corresponding ability to prevent the more insidious development of heart failure due to hypertension-related coronary artery disease.

## Possible reasons for only partial benefit — from antihypertensive therapy —

From the foregoing account, it will be apparent that despite the undoubted achievements of antihypertensive drug treatment, this has not thus far been sufficient to return the cardiovascular risk associated with high blood pressure to normal. There are several probable explanations for this relative therapeutic failure, reasons that are not mutually exclusive.[30]

### Administrative limitations

First, and most obviously, improved organizational efficiency has promoted more effective medical care. The study of the Glasgow Blood Pressure Clinic, for example,[31,32] was over a period of 15 years (1968–83). Administrative and therapeutic skills visibly improved during that time. On that basis alone, one would now expect much better results from the centre than were obtained two or more decades ago. Even so, when those patients with treated diastolic pressures below 90 mmHg were evaluated separately, morbidity still remained in excess of normal; thus the relative therapeutic failure was not attributable solely to any defects in the delivery of therapy.

### Symptomatic drug side-effects

Second, largely but not exclusively because all antihypertensive drugs have symptomatic side-effects in at least a proportion of patients, dosage is often

**Table 21.4.** Effect of antihypertensive drug treatment on complications associated with hypertension

| Corrected or prevented | Probably slowed | Less clearly or consistently prevented |
|---|---|---|
| Malignant 'accelerated' hypertension | Renal impairment | Coronary artery disease and its |
| Hypertensive encephalopathy | | consequences |
| Overt hypertensive heart failure | | Strokes due to atheroma |
| Haemorrhagic stroke | | (atherosclerosis) of large arteries |
| Lacunar brain infarcts* | | supplying the brain |

* Not all commentators agree.

constrained, or there may be frankly poor patient compliance with therapy.

## Limited antihypertensive effect

Third, there is limited antihypertensive efficacy of drugs and combinations. At least in part, this is because drugs are, perforce, prescribed unspecifically, without knowledge of, or regard to, the underlying pressor pathophysiology.

## The 'J-curve' controversy

Fourth, and of increasing prominence in recent years, is the converse issue of whether, by reducing arterial pressure too far, therapy may sometimes have increased the incidence of myocardial infarction in hypertensive patients with coronary-artery atheroma. This is the controversial affair of the so-called 'J-shaped curve',[30,33,34] which is discussed further on pages 12, 79 and 81. Clearly, there must be a level of arterial pressure below which blood pressure reduction enhances, rather than diminishes, risk. It has been suggested that this level lies, at any rate in subjects with coronary artery stenosis, rather higher than had often been supposed, possibly as high as a fifth-phase diastolic pressure of 85 mmHg. This important issue urgently requires resolution.

## Adverse biochemical and pathophysiological effects

Fifth, potentially adverse biochemical and pathophysiological accompaniments of some drug classes, for example, potassium and magnesium depletion or glucose intolerance induced by diuretics,[35,48] or distortions of plasma lipid patterns caused by diuretics or $\beta$-adrenoceptor blocking agents, may in part have offset the benefits to be obtained from blood pressure reduction.[36,37]

Some investigators have been concerned that the propensity of thiazides to cause ventricular arrhythmias and sudden death may have limited their benefits in reducing hypertension-related cardiovascular morbidity.[35,48] Others have denied this.

The issue has become prominent with the wide availability of a range of other drugs, prescribed for diverse disorders, which prolong the electrocardiographic QT interval. The conjoint ingestion of a thiazide diuretic with an agent which elongated the QT interval would be especially likely to cause serious ventricular arrhythmias. These aspects have been reviewed in detail.[35]

## Ancillary benefits of antihypertensive drugs

Sixth, and potentially of greatest future exploitation, is that antihypertensive drug treatment hitherto has focused on blood pressure reduction *per se*, to the relative neglect of important vascular accompaniments of hypertension such as left ventricular hypertrophy, loss of compliance and distensibility in large arteries, and medial thickening in resistance arteries.[3,30] The complications of hypertension which have been most obviously corrected or prevented by therapy are those related most directly to high blood pressure as such. The atherosclerotic sequelae of a raised arterial pressure are largely due to turbulence of blood flow, to endothelial lesions, and thus to atheromatous plaque formation and progression (page 62). These aspects appear to be especially worthy of attention in the pursuit of further therapeutic advances.

Thus, currently there is much interest in the possibility that antihypertensive agents that can also facilitate regression of hypertensive left ventricular hypertrophy and medial thickening in resistance vessels, while improving distensibility and compliance in larger arteries, might offer especial advantages.[3,38,41] Relevant clinical studies are in their infancy, but do raise the hope that such developments could make antihypertensive treatment more effective than hitherto against hypertension-associated coronary artery disease and cerebral infarction. Other avenues being explored are antihypertensive agents also with antiplatelet properties; with beneficial effects on vascular endothelium; and with other specific vascular protective actions (Table 21.2).

Conversely, properties of antihypertensive drugs thought to be undesirable are elevation of serum cholesterol,[36,37] seen with many thiazide diuretics and some $\beta$-adrenoceptor blockers; potassium depletion, induced by diuretics;[35] and electrocardiographic QT prolongation, found with thiazides, some calcium antagonists such as bepridil and nicardipine, the $\beta$-blocker sotalol, and the serotonergic antagonist ketanserin.[35]

## Possible differential benefit of antihypertensive drugs

As discussed above, considerable effort has been, and is increasingly being applied, to the development of antihypertensive drugs which could be particularly effective in limiting the complications of hypertension, either because of properties additional to their capacity to lower arterial pressure, or because of fewer unwanted attributes.

So far, however, direct evaluation of such possible ancillary merits and demerits of antihypertensive therapy has been limited to comparisons of thiazide diuretics versus $\beta$-blockers as initial therapy, and the interpretation even of these studies remains, as we have seen, highly controversial.[19–21]

Thus although there are suggestions that $\beta$-blockers may have advantages over thiazide diuretics in limiting the type and range of complications when given as initial therapy for hypertension, the evidence is inconsistent and the issues remain contentious. Part at least of the controversy stems from inadequacies of trial design and execution.

## Future trials

While there are theoretical grounds for supposing that more recently introduced classes of antihypertensive agent may possess various therapeutic advantages, these have not so far been demonstrated in formal trials. Several studies have, however, been planned with the intention of clarifying these aspects, as follows.[39]

A Scandinavian trial has begun in hypertensive patients aged 25–66 years, who are to be rando-

mized either to therapy based on the ACE inhibitor captopril or to treatment not including an ACE inhibitor. It is intended to study some 7000 patients over 5 years.

In the STOP-II trial it is intended to allocate 6000 elderly hypertensive patients to one of three treatment arms: ACE inhibitor, calcium antagonist, or $\beta$-blocker.

The US National Heart, Lung and Blood Institute is planning to compare the effects of ACE inhibitors and calcium antagonists on cardiovascular mortality and morbidity in some 30 000 hypertensive subjects.

These are all ambitious projects. There have been, as has been discussed herein, some spectacular failures with similar attempts in the past.[23,27] However, these aims require to be pursued if we are to illuminate the presently obscure, but crucially important, issues of whether or not there are differential benefits associated with particular agents in the treatment of hypertension.

## Case study

See Case study 5, Appendix 2.

## References

1. Robertson JIS. The nature of hypertension. In *Handbook of Hypertension*, Vol. 15: *Clinical Hypertension* (ed. JIS Robertson). Amsterdam: Elsevier, 1992: 1–13.
2. Yeo WW, Ramsay LE. Non-pharmacological treatment of hypertension. In *Handbook of Hypertension*, Vol. 15: *Clinical Hypertension* (ed. JIS Robertson). Amsterdam: Elsevier, 1992: 709–46.
3. Robertson JIS. Antihypertensive therapy: achievements, failures, and prospects. *J. Cardiovasc. Pharmacol.* 1990; **16** (suppl. 7): 102–4.
4. Zanchetti A, Chalmers J, Arakawa K *et al.* 1993 Guidelines for the management of mild hypertension: memorandum from a WHO/ISH meeting. *J. Hypertens.* 1993; **11**: 905–18.
5. Fifth Report of the Joint National Committee on Detection, Evaluation, and Treatment of High Blood Pressure (JNCV). *Arch. Intern. Med.* 1993; **153**: 154–83.

6.  Sever P, Beevers G, Bulpitt C *et al.* Management guidelines in essential hypertension: report of the second working party of the British Hypertension Society. *Br. Med. J..* 1993; **306**: 983–7.

7.  Hamilton M, Thompson EN, Wisniewski TKM. The role of blood-pressure control in preventing complications of hypertension. *Lancet* 1964; **i**: 235–8.

8.  Wolff FW, Lindeman RD. Effects of treatment in hypertension: results of a controlled study. *J. Chron. Dis.* 1966; **19**: 227–40.

9.  MRC Working Party. Medical Research Council trial of treatment of hypertension in older adults: principal results. *Br. Med. J.* 1992; **304**: 405–12.

10. Robertson JIS. The case for antihypertensive drug treatment in subjects over the age of 60. *Cardiovasc. Drugs Ther.* 1992; **6**: 579–83.

11. Coope J. Hypertension in the elderly. *J. Hypertens.* 1987; **5** (suppl. 3): 69–77.

12. SHEP Cooperative Research Group. Prevention of stroke by antihypertensive drug treatment of older persons with isolated systolic hypertension. *J. Am. Med. Assoc.* 1991; **265**: 3255–64.

13. Dahlöf B, Lindholm L, Hansson L *et al.* Morbidity and mortality in the Swedish Trial in Old Patients with Hypertension (STOP-Hypertension). *Lancet* 1991; **338**: 1281–5.

14. Hypertension Detection and Follow-up Program Cooperative Group. Five-year findings of the hypertension detection and follow-up program: I. Reduction in mortality of persons with high blood pressure, including mild hypertension. *J. Am. Med. Assoc.* 1979; **242**: 2562–71.

15. Collins R, Peto R, MacMahon S *et al.* Blood pressure, stroke and coronary heart disease: Part 2, short-term reductions in blood pressure: overview of randomised drug trials in their epidemiological context. *Lancet* 1990; **335**: 827–38.

16. Hampton JR. Treating mild hypertension: an unnecessary luxury. *Cardiovasc. Drugs Ther.* 1989; **3**: 749–52.

17. Alderman MH. Meta–analysis of hypertension treatment trials. *Lancet* 1990; **335**: 1092–3.

18. Kaplan NM. Dredging the data on antihypertensive therapy. *Am. J. Hypertens.* 1991; **4**: 195–7.

19. Medical Research Council Working Party. MRC trial of treatment of mild hypertension: principal results. *Br. Med. J.* 1985; **291**: 97–104.

20. Medical Research Council Working Party on Mild Hypertension. Coronary heart disease in the Medical Research Council trial of treatment of mild hypertension. *Br. Heart J.* 1988; **59**: 364–78.

21. Green KG. British MRC trial of treatment for mild hypertension: a more favorable interpretation. *Am. J. Hypertens.* 1991; **4**: 723–4.

22. Kendall MJ. *Beta blockade and cardioprotection.* London: Science Press, 1991.

23. Wilhelmsen L, Berglund G, Elmfeldt D *et al.* Beta-blockers versus diuretics in hypertensive men: main results from the HAPPHY trial. *J. Hypertens* 1987; **5**: 561–72.

24. Wikstrand J, Warnold I, Olsson G *et al.* Primary prevention with metoprolol in patients with hypertension: mortality results from the MAPHY study. *J. Am. Med. Assoc.* 1988; **259**: 1976–82.

25. Wikstrand J. Warnold I. Tuomilehto J *et al.* Metoprolol versus thiazide diuretics in hypertension: morbidity results from the MAPHY study. *Hypertension* 1991; **17**: 579–88.

26. Olsson G, Tuomilehto J, Berglund G *et al.* Primary prevention of sudden cardiovascular death in hypertensive patients: mortality results from the MAPHY study. *Am. J. Hypertens.* 1991. **4**: 151–6.

27. The IPPPSH Collaborative Group. Cardiovascular risk and risk factors in a randomized trial of treatment based on the beta-blocker oxprenolol: the International Prospective Primary Prevention Study in Hypertension (IPPPSH). *J. Hypertens.* 1985; **3**: 379–92.

28. Zanchetti A, Sleight P, Birkenhäger WH. Evaluation of organ damage in hypertension. *J. Hypertens.* 1993; **11**: 875–82.

29. Amery A, Birkenhäger W, Brixko P *et al.* Mortality and morbidity results from the European Working Party on High blood pressure in the Elderly trial. *Lancet* 1985; **i**: 1349–54.

30. Robertson JIS. Should the costs of development inhibit research into new antihypertensive drugs? *Cardiovasc. Drugs Ther.* 1989; **3**: 757–9.

31. Isles CG, Walker L, Beevers DG *et al.* Mortality in patients of the Glasgow Blood Pressure Clinic. *J. Hypertens.* 1986; **4**: 141–56.

32. Robertson JIS. Editorial: Antihypertensive drug therapy: achievements, failures and prospects. *Neth. J. Med.* 1990; **37**: 89–94.

33. Zanchetti A, Amery A, Berglund G *et al.* How much should blood pressure be lowered? The problem of the J-shaped curve. *J. Hypertens.* 1989; **7** (suppl. 6): 338–48.

34. D'Agostino RB, Belanger AJ, Kannel WB, Cruick-

shank JM. Relation of low diastolic pressure to coronary heart disease death in presence of myocardial infarction: the Framingham study. *Br. Med. J.* 1991; **303**: 385–9.

35. Singh BN, Hollenberg NK, Poole-Wilson PA, Robertson JIS. Diuretic-induced potassium and magnesium deficiency: relation to drug-induced QT prolongation, cardiac arrhythmias and sudden death. *J. Hypertens.* 1992; **10**: 301–16.

36. Ames RP. the effects of antihypertensive drugs on serum lipids and lipoproteins. I. Diuretics. *Drugs* 1986; **32**: 260–78.

37. Ames RP. The effects of antihypertensive drugs on serum lipids and lipoproteins. II. Non-diuretic drugs. *Drugs* 1986; **32**: 335–7.

38. Spence JD, Arnold JMO, Gilbert JJ. Vascular consequences of hypertension and effects of antihypertensive therapy. In *Handbook of Hypertension*, Vol. 15: *Clinical Hypertension* (ed. JIS Robertson). Amsterdam: Elsevier, 1992: 621–54.

39. Hansson L, Dahlöf B, Himmelman A *et al.* Angiotensin-converting enzyme inhibitors in the treatment of essential hypertension. In *The Renin–Angiotensin System* (eds JIS Robertson and ME Nicholls). London: Gower Medical, 1993: chapter 91.

40. Robertson JIS. The large studies in hypertension: what have they shown? *Br. J. Clin. Pharmacol.* 1987; **24** (suppl.): 3–14.

41. O'Rourke M. Arterial haemodynamics and ventricular–vascular interaction in hypertension. *Blood Pressure* 1994; **3**: 33–7.

42. Staessen JA, Amery A, Birkenhäger W. Inverse association between baseline pressure and benefit from treatment in isolated systolic hypertension. *Hypertension* 1994; **23**: 269.

43. VA Cooperative Study Group. Effects of treatment on morbidity in hypertension: results in patients with diastolic blood pressures averaging 115 through 129 mmHg. *J. Amer. Med. Ass.* 1967; **202**: 116–22.

44. VA Cooperative Study Group. Effects of treatment on morbidity in hypertension, II: results in patients with diastolic blood pressures averaging 90 through 114 mmHg. *J. Amer. Med. Ass.* 1970; **213**: 1143–52.

45. Doyle AE. Hypertension and vascular disease. *Am. J. Hypertens.* 1991; **4** (suppl.): 103–6.

46. Fisher M, Minematsu L. Lacunar stroke: diagnosis, evaluation and management. *Heart Dis. Stroke* 1992; **1**: 353–5.

47. Ikeda T, Gomi A *et al.* Role of hypertension in asymptomatic cerebral lacunae in the elderly. *Hypertension* 1994; **23** (suppl. 1): 259–62.

48. Siscovick DS, Raghunathan TE, Psaty BM *et al.* Diuretic therapy for hypertension and the risk of primary cardiac arrest. *N. Engl. J. Med.* 1994; **330**: 1852–7.

49. Ramsay LE, Waller PC. Strokes in mild hypertension: diastolic rules. *Lancet* 1986; **ii**: 854–6.

50. Wright BM. Diastolic versus systolic. *Lancet* 1986; **ii**: 1041–2.

51. Peart WS, Greenberg G. Diastolic versus systolic. *Lancet* 1986; **ii**: 1042.

52. Bulpitt CJ. Is systolic pressure more important than diastolic? *J. Hum. Hyp.* 1990; **4**: 471–6.

# 22
# Antihypertensive therapy

Until recent years, antihypertensive therapy was based on the assumption that all methods were equally efficacious in correcting or preventing complications, given that the blood pressure was lowered to a similar extent.[1] Thus, treatment might be surgical, pharmacological or non-pharmacological. One of the earliest pieces of evidence that the malignant phase was simply a complication of high blood pressure, albeit a very severe one, and not a disease entity in its own right, was that it could be corrected irrespective of the method of blood pressure reduction employed.

## ——— Surgical therapy ———

The surgical treatment of essential hypertension (as contrasted with the surgical correction of a specific lesion causing secondary hypertension) is now of historic interest only. Such measures included bilateral dorsolumbar sympathectomy or adrenalectomy. These were formidable procedures, with a high rate of complications and usually unpleasant side-effects. However, they did demonstrate the value of blood pressure reduction in correcting the most severe complications of high blood pressure, such as the malignant phase and hypertensive heart failure, thereby providing a scientific basis for drug therapy.

## ——— Antihypertensive drugs ———

The use of antihypertensive drugs has dominated the treatment of hypertension for the past four decades and will provide the mainstay of therapy in the immediate future at least, although non-pharmacological means are being increasingly enthusiastically explored (page 129).[2,3] Details of the wide range of individual drugs and of dosage are given in Appendix 1 on page 263. The principal classes are summarized here. Further details are given in the works by Doyle,[3] Dollery et al.[4] and Hansson et al.[5] The use of antihypertensive drugs in pregnancy is dealt with in Chapter 47, pages 251–254.

### Autonomic ganglion-blocking agents

The development of the earliest effective antihypertensive drugs, the autonomic ganglion-blocking agents, followed logically from bilateral dorsolumbar sympathectomy. The introduction of these compounds represented one of the major therapeutic advances this century. However, the sympathetic blockade meant that ganglion blockers, to be effective, had a marked postural hypotensive effect; moreover, their parasympathetic blocking actions induced constipation, dryness of the mouth and occasional paralytic ileus.

### Adrenergic neurone-blocking drugs

The successors to ganglionic blockers, the sympatholytic agents such as bretylium, guanethidine, bethanidine and debrisoquine, are highly concentrated in adrenergic neurones, blocking neurotransmitter release. Thus, they combine the disadvantages of unopposed parasympathetic discharge with sympathetic blockade. Their administration is therefore characterized by postural hypotension and diarrhoea.

Both the ganglion blockers and the adrenergic neurone-blocking agents have now passed out of clinical use.

### Centrally acting drugs

This class now contains principally three drugs, $\alpha$-methyldopa (methyldopa), clonidine and reserpine; the clonidine derivative rilmenidine also deserves mention. These agents have important similarities and also some differences of action.

#### Methyldopa

Methyldopa has been most valuable in the treatment of hypertension and, despite its obsolescence, is still widely used. Its mode of action remains imperfectly understood. Methyldopa was thought to lower blood pressure by inhibiting the enzyme dopa-decarboxylase, thereby limiting the generation of catecholamines. Additionally, with methyldopa therapy, noradrenaline in sympathetic nerve terminals is replaced by $\alpha$-methyl noradrenaline, a much weaker agonist than noradrenaline itself and thus a so-called 'false transmitter'. Third, the methyldopa metabolite, $\alpha$-methyl noradrenaline, has central nervous system effects, prominent among which is probably $\alpha_2$-adrenergic agonism, depressing sympathetic nerve discharge. All three of these actions could contribute to the reduction of arterial pressure.

Methyldopa lowers blood pressure with a mild but usually distinct additional fall in pressure on standing. Heart rate is modestly slowed.

Side-effects include drowsiness, dryness of the mouth, nasal stuffiness, postural hypotension, rashes and diarrhoea. Rarer but more serious is toxic hepatitis, which occurs in one of two forms, either early or during chronic therapy; in these patients serious liver damage can occur if there is re-exposure to the drug. A positive Coombs test is found in about 20% of patients. More rarely, haemolytic anaemia may be a problem. The initial days and weeks of treatment with methyldopa can be accompanied by salt and water retention, which may limit the antihypertensive effect (so-called

'false tolerance'). This often requires methyldopa to be given in combination with a diuretic to obtain a better therapeutic result.

Marked rebound hypertension when methyldopa is discontinued is not usually a feature, and this is an important aspect of distinction and advantage in comparison with clonidine (see below).

Methyldopa has been extensively employed in the treatment of pregnancy hypertension, and the demonstration of this aspect of its safety is reassuring. This is discussed further in Section 5 on hypertension in pregnancy (page 251). Methyldopa was also studied and its value shown as a supplementary drug in various controlled trials, including the European trial of antihypertensive treatment in the elderly, and in the Australian and the British (MRC) trials of treatment of mild hypertension.

Oral treatment is usually begun with 250 mg twice daily for at least 2 days (125 mg twice daily in elderly subjects). The dose can then be adjusted upwards if necessary by 250–500 mg daily at intervals of not less than 2 days, depending on the response. The maximum daily dose is 3 g.

#### Clonidine

The mode of action of clonidine appears to be a centrally mediated $\alpha_2$-adrenergic agonism, which depresses sympathetic discharge. Clonidine effectively lowers arterial pressure with, like methyldopa, a distinct reduction of heart rate but probably less of a postural component. The most prominent side-effects are somnolence, dryness of the mouth and constipation.

The starting dose is 50 $\mu$g twice or thrice daily, with dose increases at intervals of not less than 2 days to a maximum of 600–1200 $\mu$g daily. Slow-release capsules provide 250 $\mu$g once daily.

If clonidine therapy is suddenly stopped, there follows excessive sympathetic discharge for 1–2 days, with a surfeit of circulating catecholamines, tachycardia, rebound hypertension and headache. The attack has all the features of a paroxysm of phaeochromocytoma, which it closely resembles pathophysiologically (see also page 214). These attacks can be treated by promptly re-starting clonidine, or, as for phaeochromocytoma, giving α-blockers alone, or both α- and β-adrenergic antagonists.

More recently, clonidine has been given trans-dermally rather than orally, an adhesive polymer designed to release 100 μg of clonidine daily over 1 week being applied to the chest or upper arm. However, skin reactions have been reported in up to 25% of patients given clonidine by such patch application. Rebound hypertension has also been noted after removal of the clonidine patch.

### Rilmenidine

Rilmenidine is a clonidine-like drug which appears to have an additional property counteracting the usual sedative effect of $\alpha_2$-agonists. It has been shown to lower arterial pressure effectively over 24 h at a dose of 1 mg daily, without causing seda-tion or dryness of the mouth. The latter side-effects can, however, appear at higher doses.

### Reserpine

Reserpine is a rauwolfia alkaloid that depletes nor-adrenaline stores in sympathetic nerve terminals both within the central nervous system and periph-erally. The effect is cumulative and may persist for several weeks after stopping therapy.

Blood pressure lowering is accompanied by some cardiac slowing, but there is minimal postural hypotensive effect.

Side-effects include nasal stuffiness, diarrhoea, drowsiness, lethargy and occasional frank de-pression.

Reserpine is now rarely employed alone.

The recommended initial dose is 0.25 mg daily for 1 week, then reducing to 0.1 mg daily.

Although its use is widespread in some coun-tries, notably the USA, Germany and Switzerland, reserpine has never been widely employed in the UK, largely because of the depression it can cause, although this is an unusual occurrence at the doses now prescribed.

### Diuretics: benzothiadiazines (thiazides); loop-acting drugs; potassium-conserving agents

The antihypertensive effect of the orally acting diuretics has been shown for all of the commonly used thiazides and related drugs, as well as for the more powerful loop-acting diuretics frusemide, bumetamide, ethacrynic acid and piretanide, and the potassium-conserving agents amiloride, spiro-nolactone, canrenoate and triamterene.

Diuretics, and especially the thiazides, have pro-vided the backbone of therapy in most of the major therapeutic trials, and experience of several decades of their use, together with their comparative cheap-ness, has given a confidence in their employment to many physicians, who regard them often as the first choice in antihypertensive treatment.

Generally, the longer acting thiazides, such as bendrofluazide or hydrochlorothiazide, which do not have an abrupt and severe diuretic effect, are those most appropriate in the treatment of essential hypertension, unless there are particular features such as renal or cardiac impairment or resistant hypertension which require a loop-acting diuretic.

The potassium-conserving agents also have an antihypertensive action, and have been employed as monotherapy in essential hypertension. More usually, however, potassium-conserving drugs are reserved for use in conjunction with a thiazide, when they add to the blood pressure lowering action while helping to sustain plasma potassium. All of the commonly used potassium-conserving diuretics have the capacity also to promote conser-vation of magnesium; this has been regarded as an additional merit. Moreover, potassium-conserving diuretics are invaluable as pre-operative therapy in patients with aldosterone-secreting tumours. This latter use is described in detail on page 199.

The mode of action of diuretics in lowering arterial pressure in essential hypertension remains uncertain. One obvious possibility is a diuretic and natriuretic effect, with reduction of plasma and extracellular fluid volumes. Since, as has been described on page 29, body sodium content is expanded in older, more severely hypertensive patients (in contrast to young hypertensives, who are deficient in body sodium), this accords with the claims made by some authors for a superior antihypertensive action of diuretics with advancing age. Unfortunately for comfort, however, such claims are not well-founded.[50] Moreover, while the notion that diuretics lower blood pressure by diminishing body sodium content is consistent with the sustained elevations of renin and angiotensin II they produce, it has been difficult to confirm. For example, in one experimental study of chlorothiazide in the spontaneously hypertensive rat, the blood pressure reduction and diminution of exchangeable sodium were dissociated.[66]

Exchangeable body potassium content is consistently lowered, together with plasma potassium concentration, with long-term thiazide or loop-acting diuretic treatment of essential hypertension (Figure 7.6, page 32).[6] These changes are likely to diminish, not enhance, the antihypertensive effect and provide one reason for giving potassium-conserving agents with thiazides. Potassium salts, in the doses usually employed, are ineffective in this respect.[6]

Diuretic-induced loss of sodium and water from the wall of resistance vessels could alter the wall-to-lumen ratio and thus facilitate blood pressure reduction (page 62). A further possibility is that diuretics lower blood pressure by causing, via a direct effect on arterial smooth muscle, dilatation in resistance vessels. This notion is given some credence by the observation that a closely related but non-diuretic drug, diazoxide, is a powerful vasodilator.

Further, indapamide, derived chemically from thiazides, can lower blood pressure at doses below those causing natriuresis, although diuresis is seen also with higher doses. In treating hypertension, indapamide is recommended to be given as a single daily dose of 2.5 mg, which should not be exceeded.

### Thiazide diuretics, including chlorthalidone and xipamide

The thiazide diuretics carry a substantial burden of side-effects, endorsed by findings from the same trials as have confirmed their value. Thiazides impair glucose tolerance; raise serum uric acid and cause gout; elevate serum cholesterol; sometimes depress serum sodium; cause muscle cramps, constipation and lethargy; and provoke male sexual impotence. More rare but serious problems are bone marrow depression, hepatitis and necrotizing vasculitis.

Most importantly, diuretic-induced hypokalaemia, which, as mentioned, accompanies depletion of body potassium content,[6] has been considered by some critics to be a cause of serious ventricular arrhythmias, perhaps especially likely if there is accompanying left ventricular hypertrophy. Thiazide-induced ventricular ectopy is more prevalent in older patients. The critics have cited a number of trials in which thiazide use in hypertension has been accompanied by an excess of sudden deaths in comparison with other therapies, and they have postulated that such problems may have limited the benefits of blood pressure reduction with diuretic treatment. Other writers have denied this. There is little doubt that in some trials, the dose of thiazide was too high; more modest doses would alleviate certain of the problems, as would the conjoint prescription of a potassium-conserving diuretic. However, as discussed earlier, potassium supplements are likely to be inadequate.[6]

Of the most commonly used drugs of this type, bendrofluazide is given at 2.5–5.0 mg; chlorothiazide at 125–500 mg; hydrochlorothiazide at 12.5–50 mg; chlorthalidone at 25–50 mg; and xipamide at 20 mg, once daily.

### Loop-acting diuretics: frusemide, ethacrynic acid, bumetanide

Several of the above side-effects of thiazides are shared by the loop-acting diuretics, but generally the metabolic disturbances with the latter are less marked than those with the thiazides. Deafness is a rare but well-recognized problem with frusemide and ethacrynic acid. The diuresis and natriuresis caused by loop diuretics is too acute in onset and often too brief for these to be generally suitable for the treatment of hypertension. However, they can be valuable with accompanying renal or cardiac failure. Much larger doses are given with renal failure.

Frusemide is usually given as 20–40 mg doses (although up to 2 g or more daily can be employed if necessary); ethacrynic acid in 50–100 mg doses; and bumetanide at 0.5–2 mg daily.

### Potassium-conserving diuretics: amiloride, canrenoate, spironolactone, triamterene

With the use of potassium-conserving agents, hyperkalaemia is conversely a potential danger, especially if there is impairment of renal function. This is more likely in elderly patients. In addition, flatulence has been reported with amiloride; impotence, gynaecomastia, menstrual irregularities and peptic ulceration with spironolactone; and rashes and megaloblastosis with triamterene.

In the treatment of essential hypertension, potassium-conserving drugs are usually employed as adjuncts to thiazides: amiloride at 2.5–20 mg once daily; triamterene at 75–125 mg twice daily. Spironolactone, earlier given at 50–100 mg once daily, is no longer recommended in the UK for the treatment of essential hypertension. Much higher doses of potassium-conserving diuretics are given as monotherapy in cases of aldosterone-secreting adenoma (page 199).

## Vasodilators

Dilatation in resistance arteries is a feature of the action of several classes of antihypertensive agent. However, the term is usually reserved for those drugs that cause vasodilatation by a presumed direct action on vascular smooth muscle.

### Hydralazine

Hydralazine especially has been a mainstay of antihypertensive therapy for many years, often being given in conjunction with a diuretic and β-adrenergic blocking agent as what is termed in the USA 'standard triple therapy'. The full potential of hydralazine was realized only after the introduction of the β-blockers, with their action in slowing heart rate. Before that, tachycardia reflexly caused by the vasodilatation limited the application of hydralazine. Postural hypotension is unusual.

Hydralazine can cause fluid retention. This can hinder the antihypertensive action (so-called 'false tolerance'; see also page 113) and requires the introduction of a diuretic. If doses in excess of 200 mg are given daily a syndrome akin to lupus erythematosus can occur, with fever, weight loss, joint pains, arthritis and rashes; more rarely, splenomegaly, pleurisy and pericarditis appear. The haemoglobin level can fall, lupus cells can appear in the blood, and the erythrocyte sedimentation rate is increased. Renal involvement is, however, unusual. Individuals who acetylate hydralazine only slowly are particularly prone to this syndrome, which has been estimated to appear in as many as 12% of women and 3% of men during long-term treatment. Sometimes, hirsutism can be an unwanted feature of hydralazine therapy.

Hydralazine remains, nevertheless, a most valuable drug and, in one comparative trial of a range of adjuncts to β-blocker plus thiazide treatment, it was found to be best in terms of superior efficacy with relatively few side-effects.[7]

The usual starting oral dose is 25 mg twice daily (although a 10 mg starting dose is available), proceeding if necessary to a maximum of 300 mg in a total daily dose. However, as mentioned, daily doses above a total of 200 mg can provoke a lupus-like syndrome. The use of hydralazine in pregnancy is described on pages 252 and 253.

### Minoxidil

A much more powerful vasodilator is minoxidil, reserved for resistant hypertension, in which it is very effective. This drug causes more marked fluid retention and tachycardia than does hydralazine, and therefore should always be given in conjunction with a β-blocker and a loop diuretic. In patients unable to tolerate a β-blocker for any reason, methyldopa or an angiotensin-converting enzyme (ACE) inhibitor or verapamil can sometimes control minoxidil-induced tachycardia.

A major disadvantage of minoxidil treatment is the severe hirsutism. This can lead to refusal to take the drug, particularly by female patients, despite its efficacy.

The initial oral dose is 2.5 mg once daily, proceeding as needed in maximum increments of 10 mg to a usual ceiling of 25 mg twice daily (exceptionally 100 mg daily).

### Diazoxide

Diazoxide, a powerful vasodilator, although very effective in lowering blood pressure, is now little used other than for hypertensive emergencies in pregnancy (page 253), because with continued administration it almost always causes diabetes mellitus. Other side-effects include tachycardia and hirsutism.

## β-Blockers

The antihypertensive effect of the β-adrenoceptor blocking agents was discovered by an astute clinical observation. Their mode of action in lowering blood pressure remains obscure. With the thiazide diuretics they are the agents of first choice for many physicians, and they have the additional advantage of combining well with diuretics. The triple combination of β-blocker with a diuretic and a vasodilator, such as hydralazine, is often a standard form of treatment ('triple therapy').

A range of β-adrenoceptor blocking agents has been used in the treatment of hypertension, and these vary widely in their individual characteristics (see also Appendix 1).

Amongst the very many β-blockers, atenolol, acebutolol, metoprolol and nebivolol are relatively selective for the $\beta_1$ receptor ('cardioselective'); carvedilol, nadolol, oxprenolol, pindolol, propranolol, timolol and labetalol are unselective; oxprenolol modestly and pindolol markedly show agonistic properties ('intrinsic sympathomimetic activity'); carvedilol and labetalol also block α

receptors (see later). The common feature apparently necessary for blood pressure reduction is $\beta_1$-receptor antagonism.

At least four possible modes of action of β-blocking agents have been considered in attempting to explain their ability to lower arterial pressure: a central nervous system effect diminishing sympathetic outflow; reduction in cardiac output; diminution of renin secretion; and a presynaptic action inhibiting neurotransmitter release. None is entirely convincing as a single explanation.

A central nervous effect may contribute but, as a wide range of β-adrenoceptor blocking agents lower arterial pressure irrespective of the capacity to enter the brain, this seems at best to provide only a partial explanation.

The possibility that β-blockers could reduce blood pressure by diminishing cardiac output has been studied in detail by several workers. When a drug such as propranolol is administered, there is an initial fall in cardiac output and in arterial pressure, with a rise in calculated peripheral resistance. With continued therapy, although blood pressure stays down, cardiac output rises once more and peripheral resistance falls. Thus, there is evidently no simple relationship between any changes in cardiac output and alterations in arterial pressure.

Renin secretion from the kidney is partially under adrenergic control, being stimulated by β-adrenergic agonism and inhibited by α-adrenergic agonism. Thus, most β-blockers have an inhibitory effect on renin release, and plasma angiotensin II falls in consequence. Since in many patients with hypertension, as well as in normal subjects, peripheral concentrations of plasma angiotensin II are within a range having a direct immediate effect on arterial pressure, any inhibition of renin secretion induced by β-blockade must make a contribution to the fall in blood pressure. The results of several studies have demonstrated a correlation between blood pressure reduction achieved by β-blockers and changes in plasma renin. However, this seems unsatisfactory as a full explanation for the mode of action of this class of drugs. For example, pindolol, a β-blocker with marked intrinsic sympathomimetic activity, has been shown to lower arterial pressure while plasma renin levels are rising. Further, the inhibitory effect of $\beta$-blockade on renin release is limited, and is readily overcome, for example, by concurrent diuretic administration or by upright tilting, although blood pressure reduction is sustained through such manoeuvres.

A fourth possibility links the antihypertensive action of $\beta$-blockers to the proposed presynaptic pressor effect of catecholamines, especially adrenaline (page 43). It has been suggested that circulating adrenaline can be taken up and accumulate in sympathetic nerve terminals, subsequently being released and, by stimulating presynaptic $\beta_2$-receptors, promoting the discharge of neurotransmitter noradrenaline, thus elevating arterial pressure. Stored adrenaline may also be released as a co-transmitter. $\beta$-Blockers could inhibit these effects. However, it is not clear why a $\beta_2$-dependent mechanism should explain the antihypertensive action which is clearly linked to $\beta_1$ antagonism.

The $\beta$-adrenoceptor blocking drugs have become established, together with the thiazides, as one of the two major classes of drug employed in the initial therapy of hypertension (pages 148 and 303). Several, but by no means all of the trials which have demonstrated benefit in limiting morbidity with the treatment of high blood pressure, have employed $\beta$-blockers or thiazides, separately or in conjunction. Indeed some,[8-12] but not all studies have indicated a superior effect of $\beta$-blocker therapy over treatment with thiazides (see also Chapter 21, page 106).

$\beta$-Blockers lower blood pressure rapidly, and maintain control indefinitely, with little or no postural component. Heart rate is reduced, an effect that is less marked with those $\beta$-blockers possessing intrinsic sympathomimetic action.

Older, unselective $\beta$-blockers such as propranolol or timolol have been thought by some workers to be hazardous in patients with impending cardiac failure, although both of these agents have nevertheless been used in trials showing limitation of morbidity and mortality when given after acute myocardial infarction.[13,14] The dangers of causing heart failure are less with newer $\beta$-blockers,

especially those possessing vasodilator properties. Indeed there is increasing interest in the use of $\beta$-blockade in the treatment of cardiac failure.[15]

Side-effects of $\beta$-blockade are not negligible, and can vary greatly among patients. Included are physical and mental fatigue, bad dreams, nausea, rashes, impotence and cold extremities. $\beta$-Blockers are unsafe in patients who have reversible airflow obstruction, especially asthma; because selectivity is relative only, so-called $\beta_1$-selective agents, even when possessed also of partial $\beta_2$ agonism, should not be given to such subjects. As insulin secretion is partly under $\beta$-adrenergic control, $\beta$-blockers could destabilize control of diabetes mellitus, although these drugs have been widely used in such patients without apparently causing major problems; however, tachycardia and other features of hypoglycaemia can be obscured. Bradycardia caused by $\beta$-blockers can also mask internal bleeding.

Whilst two trials which compared propranolol with captopril found the quality of life to be less with propranolol,[16,17] this has not been the case when newer and more cardioselective $\beta$-blockers have been studied. Atenolol, for example, has been found to be indistinguishable from, or even superior to, various ACE inhibitors in the preservation of life quality.[17-19]

Despite the problems and the continuing uncertainties concerning their antihypertensive mode of action, the $\beta$-blockers have made, and will continue to make, a major contribution to the treatment of hypertension. A wide range of such drugs has been, and still continues to be, developed.

Doses of some $\beta$-blockers are: atenolol 25–100 mg once daily; acebutolol 200–400 mg twice daily; bisoprolol 5–20 mg once daily; carvedilol 12.5 mg once daily to 50 mg twice daily; metoprolol 50–200 mg twice daily; nadolol 80–240 mg once daily; nebivolol 2.5–5 mg once daily; oxprenolol 40–160 mg twice to thrice daily (or 160 mg slow-release one or two once daily); pindolol 5–15 mg twice or thrice daily; propranolol 40–160 mg twice daily (slow-release form given once daily); timolol 5–30 mg twice daily. The $\beta$- and $\alpha$-blocker labetolol is given at 100–800 mg twice daily.

## α-Blockers

α-Adrenergic blockade was initially unimpressive in the treatment of essential hypertension. Non-selective agents such as phentolamine had a modest and poorly sustained antihypertensive effect, and could provoke marked postural hypotension, tachycardia and diarrhoea.

### *Prazosin, terazosin, doxazosin*

An important advance was the development of prazosin, a selective postsynaptic $\alpha_1$-blocking agent, although, perhaps surprisingly, the mode of action of prazosin was not at first clearly recognized. Further agents have been developed along the prazosin genealogy, including the longer acting drugs terazosin and doxazosin.

The major problem with agents such as prazosin is frequent and unpredictable severe hypotension following the first dose when other than very small quantities are administered. With continued treatment mild postural hypotension can occur, and heart rate may be elevated. These features have limited the popularity of this drug class, especially in older patients, although side-effects are otherwise light, and the lack of disturbance of serum lipids has been regarded by many, but not all, workers as an advantage.

α-Blockers such as prazosin are generally utilized as supportive therapy, rather than as monotherapy, in essential hypertension. Their use in phaeochromocytoma is described on page 218.

Prazosin is started at 0.5 mg twice daily, proceeding as needed to 10 mg twice daily. Doxazosin is started at 1 mg once daily, increasing as needed to 16 mg once daily; terazosin at 1 mg, increasing to 2–10 mg once daily.

### *Indoramin*

Indoramin is an $\alpha_1$-blocking antihypertensive agent unrelated to prazosin. Drowsiness, nasal stuffiness and dryness of the mouth are reported with indoramin. The dose is 25–100 mg twice daily.

### *Urapidil*

Urapidil lowers blood pressure by peripheral $\alpha_1$-blockade combined with stimulation of central serotonergic type 1A (5-HT$_{1A}$) receptors. Urapidil has been shown to be similarly effective to prazosin.

### *Ketanserin*

Ketanserin possesses weak $\alpha_1$-blocking activity together with powerful blockade of serotonergic type 2 (5-HT$_2$) receptors peripherally. It may be questioned whether it is most appropriately discussed under this heading; clearly it differs greatly from prazosin, indoramin or urapidil.

The mode of action of ketanserin in lowering blood pressure is disputed. A central effect is not excluded. A major influence of a change of baroreceptor function is unlikely. Some $\alpha_1$-blockade can usually be demonstrated, especially during prolonged therapy; however, blood pressure lowering has been shown in the absence of demonstrable α-blockade. It has been proposed that a combination of powerful 5-HT$_2$ blockade with some weaker $\alpha_1$-blockade may be needed for its sustained antihypertensive effect. Another attractive possibility is depletion of peripheral neuronal catecholamine stores.

Ketanserin given orally has a gradually increasing effect on blood pressure over 2–3 months. Blood pressure reduction is also often greater in older subjects. There is little or no postural effect, and first-dose hypotension seems rare.

The drug does not cause changes in serum electrolytes or urea, although minor increases in serum creatinine have been reported in some series. Ketanserin does have mild class III antiarrhythmic action and has been shown in both volunteers and patients with hypertension to prolong the QT interval in a dose-related fashion. As, in these circumstances, potassium depletion could predispose to ventricular rhythm disorders, it seems prudent when combining ketanserin and diuretic therapy to include a potassium-conserving agent.[6] For similar reasons, ketanserin should be used with caution if there is atrioventricular block of grade II or higher, or together with antiarrhythmic agents. Other side-effects include drowsiness, which is usually most prominent in the early days of treatment then receding, dizziness, dryness of the mouth and mild pedal oedema.

Serotonin is under some circumstances a powerful peripheral vasoconstrictor, which can additionally amplify the constrictor effect of other agents, such as angiotensin II and noradrenaline. Furthermore, serotonin can cause platelet aggregation. These various peripheral actions of serotonin are mediated by the serotonin type 2 (5-HT$_2$) receptor. The use of an antihypertensive drug which also moderates these effects of serotonin might, it is proposed, help to limit vascular and cardiac complications of hypertension. Despite some suggestive evidence, this is not so far proved. The place of ketanserin in the therapeutic repertoire is not yet established and it is not available in the UK for treating essential hypertension.

### Carvedilol and labetalol

The $\beta$-blockers carvedilol and labetalol, which also block $\alpha$-receptors, have been described earlier (page 117).

### Calcium antagonists

This large and heterogeneous group of drugs has become increasingly employed in the treatment of hypertension in recent years.

Several groups of calcium antagonist have been recognized[20] and include class I agents, typified by verapamil; class II agents, the dihydropyridines, typified by nifedipine; class III agents, typified by diltiazem; and class IV agents, typified by flunarizine. Classes I–III contain those drugs most valuable in treating hypertension. Interestingly, flunarizine, a class IV calcium antagonist, has been shown to limit arterial lesions in experimental hypertension although having little effect on blood pressure.[21]

Calcium antagonists preferentially block the transport of calcium into the cells of vascular smooth muscle, and the myocardium. They reduce blood pressure mainly by lowering peripheral vascular resistance.

Not surprisingly, there has been much attention also towards the possibility that the use of various calcium antagonists could be especially valuable in preventing vascular damage in hypertension. This remains controversial (see later).

### Class I, e.g. verapamil

Verapamil lowers blood pressure without a postural effect. Verapamil depresses atrioventricular conduction, and heart rate is reduced. It must be used cautiously, if at all, in combination with $\beta$-blockers, because profound bradycardia or cardiac arrest may occur, especially in older patients. The other principal complication is constipation. These several problems have led some authorities[22] to advise against its use in elderly patients.

Verapamil is given orally as 80–240 mg twice daily in the regular preparation, or as 160–480 mg once daily in the slow-release form.

### Class II, e.g. nifedipine

Thus far, the dihydropyridines, typified by nifedipine, have been the most extensively used calcium antagonists in the treatment of hypertension, and a wide range has been introduced (see Appendix 1, page 263). Individual drugs differ in the extent of arterial dilatation achieved in various organs, and most importantly, in their duration of action.

A considerable problem with the earlier agents of this type, e.g. nifedipine and nicardipine, was their usually rapid absorption and short duration of action. If a sufficient dose to give a prolonged effect was administered, excessively high blood levels were reached, with consequent marked side-effects. Attempts were made to produce sustained-release formulations, which succeeded in enhancing the convenience of use and in moderating the occurrence of side-effects. Subsequently, class II calcium antagonists such as felodipine and amlodipine have been developed; these have a longer action, and hence the antihypertensive effect can be sustained, whilst transient severe elevations of blood level are avoided and side-effects are lessened.

The main adverse reactions of the class II calcium antagonists comprise headache, nausea and tachycardia, which are prominent in the early days and weeks of therapy and tend to subside later; facial flushing, which may persist; and ankle or pedal oedema. The lower limb oedema is held to be usually unaccompanied by weight gain and hence to be independent of overall fluid retention. However, this would necessitate the operation of complex internal redistributions of water and electrolytes, which have so far not been defined. A possibility which seems at least as likely to the present authors is that the extracellular fluid retention induced by drugs such as nifedipine is usually modest, and consequently often insufficient to be reflected in the frequently crude measurements of body weight made in outpatient clinics. One careful study showed that the oedema was accompanied by a significant increase in weight (Table 22.1).[23] Moreover, whilst it is often stated that nifedipine-induced pedal oedema is not responsive to diuretic therapy,[24] careful observations have shown that the addition of diuretics can afford relief.[23]

A related and attractive feature of some of the class II calcium antagonists is an early modest diuresis and natriuresis. It has been suggested that at least a brief effect of this kind is apparent after each daily dose of nifedipine as late as the third month of therapy; this must, however, imply some compensatory salt and water retention between doses for the therapy to be compatible with life. Further,

Pevahouse et al. reported[25] that the cessation of long-term nifedipine treatment in essential hypertension was followed by sodium and water retention over the next few days. However, the possible confounding influence of any concomitant drug treatment was not excluded.[26]

Pevahouse et al. claimed[25] that their observations supported the concept of a sustained contraction of body sodium and fluid content with long-term nifedipine treatment in essential hypertension. This conclusion does not, however, follow from the data they provided.[26] Indeed, direct measurements have given contrary findings. Marone et al. observed[23] that nifedipine monotherapy for hypertension was accompanied by a highly significant average 24% expansion of total exchangeable body sodium at 12 weeks (Table 22.1). This nifedipine-induced expansion of body sodium was corrected with the addition of chlorthalidone. Murray et al. found[27] no change in total body sodium at the third month of treatment with nicardipine.

Not surprisingly, the foregoing disputes are paralleled by related arguments concerning whether or not the addition of diuretics to class II calcium antagonist therapy causes a useful further lowering of arterial pressure. Some workers hold that it does; others that it does not. The detailed study of Marone et al.[23] showed that the addition of chlorthalidone to nifedipine both corrected the nifedipine-induced expansion of total exchangeable body sodium and caused a substantial additional reduction of blood pressure (Table 22.1).

**Table 22.1.** Some effects of nifedipine 3 × 10–20 mg three times daily and of nifedipine combined with chlorthalidone 25–50 mg daily, each for 6–8 weeks, in 10 patients with essential hypertension (means ± SEM). * = Significantly different from placebo, † = significantly different from nifedipine

|  | Placebo | Nifedipine | Nifedipine plus chlorthalidone |
|---|---|---|---|
| Supine BP (mmHg) | 151/97 (5/2) | 132/88 (6/20)* | 124/83 (7/3)* |
| Body weight (kg) | 72.7 (3.9) | 73.9 (4.0)* | 72.1 (3.9)† |
| Exchangeable sodium (mmol) | 2624 (237) | 3360 (266)* | 2638 (248)† |

*Source:* From Ref. 23.

Resnick et al.[28] have found that dietary calcium supplementation did not diminish the antihypertensive effect of isradipine, but, perhaps surprisingly, rather enhanced it.

The effect of nifedipine is enhanced by concurrent cimetidine administration or by the ingestion of grapefruit juice.[29]

Other arguments surround the alleged sublingual bioavailability of nifedipine. Some workers have reported rapid blood pressure reduction with ingested nifedipine, and have attributed this to sublingual absorption of the drug. Other workers, however, have found the sublingual absorption of nifedipine to be negligible, and have emphasized that the drug has to be swallowed to be effective.[30,31]

Nifedipine can worsen angina in patients with coronary artery lesions and a distinctly developed collateral circulation, probably by diverting blood away from the ischaemic myocardium ('steal effect').[32]

Nifedipine is available orally in four varieties: adalat retard tablets 10–40 mg twice daily; adalat long-acting (LA) tablets 30–90 mg once daily; adalat capsules 5–20 mg three times daily; and coracten capsules 10–40 mg twice daily. Nicardipine is given at 20–40 mg thrice daily; amlodipine at 5–10 mg once daily; isradipine at 2.5–5 mg twice daily; and felodipine at 5–10 mg once daily.

### Class III, e.g. diltiazem

Although calcium antagonists of class III tend to share the range of side-effects of both classes I and II, these are usually less severe with class III drugs, which constitutes a clear advantage for agents such as diltiazem. Rarely, a severe rash has been reported.

The dose of diltiazem is 60–180 mg twice to thrice daily, with a maximum daily dose of 480 mg usually. Slow-release preparations provide 90–180 mg once to twice daily.

### Calcium antagonists and vascular or cardiac protection

An attractive theoretical feature of calcium antagonists is their potential to limit the vascular complications of hypertension. This has been supported by a wealth of experimental data summarized notably by Fleckenstein and his colleagues.[33] The ability of flunarizine, a class IV calcium antagonist with little antihypertensive effect, to limit vascular damage accompanying severe experimental hypertension, has already been noted.[21]

This theoretical and laboratory-based promise has so far been incompletely fulfilled in the clinic. Thus while limited protection, in restricted numbers of patients, has been found after myocardial infarction employing verapamil[34] and diltiazem,[35] these are exceptional observations. Overall surveys of the use of calcium antagonists of classes I, II and III following acute myocardial infarction have revealed that they are at best ineffectual, and might well be adverse.[36,37] As mentioned above, nifedipine can exacerbate angina pectoris.[32] Thus the calcium antagonists contrast unfavourably with the β-blockers, which have proved clearly beneficial in these indications.

Similarly, while there are hints that the class II agent nimodipine or the class IV agent flunarizine[38,61,64] can be protective following stroke, the findings require confirmation and extension.

Despite the reservations and some disappointments, the possible vascular and cardiac protective properties of the various classes of calcium antagonists continue to be explored with vigour. These potential benefits constitute a major explanation for the undiminished popularity of calcium antagonists, notwithstanding their substantial burden of side-effects and disadvantages.

## Drugs acting on the renin system

Of the several classes of drugs that have been designed to act against the renin–angiotensin system (Figure 9.3), only the ACE inhibitors have so far become established in the therapeutic repertory, although the orally active non-competitive angiotensin II antagonists hold much promise. By contrast, the poor oral absorption and brief duration of action of renin inhibitors have so far prevented them from realizing their considerable potential, despite their theoretical advantages.

*Angiotensin II analogue antagonists*

Peptide analogues which are competitive antagonists of angiotensin II are typified by saralasin, which is so named because sarcosine has been substituted in position 1, and alanine in position 8, of natural bovine angiotensin II.[39] These competitive octapeptides require to be given parenterally, which is a serious therapeutic limitation. A more minor, but still distinct, concern is the partial agonism possessed by a number of these agents. Use of such drugs has nevertheless provided a wealth of information clarifying the physiology and pathophysiology of the renin–angiotensin system. However, they have little or no therapeutic value. They did enjoy a transient, if controversial, role in the diagnosis and evaluation of clinical renovascular hypertension (see also page 188).

*Non-peptide angiotensin II receptor antagonists*

A subsequent and exciting advance was the development of orally active long-acting non-peptide antagonists of the angiotensin II receptor.[39] The first of many agents of this type to be widely employed clinically was losartan; its definitive dose as an antihypertensive drug has yet to be agreed. Introduction of non-peptide angiotensin II antagonists led to the recognition of heterogeneity of angiotensin II receptor subtypes; the major population responsible for mediating angiotensin II-regulated blood pressure and aldosterone secretion is the type I ($AT_1$) receptor. Losartan is apparently specific for the $AT_1$ receptor.

At the time of writing, the orally active angiotensin II antagonists are being widely studied in the treatment of hypertension and heart failure. They offer the prospect of selective, specific blockade of the renin–angiotensin system. However, their place in the therapeutic repertoire remains to be defined.

*Renin inhibitors*

Inhibitors of the enzyme renin also offer considerable therapeutic promise, especially because renin is a fastidious substrate-specific enzyme.[40] Thus its inhibition should provide a precise means of lowering angiotensin II. Both parenterally administered and orally active renin inhibitors have been tested in humans, and shown to be effective. However, their oral bioavailability has been mainly disappointing, and the duration of action transient.

While renin inhibitors continue to offer the possibility of major therapeutic advance, their considerable promise has so far been largely unrealized.

*Angiotensin-converting enzyme (ACE) inhibitors*

The orally active inhibitors of angiotensin-converting enzyme (ACE) have provided the major impetus to this area of therapy. A wide range of these agents is now available.[41,42] Some, such as captopril and lisinopril, are ingested in the active form; others, like enalapril and ramipril, are administered as a largely inactive pro-drug, which is then de-esterified in the liver to the active forms (enalaprilat and ramiprilat, respectively). All four of these agents (and indeed most other ACE inhibitors) depend mainly on the kidney for elimination, and the dose needs to be lowered in the presence of renal functional impairment. An exception is spirapril, which is excreted mainly in bile.

All ACE inhibitors studied in detail have been shown in humans to cause dose-dependent and sustained falls in circulating plasma angiotensin II; this appears to be a major, but not necessarily the sole, mode of action in lowering blood pressure. Reduction of angiotensin II formation in other tissues, notably in arterial smooth muscle, could also be important. There are converse increases in the circulating concentrations of the enzyme renin and of the inactive precursor peptide angiotensin I (Figure 22.1).

Angiotensin-converting enzyme, also known as kininase II (page 47), is furthermore capable of breaking down kinins into smaller peptide fragments. Thus, ACE inhibition may lower blood pressure not only by limiting the generation of angiotensin II, but also by promoting the accumulation of kinins in various tissues. Such kinin accumulation could less advantageously contribute to certain of the side-effects of ACE inhibitors.

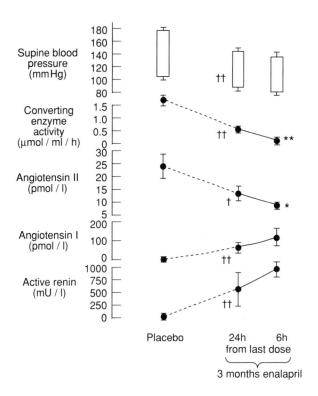

**Figure 22.1.** Comparison of blood pressure and various plasma values after 3 months of continuous once-daily enalapril monotherapy in 10 hypertensive patients with renal artery stenosis with last day of placebo. Measurements on enalapril show values 24 h and 6 h from the preceding dose. Comparison with placebo: † $P < 0.05$; †† $P < 0.01$; comparison with 24 hour values: * $P < 0.05$, ** $P < 0.01$. (Redrawn from Ref. 43, with permission.)

The development of orally active angiotensin II antagonists and renin inhibitors has been partly motivated by the possibility thereby of avoiding this kinin accumulation.

The use of ACE inhibitors in essential hypertension will be considered here; their employment in renovascular hypertension is described on page 191.

Considerable evidence exists that in many patients with essential hypertension, peripheral plasma concentrations of angiotensin II are within a range that has an immediate direct effect on arterial pressure. ACE inhibitors thus cause an instant reduction in blood pressure, in proportion to the fall in plasma angiotensin II they induce. The longer term elimination by ACE inhibition of other physiological actions of angiotensin II, such as sympathetic stimulation, enhancement of vagal tone, promotion of aldosterone secretion; and possibly also therapeutic diminution of angiotensin II generation in cardiac and arterial walls, can cause further blood pressure lowering.

The initial fall in pressure is usually modest, as many patients with essential hypertension have low levels of plasma renin and angiotensin II. However, in elderly subjects, steep and severe falls in blood pressure have been reported, occasionally with the initial dose of ACE inhibitor, sometimes despite low pre-treatment plasma renin values. ACE inhibitors do not usually cause postural hypotension or changes in heart rate, in part because of concomitant diminution of sympathetic and elevation of vagal, nervous tone. Sometimes, however, sinus tachycardia does occur, especially with conjoint diuretic use, and can be sustained.

As diuretics cause rises in renin and angiotensin II, which then limit their antihypertensive effect, the combination of a diuretic with an ACE inhibitor, the latter lowering circulating angiotensin II, is particularly efficacious. The concurrent administration of ACE inhibitors with a thiazide is thus a valuable approach to the treatment of essential hypertension. Similar considerations have led to the use of dietary salt restriction with ACE inhibition. Severe and previously intractable hypertension has also been reported often as responding to the combination of ACE inhibitor with a loop diuretic.

As aldosterone secretion is largely under the regulatory control of angiotensin II, plasma levels of aldosterone will typically remain low with ACE inhibition, even with concurrent diuretic therapy. Thus, hypokalaemia does not usually develop, and neither potassium supplements nor potassium-conserving diuretics are usually needed with this combination. Indeed, their administration with ACE inhibition might provoke dangerous hyperkalaemia, especially in the presence of renal impairment. Renal impairment may also be worsened if aggressive diuretic therapy is combined with ACE inhibition.

ACE inhibitors have also been reported as combining effectively with calcium antagonists or other vasodilating drugs in treating only partially responsive cases of hypertension. The combination of ACE inhibitor with $\beta$-blocker, by contrast, would be expected to be less potent, probably because these two drug classes partly share a mode of action in suppressing the renin system. However, in some reports, an added lowering of pressure when combining these two classes of drug has been described.[60]

Side-effects shared by ACE inhibitors as a class[44] include unproductive cough, which occurs in some 5% of patients (see page 47), urticarial or morbilliform rash, headache, syncope, Raynaud's phenomenon, and, more rarely, angioneurotic oedema, this last appearing usually early in therapy. Guillain–Barré neuropathy is a very rare complication, thought earlier to be restricted to captopril; however, it has been seen also with enalapril treatment (Chapter 44). Side-effects apparently peculiar to captopril were seen most often when large doses of the drug were employed, and have become less prominent or absent since the dose was limited to 150 mg/day, with further limitation in the presence of renal impairment. It is suspected that these captopril-specific side-effects may be due to the presence of a sulphydryl group in the molecule. They include taste loss or disturbance, proteinuria (with occasional instances of nephrotic syndrome), and leucopenia. The sulphydryl group may confer on captopril its property to generate prostacyclin, which *per contra* could be beneficial.

Caution is needed in introducing ACE inhibitors in patients likely to have high plasma levels of renin and angiotensin II, because a steep initial fall in blood pressure may occur in these circumstances. If diuretics (with or without additional drugs) are being given, it is advisable, wherever possible, to withdraw them before initiating ACE inhibition. Elderly subjects may be susceptible to first-dose hypotension with ACE inhibitors, apparently irrespective of the plasma renin value. Reducing the dose, or selecting an ACE inhibitor with a short action, such as captopril, is unlikely to prevent first-dose hypotension, but may limit its duration and so facilitate management.

Despite these various occasional side-effects and dangers, ACE inhibitors seem often to be well-accepted by many patients.

An added attraction is that ACE inhibitors, when added to digoxin plus diuretic, relieve symptoms and extend prognosis in cardiac failure.[45] Moreover, both ramipril and captopril have been shown to be clearly beneficial when introduced after stabilization following acute myocardial infarction.[46,67] As many hypertensive patients suffer from coronary artery disease and its sequelae, including heart failure, these are cogent reasons for the employment of converting enzyme inhibitors in the treatment of hypertension.

Captopril is given in oral doses of 12.5–50 mg twice daily; enalapril 2.5–40 mg once daily; lisinopril 2.5–40 mg once daily; and ramipril 1.25–10 mg once daily. With all of these four agents, lower doses are needed with renal functional impairment.

## 'Stepped care' and the concept of drug combinations

In the 1970s, both the World Health Organization and the American Heart Association set out detailed proposals for what came to be termed 'stepped care' in the treatment of hypertension.[47] In these schedules, drugs were introduced in set combinations, additions being made to therapy as needed in order to reduce the arterial pressure adequately. These stepped care programmes served well in encouraging and instructing practitioners in the therapy of hypertension, and the ways in which drugs with different modes of action could usefully be combined. However, such formal programmes of treatment are now not as popular. A more enlightened and enterprising approach is progressively being adopted, with drugs being selected with the specific needs of the individual patient in mind. If a drug given alone is ineffective, the present tendency is to withdraw it and replace it with an alternative, also given as monotherapy. There is increasing reluctance to proceed to multiple drugs in combination unless a distinct need has been demonstrated. Even so, it has to be accepted that less than 50% of hypertensive patients will be adequately controlled by monotherapy.

Moreover, it has also to be recognized that the use of two agents together can minimize the side-effects that the employment of one drug alone, in larger dose, might incur. Further, an additional agent can sometimes eliminate an adverse effect imposed by a previous one; a typical example would be the fluid retention due to methyldopa

being corrected by the introduction of a diuretic (page 113).

Few physicians now favour the administration of drugs more than once or twice daily, and elaborate titration is to be avoided if possible. Agents that can be given in one or two increments have obvious attractions. Although firm data are elusive, albeit not absent, it appears likely that simple dose schedules, with once or at most twice daily dosing, will aid patient compliance. They should certainly facilitate convenience.

For these reasons, prejudices of only a few years ago against fixed drug combinations, made up in a single preparation, are declining. Many doctors and patients appreciate the rationale and simplicity of such an approach.

It is useful in these circumstances to indicate which drugs when given together are likely to be effective, and which are contraindicated. A more detailed summary is provided in Appendix 1 on page 263.

### Some suitable and some unsuitable drug combinations

Twin combinations likely to be useful include $\beta$-blocker plus diuretic; $\beta$-blocker plus class II (dihydropyridine) calcium antagonist; $\beta$-blocker plus prazosin; $\beta$-blocker plus ketanserin; ACE inhibitor plus diuretic; ACE inhibitor plus calcium antagonist; ACE inhibitor plus ketanserin; and diuretic plus methyldopa (Table 22.2).

Combinations less likely to be effective are $\beta$-blocker plus ACE inhibitor (although not all agree on this[60]); and diuretic plus calcium antagonist (Table 22.2).

Contraindicated either because the drugs are too similar in action and/or because the combination might be dangerous are methyldopa, clonidine, rilmenidine or reserpine in any conjoint grouping because of their common central effects; ACE inhibitors and potassium-conserving diuretics, because of the danger of hyperkalaemia; and verapamil and $\beta$-blocker, because of the danger of cardiac conduction defects.

**Table 22.2.**   Some suitable and unsuitable antihypertensive drug combinations

*Suitable two-drug combinations:*
    Diuretic/$\beta$-blocker
    Diuretic/$\alpha$-blocker
    Diuretic/methyldopa
    Diuretic/clonidine
    Diuretic/reserpine
    Diuretic/class I calcium antagonist (e.g. verapamil)
    Diuretic/class II calcium antagonist (e.g. nifedipine)[a]
    Diuretic/class III calcium antagonist (e.g. diltiazem)[a]
    $\beta$-Blocker/$\alpha$-blocker
    $\beta$-Blocker/class II or class III calcium antagonist
    $\beta$-Blocker/hydralazine
    $\beta$-Blocker/methyldopa
    $\beta$-Blocker/clonidine
    $\beta$-Blocker/reserpine
    $\beta$-Blocker/ketanserin
    ACE inhibitor/diuretic
    ACE inhibitor/calcium antagonist
    ACE inhibitor/ketanserin

*Suitable three-drug combinations:*
    Diuretic/$\beta$-blocker/hydralazine
    Diuretic/$\beta$-blocker/methyldopa
    Diuretic/$\beta$-blocker/$\alpha$-blocker
    Diuretic/$\beta$-blocker/ACE inhibitor
    Diuretic/$\beta$-blocker/class II or class III calcium antagonist
    Diuretic/ACE inhibitor/class III calcium antagonist
    Loop diuretic/$\beta$-blocker/minoxidil
    Loop diuretic/methyldopa/minoxidil
    Loop diuretic/clonidine/minoxidil

*Unsuitable combinations:*
    $\beta$-Blocker/class I calcium antagonist (e.g. verapamil)
    $\beta$-Blocker/ACE inhibitor[a]
    Reserpine/methyldopa/clonidine in any conjoint grouping

[a] Not all workers agree.

Should a triple grouping be necessary, one of the best established is that comprising $\beta$-blocker, diuretic and hydralazine (so-called 'standard triple therapy' in the USA). In more resistant patients, minoxidil may be substituted for hydralazine, but the diuretic then needs to be a powerful loop-acting agent; an ordinary thiazide will usually be insufficient to counteract the fluid retention caused by minoxidil.[7] The combination of $\beta$-blocker plus diuretic plus prazosin has also been shown to work well,[7] as also, perhaps surprisingly, has the combination of $\beta$-blocker plus diuretic plus captopril.[60]

## 'Specific' antihypertensive drug therapy

An attractive, but still elusive, goal is the deployment of antihypertensive drugs which would correct a specific pathophysiological abnormality underlying or accompanying hypertension. This problem has been mentioned in some detail above (pages 20 and 59). Despite the attraction, this remains for future achievement. At present, prescription schedules in essential (primary) hypertension are according to the principles set out herein.

## Preservation of quality of life

An underlying, insistent, and very proper concern with antihypertensive treatment is effective control of arterial pressure together with preservation of the quality of life. Such considerations have led to the development of methods (sometimes referred to as 'instruments') for the evaluation of life quality.[48]

The assessments embrace globally the burden of drug effects and side-effects; constraints imposed by dosage schedules; the psychological impact of knowledge of hypertension, its risks and need for therapy; and the discomforts which may well accompany non-pharmacological interventions and modifications, achieved or attempted, in lifestyle. Comparative trials assessing quality of life with different antihypertensive regimes are discussed below.

## Studies of comparative efficacy and tolerability: single drugs

It is probably true to state that different antihypertensive drugs, prescribed singly, are broadly similarly effective in lowering blood pressure.

American black patients often respond less well than do white subjects.[49] Generally, diuretics appear more suitable and more potent than β-blockers in black American subjects.[49]

Claims for age-related differential efficacy, with, for example, β-blockers and ACE inhibitors being more useful in young hypertensives, and calcium antagonists and diuretics more valuable in the elderly, have not withstood critical analysis.[50] While β-blockers are less effective than some other drug classes in lowering systolic pressure, and systolic pressure elevation is prominent with ageing,[62] three major trials[51-53] showing benefit from the treatment of hypertension in patients over 60 featured β-blockade.

A multicentre American trial in men,[54] comparing various drugs as monotherapy, showed that success (defined as a diastolic pressure below 95 mmHg) was most frequent with diltiazem (59%), followed by atenolol (51%), clonidine (50%), hydrochlorothiazide (46%), captopril (42%) and prazosin (42%). Twenty-five per cent of those given only placebo had diastolic pressures which fell below 95 mmHg. Antihypertensive efficacy was best in young white men taking captopril, older white men taking atenolol, and black men of various ages on diltiazem. The incidence rates of drug intolerance were highest with clonidine (14%), followed by prazosin (12%), captopril (7%), placebo (6%), atenolol (5%), diltiazem (4%) and hydrochlorothiazide (3%).

In elderly hypertensive women, little difference in the capacity to lower diastolic pressure or in physical side effects was found between atenolol, enalapril, and isradipine (hydrochlorothiazide was added in 16% of cases).[63]

## Studies of comparative efficacy and tolerability: drug combinations

McAreavey et al.[7] made a comparison of various agents added when blood pressure was inadequately controlled by the combination of atenolol 100 mg plus bendrofluazide 5 mg daily. Minoxidil was the most effective third agent and was safe in combination with bendrofluazide in the less severely hypertensive patients. For those with higher pressures, the use of minoxidil required the substitution of a loop-acting diuretic to prevent fluid retention. Added hydralazine, methyldopa, prazosin or labetalol (the last with atenolol then withdrawn) were similarly effective to one another, less effective than minoxidil, and more effective than placebo. The order of acceptability was placebo, hydralazine, prazosin, methyldopa, labetalol. In this trial, hydralazine was considered to be the most suitable third drug, with prazosin a close rival.

A later study from the same centre, and with very similar design,[60] compared hydralazine with nifedipine, captopril and placebo, each again added to the fixed combination of atenolol 100 mg plus bendrofluazide 5 mg. Blood pressures below 140/95 mmHg were achieved most often on added captopril (33%), followed by hydralazine (29%), nifedipine (17%) and placebo (10%). Intolerable side-effects leading to withdrawal occurred most often with hydralazine (24%), followed by nifedipine (22%), captopril (15%) and placebo (3%).

Thus combining the data of these two closely allied trials,[7,60] the most generally useful third drug added to β-blocker plus diuretic was the ACE inhibitor captopril.

## Non-pharmacological methods of blood ——————— pressure reduction ———————

The wide range of dietary, environmental, behavioural and other factors which can influence the phenotypic expression of essential hypertension have been considered in some detail earlier (Chapters 6 and 7). These also have obvious therapeutic implications which are considered briefly here.[2,56] (See also page 241.)

### Dietary changes

Several dietary means of lowering high blood pressure have already been discussed in Chapter 7. These include the established benefits of weight reduction and of restriction of alcohol intake, as well as the more questionable value of a vegetarian diet, the addition of fish oils, of restriction of caffeine and sodium intake, or of supplementation of potassium and calcium and fibre ingestion.[56]

The feasibility and efficacy, as well as some limitations, of a multiple dietary approach has been shown in a 4-year trial[65] of weight reduction, sodium restriction and alcohol restriction. Compliance was good, and blood pressure was lowered, although not as effectively as in a control group of patients who remained on antihypertensive drugs.

### Physical exercise

Physical exercise has been demonstrated to cause a distinct and probably clinically valuable reduction of blood pressure. This effect is independent of any associated weight reduction.

### Psychological approaches

A variety of psychological measures, including yoga, transcendental meditation, relaxation training and so-called 'biofeedback' techniques have been shown, at least in the short term, and with dedicated exponents, to lower high blood pressures. On present evidence, the use of such methods long term or for wide-scale therapy is more questionable. One prospective trial showed relaxation therapy to be ineffective.[57] Even so, these approaches deserve further attention.

### Benefit has not been evaluated

Requiring emphasis is that the capacity of the various non-pharmacological measures indicated above to diminish morbidity accompanying hypertension has not been studied, and any burdens of unwanted effects are largely unassessed.

These important caveats are necessary because some writers have assumed, unreasonably, that non-pharmacological forms of intervention, and especially dietary changes, can only be beneficial. Thus it is often implied, and occasionally stated, that such measures are inherently superior to drug therapy. The therapeutic superiority of a dietary or behavioural intervention over a particular form of drug therapy needs, it must be emphasized, to be demonstrated before it can be accepted. To claim that, say, a particular dietary habit or pattern is potentially harmful, and simultaneously to assume, blindly, that modification of that dietary behaviour can only be beneficial, is fallacious reasoning (see also Appendix 3). One clearly relevant observation is the demonstration that a reduction of dietary sodium chloride intake in patients with essential hypertension is accompanied, at least in the short-term, by a significant rise in serum cholesterol concentration (Chapter 20), and by impairment of glucose tolerance (Chapter 7).

## Cessation of smoking

The role of cigarette smoking, and of cessation of smoking, in hypertension and its therapy is important and complex. Smoking greatly compounds the adverse cardiovascular effects of hypertension and minimizes the benefits of therapy (Chapter 8).[58] For a given blood pressure level, smokers are more likely than non-smokers to suffer a stroke or heart attack, or to enter the malignant phase of hypertension. Prognosis after these events is also worse in smokers than in non-smokers. Smokers are more likely than non-smokers to have renal artery stenosis. These are all powerful reasons for combining strong antismoking measures with antihypertensive treatment. However, although smoking raises blood pressure acutely, particularly if combined with the drinking of coffee, smokers tend otherwise to have lower blood pressure than non-smokers. This may be partly explained by lower body weight in smokers.[59]

## Case studies

See Case studies 1, 2, 3, 4 and 17, Appendix 2.

## References

1. Pickering GW. *High Blood Pressure*, 2nd edn. London: Churchill, 1968.
2. Yeo WW, Ramsay LE. Non-pharmacological treatment of hypertension. In *Handbook of Hypertension*, Vol. 15: *Clinical Hypertension* (ed. JIS Robertson). Amsterdam: Elsevier, 1992: 709–46.
3. Doyle AE (ed.). *Clinical Pharmacology of Antihypertensive Drugs. Handbook of Hypertension*, Vol. 11. Amsterdam: Elsevier, 1988.
4. Dollery C, Boobis AR, Burley D *et al.* (eds). *Therapeutic Drugs*. Edinburgh: Churchill Livingstone, 1991.
5. Hansson L, Svensson A, Dahlöf B *et al.* Drug treatment of hypertension. In *Handbook of Hypertension*, Vol. 15: *Clinical Hypertension* (ed. JIS Robertson). Amsterdam: Elsevier, 1992: 655–708.
6. Singh BN, Hollenberg NK, Poole-Wilson PA, Robertson JIS. Diuretic-induced potassium and magnesium deficiency: relation to drug-induced QT prolongation, cardiac arrhythmias and sudden death. *J. Hypertens.* 1992; **10**: 301–16.
7. McAreavey D, Ramsay LE, Latham L *et al.* 'Third Drug' trial: comparative study of antihypertensive agents added when blood pressure remains uncontrolled by a beta blocker plus thiazide diuretic. *Br. Med. J.* 1984; **288**: 106–11.
8. Medical Research Council Working Party on Mild Hypertension. Coronary heart disease in the Medical Research Council trial of treatment of mild hypertension. *Br. Heart J.* 1988; **59**: 364–78.
9. Green KG. British MRC trial of treatment for mild hypertension: a more favorable interpretation. *Am. J. Hypertens.* 1991; **4**: 723–4.
10. Wikstrand J, Warnold I, Olsson G *et al.* Primary prevention with metoprolol in patients with hypertension: mortality results from the MAPHY study. *J. Am. Med. Assoc.* 1988; **259**: 1976–82.
11. Wikstrand J. Warnold I. Tuomilehto J *et al.* Metoprolol versus thiazide diuretics in hypertension: morbidity results from the MAPHY study. *Hypertension* 1991; **17**: 579–88.
12. Olsson G, Tuomilehto J, Berglund G *et al.* Primary prevention of sudden cardiovascular death in hypertensive patients: mortality results from the MAPHY study. *Am. J. Hypertens.* 1991; **4**: 151–6.
13. The Norwegian Multicenter Study Group. Timolol-induced reduction in mortality and reinfarction in patients surviving acute myocardial infarction. *N. Engl. J. Med.* 1981; **304**: 801–7.
14. Beta-blocker Heart Attack Trial Group. A randomized trial of propranolol in patients with acute myocardial infarction. I. Mortality results. *J. Am. Med. Assoc.* 1982; **247**: 1707–14.
15. Andersson B, Waagstein F. Improved exercise hemodynamics in dilated cardiomyopathy following adrenergic beta-blocker treatment. *Eur. Heart J.* 1993; **14** (abstr. suppl.): 11.

16. Croog SH, Levine S, Testa MA *et al.* The effects of antihypertensive therapy on the quality of life. *N. Engl. J. Med.* 1986; **314**: 1657–64.

17. Steiner SS, Friedhoff AJ, Wilson BL *et al.* Antihypertensive therapy and quality of life: a comparison of atenolol, captopril, enalapril and propranolol. *J. Human Hypertens.* 1990; **4**: 217–25.

18. Herrick AL, Waller PC, Berkin KE *et al.* Comparison of enalapril and atenolol in mild to moderate hypertension. *Am. J. Med.* 1989; **86**: 421–6.

19. Palmer AJ, Fletcher AE, Rudge PJ *et al.* Quality of life in hypertensives treated with atenolol or captopril: a double-blind crossover trial. *J. Hypertens.* 1992; **10**: 1409–16.

20. Vanhoutte PM, Paoletti R. The WHO classification of calcium antagonists. *Trends Pharmacol. Sci.* 1987; **8**: 4–5.

21. Verheyen A, Schwabedal PE, Pulina M *et al.* Dose-dependent supression of arteriosclerosis by the calcium antagonist flunarizine in Skelton-hypertensive rats without reduction in blood pressure. In *Atherosclerosis and Cardiovascular Disease*, Vol. 4 (eds CG Descovich *et al.*). Bologna: Editrice Compasitori, 1989: 813–18.

22. Doyle AE. Side effects of calcium antagonists. *J. Cardiovasc. Pharmacol.* 1988; **12** (suppl. 8): 175–6.

23. Marone C, Luisoli S, Bomio F *et al.* Body sodium-blood volume state, aldosterone, and cardiovascular responsiveness after calcium entry blockade with nifedipine. *Kidney Int.* 1985; **28**: 658–65.

24. Maclean D, MacConnachie AM. Selected side-effects: peripheral oedema with dihydropyridine calcium antagonists. *Prescribers J.* 1992; **32**: 4–6.

25. Pevahouse JB, Markandu ND, Cappuccio FP *et al.* Long term reduction in sodium balance: possible additional mechanism whereby nifedipine lowers blood pressure. *Br. Med. J.* 1990; **301**: 580–4.

26. Robertson JIS. Long-term reduction in sodium balance. *Br. Med. J.* 1990; **301**: 1159–60.

27. Murray TS, East BW, Robertson JIS. Nicardipine versus propranolol in the treatment of essential hypertension: effect on total body elemental composition. *Br. J. Clin. Pharmacol.* 1986; **22** (suppl. 3): 249–66.

28. Resnick LM, Nicholson JP, Gupta RK, Laragh JH. Interactive effects of oral calcium supplementation with calcium channel antagonist therapy in essential hypertension. Abstracts, 6th European Meeting on Hypertension, Milan, 1993, no. 612.

29. Bailey DG, Spence JD, Munoz C, Arnold JMO. Interaction of citrus juices with felodopine and nifedipine. *Lancet* 1991; **337**: 268–9.

30. Spence JD, Arnold JMO, Gilbert JJ. Vascular consequences of hypertension and effects of antihypertensive therapy. In *Handbook of Hypertension*, Vol. 15: *Clinical Hypertension* (ed. JIS Robertson). Amsterdam: Elsevier, 1992: 621–54.

31. Van Harten J, Burggraaf K, Danhof M *et al.* Negligible sublingual absorption of nifedipine. *Lancet* 1987; **ii**: 1363–5.

32. Egstrup K, Andersen PE. Transient myocardial ischemia during nifedipine therapy in stable angina pectoris, and its relation to coronary collateral flow and comparison with metoprolol. *Am. J. Cardiol.* 1993; **71**: 177–83.

33. Fleckenstein A, Fleckenstein-Grün G, Frey M *et al.* Future directions in the use of calcium antagonists. *Am. J. Cardiol.* 1987; **59**: 117–87B.

34. The Danish Study Group on Verapamil in Myocardial Infarction (DAVIT II). Effect of verapamil on mortality and major events after acute myocardial infarction. *Am. J. Cardiol.* 1990; **66**: 779–85.

35. The Multicenter Diltiazem Postinfarction Trial Research Group. The effect of diltiazem on mortality and reinfarction after myocardial infarction. *N. Engl. J. Med.* 1988; **319**: 385–92.

36. Held PH, Yusuf S, Furberg CD. Calcium channel blockers in acute myocardial infarction and unstable angina: an overview. *Br. Med. J.* 1989; **299**: 1187–92.

37. Fischer Hansen J. Calcium antagonists and myocardial infarction. *Cardiovasc Drugs Ther.* 1991; **5**: 665–70.

38. Gheuens J, De Ryck M, Van Reempts J *et al.* Treatment of acute ischemic stroke with calcium antagonists. In *Calcium Antagonists* (eds T Godfraind *et al.*). Dordrecht: Kluwer, 1993: 257–63.

39. Brunner HR, Nussberger J, Waeber B. Angiotensin antagonists. In *The Renin–Angiotensin System* (eds JIS Robertson and MG Nicholls). London: Gower Medical, 1993: chapter 86.

40. Hui KY, Haber E, Renin inhibitors. In *The Renin–Angiotensin System* (eds JIS Robertson and MG Nicholls). London: Gower Medical, 1993: chapter 85.

41. Hansson L, Dahlöf B, Himmelman A *et al.* Angiotensin-converting enzyme inhibitors in the treatment of essential hypertension. In *The Renin–Angiotensin System* (eds JIS Robertson and ME Nicholls). London: Gower Medical, 1993: chapter 91.

42. Johnston CI. Angiotensin-converting enzyme in-

hibitors. In *The Renin–Angiotensin System* (eds JIS Robertson and MG Nicholls) London: Gower Medical, 1993: chapter 87.

43. Robertson JIS. Angiotensin-converting enzyme inhibitors in clinical renovascular hypertension. In *The Renin–Angiotensin System* (eds JIS Robertson and MG Nicholls). London: Gower Medical, 1993: chapter 88.

44. Fletcher AE, Dollery CT. Side effects associated with inhibitors of angiotensin-converting enzyme. In *The Renin–Angiotensin System* (eds JIS Robertson and MG Nicholls). London: Gower Medical, 1993: chapter 99.

45. Crozier IG, Ikram H, Nicholls MG. Angiotensin-converting enzyme inhibitors in the treatment of heart failure. In *The Renin–Angiotensin System* (eds JIS Robertson and MG Nicholls). London: Gower Medical, 1993: chapter 93.

46. Nicod P, Waeber B, Brunner HR. Renin in myocardial infarction. In *The Renin–Angiotensin System* (eds JIS Robertson and MG Nicholls). London: Gower Medical, 1993: chapter 77.

47. Zanchetti A. Which drug to which patient? *J. Hypertens.* 1987; **5** (suppl. 2): 57–61.

48. Testa MA. Quality of life during antihypertensive therapy: technique for clinical assessment and evaluation. *Br. J. Clin. Pharmacol.* 1987; **23** (suppl.): 9–13.

49. Fifth Report of the Joint National Committee on Detection, Evaluation, and Treatment of High Blood Pressure (JNCV). *Arch. Intern. Med.* 1993; **153**: 154–83.

50. Robertson JIS, Doyle AE, Vanhoutte P. (eds) Age-related effects of antihypertensive therapy: the Corsendonk Symposium. *J. Cardiovasc. Pharm.* 1988; **12** (suppl. 8).

51. MRC Working Party. Medical Research Council trial of treatment of hypertension in older adults: principal results. *Br. Med. J.* 1992; **304**: 405–12.

52. SHEP Cooperative Research Group. Prevention of stroke by antihypertensive drug treatment of older persons with isolated systolic hypertension. *J. Am. Med. Assoc.* 1991; **265**: 3255–64.

53. Dahlöf B, Lindholm L, Hansson L *et al.* Morbidity and mortality in the Swedish Trial in Old Patients with Hypertension (STOP-Hypertension). *Lancet* 1991; **338**: 1281–5.

54. Materson BJ, Reda DJ, Cushman WC. Single-drug therapy for hypertensive men: a comparison of six antihypertensive agents with placebo. *N. Engl. J. Med.* 1993; **328**: 914–21.

55. Beilin LJ. Environmental and dietary aspects of primary hypertension. In *Handbook of Hypertension*, Vol. 15: *Clinical Hypertension* (ed. JIS Robertson). Amsterdam: Elsevier, 1992: 95–140.

56. Eliasson K, Ryttig KR, Hylander B. *et al.* A dietary fibre supplement in the treatment of mild hypertension: a randomized, double-blind, placebo-controlled trial. *J. Hypertens.* 1992; **10**: 195–9.

57. Johnston DW, Gold A, Kentish J *et al.* Effect of stress management on blood pressure in mild primary hypertension. *Br. Med. J.* 1993; **306**: 963–6.

58. Materson BJ, Reda D, Freis ED, Henderson WG. Cigarette smoking interferes with treatment of hypertension. *Arch. Intern. Med.* 1988; **148**: 2116–19.

59. Wannamethee G, Shaper AG. Body weight and mortality in middle aged British men: impact of smoking. *Br. Med. J.* 1989; **299**: 1497–502.

60. Bevan EG, Pringle SD, Waller PC *et al.* Comparison of captopril, hydralazine and nifedipine as third drug in hypertensive patients. *J. Human Hypertens.* 1993; **7**: 83–8.

61. Langley MS, Sorkin EM. Nimodipine: a review of its pharmacodynamic and pharmacokinetic properties, and therapeutic potential in cerebrovascular disease. *Drugs* 1989; **37**: 669–99.

62. Avanzini F, Alli C, Betteli G *et al.* Antihypertensive efficacy and tolerability of different drug regimens in isolated systolic hypertension in the elderly. *Eur. Heart J.* 1994; **14**: 206–12.

63. Croog SH, Elias MF, Colton T *et al.* Effects of antihypertensive medications on quality of life in elderly hypertensive women. *Am. J. Hypertens.* 1994; **7**: 329–39.

64. Kornhuber HH, Hartung J, Herrlinger JD *et al.* Flunarizine in ischemic stroke: a randomised multicentre, placebo-controlled, double-blind study. *Neurol. Psychiatr. Brain Res.* 1993; **1**: 173–80.

65. Stamler R, Stamler J, Grimm R *et al.* Nutritional therapy for high blood pressure: final report of a four-year randomized controlled trial. *J. Amer. Med. Ass.* 1987; **257**: 1484–91.

66. Manhem PJ, Clark SW, Brown WB *et al.* Effect of chlorothiazide on serial measurements of exchangeable sodium and blood pressure in spontaneously hypertensive rats. *Clin. Sci.* 1985; **69**: 511–15.

67. Acute Infarction Ramipril Efficacy (AIRE) Study Investigators. Effect of ramipril on mortality and mobidity of survivors of acute myocardial infarction with evidence of heart failure. *Lancet* 1993; **342**: 821–8.

# 23
# The detection of hypertension

## —— Clinical features in hypertension ——

The majority of subjects with essential hypertension will be free of symptoms and clinical signs. These latter features appear only with the pathological involvement of arteries and of various organs, particularly the heart, brain, eye and kidney (Chapters 13–18), or with diagnosis and treatment. Thus, an initial problem comprises the recognition of latent hypertension. The clinical evaluation of the identified hypertensive patient is then directed particularly to the detection and assessment of organ function and damage. A further, less frequent, but important requirement is the recognition of evidence of secondary forms of hypertension. The appreciation of hypertension is therefore dependent first on effective screening, and then on supplementary investigations of varying complexity.

## —— Screening for hypertension ——

As raised arterial pressure is not usually accompanied by symptoms or signs, if it is to be detected, and preventive therapy initiated, asymptomatic subjects need to be screened.

If a formal screening programme is undertaken, for example, by inviting inhabitants of a town to attend at a specified date and time, coverage up to about 80% is usually achieved.

Alternatively, if a primary care physician takes the opportunity of routinely measuring blood pressure whenever he or she sees a patient, for whatever reason, coverage of around 80% is attained within 3 years. Almost 100% coverage can be achieved if the physician invites all patients on list to attend for screening. It is therefore recommended that a primary care physician should make every effort to record the blood pressure of all patients on list and to update the information regularly.

Screening of factory employees can also be usefully undertaken.

Blood pressure measurement in children should not be neglected, and, for example, can be part of routine medical examinations in schools where these are done. Those with above-average blood pressure in childhood are more likely to progress to distinct hypertension later in life.

## —— Blood pressure measurement ——

### Routine measurement

The measurement of blood pressure, although simple, is prone to inaccuracies.[1,26] Incorrect readings can easily lead to errors of diagnosis and thus to inappropriate or deficient therapy.

For routine clinical use, a mercury sphygmomanometer is preferable to an aneroid model. The mercury and glass should be clean, and the meniscus clearly visible at zero before inflation. An aneroid machine should be calibrated regularly against a mercury instrument. The cuff, consisting of an inflatable bladder within a restrictive cloth or plastic sheath, should be sufficiently long to wrap around the arm fully, and to be firmly secured. The inflatable bladder should not be too short or too narrow, otherwise the blood pressure will be over-estimated. The bladder length should be at least 80%, and the bladder width at least 40%, of the arm circumference. The centre of the bladder should be marked on the cuff so that it may be placed accurately over the brachial artery. The bladder must be capable of smooth swift inflation and the release valve (very frequently a faulty part) should permit smooth deflation.

Measurements in children present especial, but not insuperable, problems. To cover the age range 0–14 years, a minimum of three cuffs, with bladder dimensions 4 × 13, 8 × 18 and 12 × 35 cm (adult size) is recommended. Especially in children under 1 year of age, Korotkoff sounds may be aberrant, and instruments utilizing ultrasound, based on the Doppler principle, and focusing on systolic pressure, are then preferable.

It is recommended that before blood pressure is measured, the subject sits or lies quietly for 5 min. The procedure should be explained, emphasizing that it may be necessary to repeat the measurement several times, and especially warning that minor discomfort may be caused. Even so, higher values are likely to be obtained in many subjects initially, with lower readings after several visits and familiarity with the procedure. Conversation should be avoided during the measurement.

In hypertensive patients, and particularly when assessing drug therapy, it is advisable to measure the pressure after at least 5 min of lying (or sitting), and again after 1 min of standing.

The arm should be close to horizontal and supported so that it is at the level of the midsternum. With the subject in a suitably warm environment, the arm should be freed from restrictive clothing and the point of maximal pulsation of the brachial artery just above the antecubital fossa identified. A cuff of the dimensions already defined should be applied to the upper arm, and firmly secured. The centre of the cuff should overlie the brachial artery which runs along the medical aspect of the upper arm. Preferably, the tubing should be at the upper (axillary) side of the cuff so as not to interfere with auscultation. The lower edge of the cuff should be at least 2 cm above the site over the brachial artery

identified for auscultation. The mercury column must be vertical and at eye level.

Systolic pressure should be estimated by palpation before using the stethoscope. For this purpose, the brachial or radial artery is felt and the bladder inflated until the pulse is obliterated. This gives a measure of the systolic pressure, and enables the observer to avoid errors associated, for example, with a 'silent gap' with no Korotkoff sounds on auscultation at less than systolic pressure. The cuff is then deflated.

A stethoscope is applied gently over the site of the brachial artery previously identified, care being taken to avoid contact with the cuff. The bladder is inflated to a pressure about 10 mmHg above the previously determined systolic pressure, and deflated at an even rate of 2–3 mmHg/s. The point at which clear repetitive tapping sounds become audible is the systolic pressure; the point at which these suddenly fade is the fourth phase diastolic value; the point at which the sounds become inaudible is the fifth phase diastolic. The fifth phase is now used routinely in clinical practice in preference to the fourth phase, which is usually slightly higher than true (intra-arterial) diastolic pressure. However, fourth phase measurements are valuable in some circumstances, for example, in children, in pregnancy (page 237), or in occasional subjects where the sounds may continue down to a cuff pressure near zero.

At an initial visit, blood pressure should be measured in both arms and if an appreciable difference exists (e.g. more than 20 mmHg systolic or 10 mmHg diastolic), the arm with the higher reading should be used on that and subsequent occasions. Aortic coarctation (page 168) proximal to the origin of the subclavian artery may be responsible for substantially lower pressures in the left arm.

It is emphasized that blood pressure is continuously variable, being influenced, *inter alia*, by the circumstances of measurement, conversation, ambient temperature, meals, drinks, smoking, anxiety, the menstrual cycle, the season of the year, and, especially, pressor and antihypertensive drugs (Chapters 6–8 and 27).

## Pseudohypertension

There is a further aspect of blood pressure measurement that may be particularly relevant in elderly subjects. Not rarely, owing to extensive sclerosis in large arteries (page 60), they are resistant to compression by a sphygmomanometer cuff. This may give a spurious impression of hypertension and has been termed 'pseudohypertension', with a difference between cuff and intra-arterial values as great as 50 mmHg. Osler's manoeuvre consists of assessing whether the pulseless radial or brachial artery, distal to a point of occlusion achieved manually or by cuff compression, remains palpable. If it does, the patient is held to be likely to manifest falsely high sphygmomanometric readings. The reliability of Osler's manoeuvre has, however, been questioned.[2]

## 'Zero-muddler' sphygmomanometer

In epidemiological surveys and therapeutic trials, it is important for the observer to avoid preferentially recording certain terminal digits. Readings in millimetres of mercury expressed with a terminal number of 0 or 5 tend to be especially favoured in 'open' pressure measurements. One method of partially circumventing this problem is to use a 'zero-muddler' sphygmomanometer.[3] This is a conventional instrument in which, before each measurement, a wheel is spun that re-sets the mercury meniscus to a point above zero unknown to the observer. After measurements have been made, this unbiased and hidden addition to the value is ascertained, and then subtracted from the measured reading to obtain the correct value. The device is often termed, incorrectly, a 'random-zero' sphygmomanometer. The additions to zero are not random, however, but, predictably, follow a broadly Gaussian distribution.[4] The instrument is readily portable and simple to use, being basically an orthodox mercury sphygmomanometer.

This is a widely employed and potentially very useful procedure. O'Brien et al.[5] and Kronmal et al.[6] have nevertheless criticized the 'zero-muddler' sphygmomanometer, both groups reporting with

its use significant underestimation of blood pressure. Unfortunately, neither paper identified the reasons for the inaccuracy, or proposed remedies. The magnitudes of the errors were very different in these reports, a mean of up to 3.8 mmHg systolic and 7.5 mmHg diastolic in that of O'Brien et al.,[5] yet of only 1.65 mmHg systolic and 1.84 mmHg diastolic in that of Kronmal et al.[6] These divergencies between the two very similar studies raise the question of simple calibration error rather than a fundamental fault. Hayler[7] has stated that comparison of the 'zero-muddler' with any good standard sphygmomanometer, with a Y-piece and an inanimate arm substitute, will show precisely the same pressure reading for a fixed and decreasing pressure at all points on the scale. In Hayler's view, the error in the study of O'Brien et al.[5] could have been caused by a difference in pulsation of the mercury columns or an effect of the Y-piece connection on the physics of the 'zero-muddler' inflation. Garrow,[8] the inventor of the device, was also critical of the study by O'Brien et al.[5] The attacks on this machine have continued,[9–11] although without the fault being identified by the critics. The defence has been spirited, with several clinicians finding the 'zero-muddler' to be accurate and valuable when properly maintained and utilized.[12–17] Further investigation is evidently required.

## 'Rose box'

The more elaborate device of Rose, Holland and Crowley ('Rose box')[18] is now less favoured because it is heavy and therefore difficult to transport, it requires a special technique of operation and hence some training in its use, and it needs more frequent maintenance.

There have also been concerns about its accuracy, expressed especially by O'Brien and his colleagues, prominent amongst the critics also of the 'zero-muddler'[19] (see above). In one study, the 'Rose box' gave lower readings than those obtained with the 'zero-muddler';[19] this study was both criticized,[20,21] and defended.[22] Once more, the issue appears inconclusive.

## Automated sphygmomanometers and 24-h recording

In recent years, there has been increasing availability of light portable automated blood pressure monitoring equipment.[23,24] This has permitted 24-h evaluation of pressure in the circumstances of normal daily life, away from the clinic, and has provided a wealth of epidemiological and therapeutic information (see also Chapter 3).

Continuous intra-arterial recording is now less often employed than formerly, mainly because of worries about its safety. Nevertheless, this approach yielded valuable data and gave insight into many new areas of hypertension research.

Although the alternative modern non-invasive methods of continuous blood pressure recording have progressed rapidly, there remain concerns about their reliability under some circumstances, especially on movement and exercise, with arrhythmias or bradycardia, and because the noise and discomfort accompanying cuff compression with several such methods can interfere with sleep. Many of these methods still await full evaluation and acceptance.

These various techniques have consistently shown that arterial and organ involvement in hypertension correlates more closely with the whole-day blood pressure measurement than with values obtained in the clinic or surgery (see Chapter 3).

However, this seems not to be true of those patients prone to experience an alarm reaction in the presence of a doctor (so-called 'white coat' effect by the lovers of jargon). A subject not infrequently shows high blood pressure readings in the clinic, although 24-h records obtained in everyday surroundings are unremarkable. Treatment is thought not usually to be indicated in such cases, although it remains uncertain if the alarm reaction is truly benign (see page 271).[25]

Twenty-four hour recordings are also invaluable in permitting accurate assessment of the duration and magnitude of efficacy of antihypertensive therapy.

Proponents of electronic methods of monitoring blood pressure often anticipate with eagerness the demise of the mercury sphygmomanometer.[24] Their arguments have force, although their sentiments evince predilection and some will to belief.

———————— Case study ————————

See Case study 11, Appendix 2.

———————— References ————————

1. Petrie JC, O'Brien ET, Littler WA, de Swiet M. British Hypertension Society: recommendations on blood pressure measurement. *Br. Med. J.* 1986; **293**: 611–15.
2. Oliner CM, Elliott WJ, Gretler DD *et al.* Low predictive value of positive Osler's manoeuvre for diagnosing pseudohypertension. *J. Human Hypertens.* 1993; **7**: 65–70.
3. Garrow JS. Zero-muddler for unprejudiced sphygmomanometry. *Lancet* 1963; **iv**: 1205.
4. Holmes A, Beevers DG, Beevers M. The value of the Hawksley random zero sphygmomanometer. *Am. J. Hypertens.* 1993; **6**: 94–5.
5. O'Brien E, Mee F, Atkins N *et al.* Inaccuracy of the Hawksley random zero sphygmomanometer. *Lancet* 1990; **336**: 1465–8.
6. Kronmal RA, Rutan GH, Manolio TA *et al.* Properties of the random zero sphygmomanometer. *Hypertension* 1993; **21**: 632–7.
7. Hayler CR. Inaccuracy of the Hawksley random zero sphygmomanometer. *Lancet* 1991; **337**: 866.
8. Garrow JS. Inaccuracy of the Hawksley random zero sphygmomanometer. *Lancet* 1991; **337**: 866.
9. Silman AJ. Failure of random zero sphygmomanometer in general practice. *Br. Med. J.* 1985; **290**: 1781–82.
10. Lawson M, Johnston A. The Hawksley random zero sphygmomanometer: should be abandoned. *Br. Med. J.* 1993; **307**: 123.
11. Conroy RM, O'Brien E, O'Malley K *et al.* Measurement error in the Hawksley random zero sphygmomanometer: what damage has been done and what can we learn? *Br. Med. J.* 1993; **306**: 1319–22.

12. Macintyre CCA, Fowkes FGR. Potential problems with random zero sphygmomanometer. *Lancet* 1990; **335**: 727–8.

13. Hense HW. The Hawksley random zero sphygmomanometer: comparison with mercury instrument is illogical. *Br. Med. J.* 1993; **307**: 562.

14. Garrow J, Summerbell C. The Hawksley random zero sphygmomanometer: repeat experiment exonerates instrument. *Br. Med. J.* 1993; **307**: 123.

15. Dinning JA. The Hawksley random zero sphygmomanometer. *Br. Med. J.* 1993; **307**: 123.

16. Churchill D, Beevers M, Beevers DG. The Hawksley random zero sphygmomanometer: don't condemn it without proper evidence. *Br. Med. J.* 1993; **307**: 123–4.

17. Miall WE. Instrument is accurate if used properly. *Br. Med. J.* 1993; **307**: 124.

18. Rose GA, Holland WW, Crowley EA. A sphygmomanometer for epidemiologists. *Lancet* 1964; **i**: 296–300.

19. Fitzgerald D, O'Callaghan W, O'Malley K, O'Brien E. Inaccuracy of the London School of Hygiene sphygmomanometer. *Br. Med. J.* 1982; **282**: 18–19.

20. Rose G. Inaccuracy of the London School of Hygiene sphygmomanometer. *Br. Med. J.* 1982; **282**: 18–19.

21. Ramsay LE. Inaccuracy of the London School of Hygiene sphygmomanometer. *Br. Med. J.* 1982; **284**: 662.

22. Fitzgerald DJ, O'Malley K, O'Brien E. Inaccuracy of the London School of Hygiene sphygmomanometer. *Br. Med. J.* 1982; **284**: 662–3.

23. Neutel JM, Smith DHG, Weber MA. Diurnal and ambulatory blood pressure monitoring. In *Handbook of Hypertension*, Vol. 15: *Clinical Hypertension* (ed. JIS Robertson). Amsterdam: Elsevier, 1992: 51–62.

24. Stewart MJ, Padfield PL. Blood pressure measurement: an epitaph for the mercury sphygmomanometer? *Clin. Sci.* 1992; **83**: 1–12.

25. Kuwajima I, Suzuki Y, Fujisawa A, Kuramoto K. Is white coat hypertension innocent? Structure and function of the heart in the elderly. *Hypertension* 1993; **22**: 826–31.

26. Pickering TG. Blood pressure measurement and detection of hypertension. *Lancet* 1994; **344**: 31–5.

# 24
# The investigation of hypertension

## Purpose of investigating hypertension[1]

The purpose of investigating a subject with hypertension is fourfold:

1 to detect organ damage consequent upon the hypertension;
2 to diagnose a possible underlying cause for the raised blood pressure—this item is directed to the recognition of any of the wide range of secondary forms of hypertension (page 5, Table 1.1), and also, most importantly, the identification of aspects of diet and lifestyle which may affect arterial pressure;
3 to identify risk factors additional to hypertension; and
4 to recognize concomitant diseases that might influence the treatment of hypertension.

The tempo and extent of such investigation will vary greatly. Furthermore, the thoroughness of the procedures will be greater in certain occupational groups, for example, airline pilots. The present account is concerned with the initial stages of investigation. If evidence of secondary hypertension is found, the diagnosis should be pursued as detailed in the section dealing with the particular disorder. Some of the main features to be sought in relation to risk factors, tissue and organ damage and aetiology are given in Tables 24.1–24.3.

## History

The history-taking should include specific enquiries about a possible family history of hypertension or its consequences, or of familial diabetes mellitus, renal disease or multiple endocrine neoplasia. The patient's smoking and drinking habits should be ascertained, and whether excessive ingestion of liquorice is likely. Dietary patterns and predilections should be recorded. Medication of any kind must be noted, in particular the taking

**Table 24.1.** Evidence of additional risk factors to hypertension likely to be obtained from the history, physical examination or initial investigations

| History | Examination | Investigation |
|---|---|---|
| Family history of diabetes mellitus | Obesity | Diabetes mellitus |
| Family history of hypertension or its consequences, e.g. stroke | | Hypercholesterolaemia |
| Smoking | | |
| Alcohol intake | | |
| Oral contraceptives | | |
| Gout | | |

**Table 24.2.** Evidence of hypertensive organ damage as obtained from the history, physical examination or investigation

| Organ | History | Examination | Investigation |
|---|---|---|---|
| Heart | Chest pain<br>Breathlessness | Cardiomegaly<br>Cardiac failure | Electrocardiogram<br>Echocardiogram<br>Chest X-ray<br>Angiography |
| Brain | Transient ischaemic attacks<br>Strokes<br>Fits | Focal neurological signs | Electro-encephalogram<br>Computed tomography scan |
| Blood vessels | Claudication | Absent or decreased peripheral pulses | Arteriography |
| Eyes | Transient visual disturbance<br>Persistent visual disturbance<br>Retinal vascular occlusion | Arterial change | Fluorescein angiography |
| Kidney | Nocturia<br>Polyuria<br>Haematuria<br>Myoglobinuria | Anaemia<br>Skin pigmentation | Haemoglobin<br>Plasma urea, creatinine, electrolytes<br>Urinary blood, protein, casts<br>Intravenous urography<br>Digital subtraction angiography<br>Abdominal ultrasound |

of oral contraceptives, post-menopausal hormone replacements, ACTH, corticosteroids, non-steroidal anti-inflammatory agents, or analgesics (Table 24.4).

Organ damage may be sustained in the heart, reflected by anginal pain or dyspnoea; the brain, indicated by an account of stroke, dementia, fits or transient ischaemic attacks; the eyes, manifest by unilateral or bilateral transient or persistent visual disturbance; and the kidneys, as shown by nocturia, polyuria or haematuria. Alternatively, these latter features may indicate a renal lesion responsible for

**Table 24.3.** Evidence of underlying cause of hypertension as obtained from history or clinical examination

| History | Clinical examination |
|---|---|
| Oral contraceptive use | Appearance, e.g. Cushing's syndrome or acromegaly |
| Liquorice ingestion | Evidence of thyroid disorder |
| Non-steroidal anti-inflammatory drugs | Signs of catecholamine excess |
| ACTH or corticosteroid use | Multiple neurofibromata |
| Analgesic abuse | Abdominal or loin bruit |
| Alcohol excess | Enlarged kidneys |
| '4Ps' of phaeochromocytoma (pain (headache), palpitations, perspiration, pallor) | Femoral delay |
| Polyuria, nocturia or haematuria | |
| Past renal trauma | |
| Muscular weakness due to hypokalaemia | |
| Personal or family history of polycystic renal disease or phaeochromocytoma or of multiple endocrine neoplasia | |

**Table 24.4.**   Obligatory enquiries in a hypertensive patient

Family history suggestive of hypertension
Past or present cardiac, vascular or renal problems
Account of any pregnancies
Past or present drug intake (especially oral contraceptives and non-steroidal anti-inflammatory agents)
Any previous blood pressure measurements
Alcohol intake
Liquorice intake
Smoking habits

hypertension. Muscular weakness, polyuria or nocturia may indicate potassium depletion. An account of possible previous renal trauma should be sought. The physician should enquire for symptoms of intermittent claudication. Features of phaeochromocytoma often emerge in the history, and especially the 'four Ps': pain (usually headache), palpitation, perspiration and pallor.

─────── Clinical examination ───────

Obesity is the main risk indicator likely to be revealed clinically (pages 26 and 89).

Possible organ involvement and damage from hypertension should be fully explored on clinical examination (Table 24.5). Cardiomegaly may be recognized at the bedside, In more advanced cases, frank cardiac failure may be apparent, with raised central venous pressure, hepatic congestion, and peripheral or pulmonary oedema. Focal neurological signs may indicate brain lesions. Peripheral

vascular disease may be shown by diminished or absent arterial pulses. Detailed examination of the optic fundi should be undertaken in every hypertensive patient and will suggest the extent of arterial involvement, whether sectorial arterial or venous occlusion has occurred, and if lesions of the malignant phase or of diabetes mellitus are present. The physician should not disdain the use of short-acting pupillary-dilating eyedrops, which should always be available.

A diverse range of conditions possibly responsible for secondary hypertension can be revealed or indicated at the bedside. Thyroid disease, Cushing's syndrome or acromegaly may often be immediately apparent. Excessive thinness may suggest thyrotoxicosis or phaeochromocytoma. Multiple cutaneous neurofibromata may accompany simple phaeochromocytoma or multiple endocrine neoplasia. The femoral pulses should be felt in every hypertensive patient irrespective of age; delay and usually diminution will indicate aortic coarctation. An abdominal or loin bruit can

**Table 24.5.**   Obligatory aspects of clinical examination in a hypertensive patient

Check femoral pulses
Check peripheral pulses
Cardiac examination
Pulmonary examination
Ophthalmoscopy
Palpation for renal enlargement
Check evidence of endocrine disorder (acromegaly, Cushing's syndrome, thyroid disease etc.)
Body weight/obesity

**Table 24.6.** Minimum of investigations in a hypertensive patient

Urine testing
Plasma urea, creatinine, sodium, potassium, cholesterol, uric acid
ECG

signify renal artery stenosis. Renal enlargement may be due to a tumour or to polycystic disease.

## Special tests

The length to which special tests should be pursued in patients with raised blood pressure raises many issues: political, social, moral and economic as well as medical. The principles outlined should be modified for the individual patient and local circumstances. It should be remembered that, in unselected cases, secondary forms of hypertension are rare. Most physicians would feel uncomfortable without undertaking some of the simpler basic tests; few would or should be happy without, for example, measuring plasma electrolytes, lipids, urea and creatinine, or testing the urine.

A constant problem is a decision on the lengths to which more detailed investigation should be undertaken. Extensive tests may not always be in the interest of the patient. They must be done in the event of malignant hypertension (after initially controlling blood pressure), or if clear hints of secondary hypertension emerge from the history, clinical examination or routine investigations (Table 24.6). Otherwise, no absolute rules can be given. More detailed investigation is indicated in the circumstances listed in Table 24.7, arranged roughly in declining order of importance.

### Electrocardiography

Left ventricular hypertrophy may be recognized electrocardiographically, although the method has distinct limitations. Nevertheless, such changes are of particular concern because of their prognostic implications. Electrocardiography can also reveal or indicate ischaemic heart disease.

The electrocardiographic criteria for left ventricular hypertrophy are given in Table 24.8. An example of left ventricular hypertrophy is shown in Figure 24.1.

**Table 24.7.** Indications for more thorough investigation of hypertension

1  Clear evidence of secondary hypertension on history, clinical examination or routine tests
2  Malignant phase hypertension
3  Abnormal urinary analysis
4  Raised serum urea or creatinine
5  Diastolic pressure $> 120$ mmHg
6  Sudden deterioration of blood pressure control
7  Failure of hypertension to respond to three drugs given in combination
8  Youth ($< 45$ years)
9  Certain occupational groups (e.g. aircrew)

**Table 24.8.**    The recognized criteria for left ventricular hypertrophy

1    R in $V_4$, $V_5$ or $V_6$ exceeds 27 mm
2    S in $V_1$, $V_2$ or $V_3$ exceeds 30 mm
3    R in $V_4$, $V_5$ or $V_6$ plus S in $V_1$, $V_2$ or $V_3$ exceeds 40 mm
4    R in aVL exceeds 13 mm
5    R in aVF exceeds 20 mm
6    Ventricular activation time exceeds 0.04 s
7    ST-segment depression, T-wave flattening or T-wave inversion in leads facing the left
     ventricle ($V_4$, $V_5$ or $V_6$, leads I and aVL when the heart is horizontal and leads II and aVF
     when the heart is vertical)

### Echocardiography

Echocardiography is now widely available and provides more reliable and detailed evidence of cardiac hypertrophy than does electrocardiography.

### Chest radiography

Chest radiography is a less dependable means of assessing cardiac involvement, but, nevertheless, it should usually be included among the routine tests in hypertension.

### Urine examination

Dipstick testing of the urine is simple and sensitive. It can be done easily in all patients, it will identify some diabetic subjects, and it may alert the physician to a primary renal problem. Dipstick testing is sensitive particularly to albumin, but not to Bence–Jones proteose; 150 mg/litre will give a 'trace' of protein on testing and is about the upper limit of normal for 24-h excretion.

Stick testing requires lysis of cells to expose the haem pigments to the test area and thus to give a positive reaction to blood.

Microscopy of a fresh urine sample is needed to confirm the presence of red cells. A few may be present in normal urine, which may of course be contaminated at menstruation.

Red cell casts indicate glomerular bleeding and thus continuing glomerulonephritis or vasculitis; they may occur also together with granular casts in malignant hypertension. Red cell casts imply a renal cause for haematuria. However, it must be emphasized that the urine may be normal even with significant renal disease.

### Blood sampling

Blood should be taken for estimation of haemoglobin and for white cell counting. Measurement should also be made of plasma (or serum) urea, creatinine, potassium, sodium and uric acid. Fist clenching must not be employed as an aid to venepuncture, as this will raise plasma potassium concentration and may obscure diagnostically important hypokalaemia.[2] Relevant hypokalaemia may also disappear if dietary sodium intake is deficient.[2]

Elevation of plasma urea or creatinine will indicate renal impairment. Hypokalaemia may be a con-

**Figure 24.1 (opposite).**    ECG in left ventricular hypertophy. The rhythm is sinus. The mean frontal plane QRS axis is $-15°$, i.e. the heart is horizontal. The R-wave height in $V_5$ and $V_6$ is abnormal (peak R-wave height in $V_5$ is 41 mm). The S-wave depth in $V_1$ is abnormal (31 mm). The ventricular activation time in $V_5$ and $V_6$ is prolonged (0.06 s). There is ST-segment depression and T-wave inversion in the left precordial leads. As the heart is horizontal, those changes that are seen in the left precordial leads are also reflected in I and aVL. In this case, there is also evidence of left atrial hypertrophy (Reproduced from Ref. 3, with permission.)

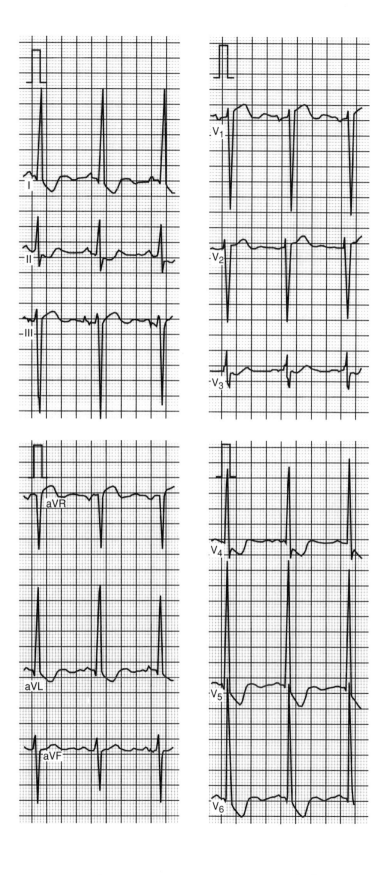

sequence of aldosterone excess, or of other forms of mineralocorticoid-induced hypertension as, for example, with liquorice ingestion. Hypokalaemia is also a feature of the rarity Liddle's syndrome.

Aldosterone excess will more frequently be secondary to stimulation of the renin–angiotensin system. Most often, this is a result of prior diuretic therapy, but it can also occur with renovascular hypertension or in the malignant phase. With secondary hyperaldosteronism, plasma sodium, as well as potassium, tends to be low. Conversely, with primary aldosterone excess, for example, that due to an aldosterone-secreting tumour, and other forms of mineralocorticoid hypertension, such as with liquorice ingestion or 17-α-hydroxylase deficiency, the renin–angiotensin system is suppressed, and a rather high value of plasma sodium accompanies the hypokalaemia.

Elevation of plasma potassium may be the result of renal failure, particularly if potassium-sparing agents have been given inappropriately. It is also a feature of the rare Gordon's syndrome (Chapter 40).

### Abdominal ultrasound

This non-invasive test can often provide information on the kidney or adrenal gland. Doppler ultrasound can indicate a renal arterial lesion.

### Intravenous urography

Intravenous urography was once regarded as part of the routine investigation of hypertension. However, several detailed studies have demonstrated that this expensive test, which is not without its discomforts and occasional hazards, is only rarely informative in unselected patients. Thus, intravenous urography (or other radiological investigation of the renal tract) is now reserved for those patients in whom there is a particular indication (Chapters 30–33).

## Case studies

See also Case studies 2 and 11, Appendix 2.

## References

1. Robertson JIS, Ball SG. The detection, assessment and management of hypertension. In *Handbook of Hypertension*, Vol. 15: *Clinical Hypertension* (ed. JIS Robertson). Amsterdam: Elsevier, 1992: 778–93.
2. Singh BN, Hollenberg NK, Poole-Wilson PA, Robertson JIS. Diuretic-induced potassium and magnesium deficiency: relation to drug-induced QT prolongation, cardiac arrhythmias and sudden death. *J. Hypertens*. 1992; **10**: 301–16.
3. Rowlands DJ. The resting electrocardiogram. In *Diseases of the Heart*, 1st edn (eds DG Julian, AJ Camm, KM Fox *et al.*). London: Baillière Tindall, 1989: 146–213.

# 25
# Management of hypertension

The pursuit and treatment of the various forms of secondary hypertension are detailed in the relevant sections. The great majority of cases, however, will have essential (primary) hypertension, and it is with the management of these patients that we are concerned here.

## Indications for investigation and treatment: comparative urgency (Table 25.1)

### Malignant hypertension

Malignant ('accelerated') hypertension, with retinal haemorrhages and exudates, irrespective of the presence of papilloedema, requires admission forthwith to hospital for urgent treatment and subsequent investigation.

### Hypertensive encephalopathy

Hypertensive encephalopathy, in which confusion, clouding of consciousness or coma, with or without epileptiform convulsions, are present, is usually but not invariably, superimposed on malig-

nant hypertension. Hypertensive encephalopathy is an immediate medical emergency requiring most urgent therapy followed by transfer to hospital. It is very rare.

### Severe hypertension

Severe hypertension, with a fifth phase diastolic pressure above 120 mmHg, especially if accompanied by other features, such as cardiac or renal functional impairment, marked proteinuria, diabetes mellitus or arterial or organ damage attributable to the raised blood pressure, requires prompt and thorough investigation, and early initiation of antihypertensive therapy.

### Mild hypertension

Most subjects found on screening to have a raised blood pressure will, however, show more mild hypertension and will be free of symptoms. In many of these, the pressure will subside on subsequent visits, or may not be raised during 24-h recording. Thus, not all subjects identified as hypertensive on screening will require treatment.

**Table 25.1.** Hypertension: comparative urgency of treatment

| | |
|---|---|
| Hypertensive encephalopathy | An immediate emergency needing most urgent therapy followed by transfer to hospital |
| Malignant ('accelerated') phase | Admission to hospital forthwith for urgent treatment and subsequent investigation |
| Overt hypertensive heart failure | Admission to hospital forthwith for urgent treatment and subsequent investigation |
| Severe hypertension (diastolic > 120 mmHg) | Prompt and thorough investigation; early initiation of treatment |
| Mild hypertension | Proceed with less haste as indicated in Table 25.2 |

The most recent (1993) recommendations made by three groups, the British Hypertension Society,[1] the American Joint National Committee,[2] and the conjoint committee of the International Society of Hypertension and the World Health Organization,[3] for starting therapy in mild hypertension are set out in Table 25.2 for comparison. American physicians in general are more aggressive in initiating antihypertensive therapy than their British counterparts, starting usually at rather lower values of blood pressure. Despite some differences of emphasis, the broad therapeutic recommendations of all three are nevertheless largely unexceptionable. However, the scientific arguments supporting these reports contain, in all cases, occasional questionable statements, which have been commented upon elsewhere.[4] (See also Appendix 3.)

The reader is reminded that there is now clear evidence of benefit in treating hypertensive subjects over the age of 60[5-9] and indeed up to 80 years of age. The STOP trial even demonstrated benefit in those aged 70–84 at entry,[8] although it is questionable whether the octogenarians in this overall group profited. Predominantly systolic pressure elevation is a feature especially of ageing, and systolic pressure is a distinct risk indicator.[5,7]

Our present proposals for initiating treatment in mild hypertension follow fairly closely, albeit with some exceptions, those of the British Hypertension Society.[1]

Drug treatment should be begun irrespective of age if the fifth phase diastolic pressure remains at or above 110 mmHg on repeated measurements over 1–2 weeks.

Drugs should also be introduced in subjects whose diastolic pressure is in the range 100–109 mmHg on three or more occasions over days or weeks and who show either evidence of hypertensive organ damage or who have cardiovascular risk factors additional to hypertension, such as glucose intolerance, previous cigarette smoking, clear hypercholesterolaemia, male gender, or a family history suggestive of hypertension or its complications.

Despite this recommendation, it is recognized that therapy limits morbidity less effectively once complications have appeared, or in the presence of other risks (see page 300).

When the diastolic pressure is in the range 100–109 mmHg, but organ damage or other risk factors are not evident, the patient should be observed initially weekly, and thereafter monthly. If the

**Table 25.2.** Recommendations for dealing with mild hypertension

| WHO/ISH | US Joint National Committee V | British Hypertension Society |
|---|---|---|
| BP measured at least twice on two different occasions<br>If average values are 140–180 mmHg systolic and/or 90–95 mmHg diastolic; repeat measurements at least twice over 4 weeks<br>If below 140/90 mmHg follow 3 monthly for a year<br>If remains 140–180/90–105 mmHg, institute non-drug measures and follow for 3 months<br>If still 140–180/90–105 mmHg, consider starting drugs, especially if organ damage or additional risk factors present | Mild hypertension defined as 90–99 mmHg diastolic and/or 140–159 mmHg systolic<br>Non-drug measures recommended initially for 3–6 months<br>Drug therapy to be started if BP remains at or above 140–159/90–99 mmHg | If systolic 160–199 mmHg and/or diastolic 90–99 mmHg start non-drug treatment and observe with repeated BP measurement over 3–6 months<br>If systolic remains over 160 mmHg and/or diastolic over 100 mmHg start drugs<br>If diastolic remains at 90–99 mmHg start drugs if additional risk factors or organ damage present |

*Sources:* From Refs 1–3.

diastolic pressure falls, under such observation, below 100 mmHg, continued monitoring should be combined with non-pharmacological antihypertensive measures despite that, as mentioned, non-pharmacological interventions have not yet been shown to limit morbidity. However, if a diastolic pressure at or above 100 mmHg is sustained, drug treatment should be begun.

For those subjects whose diastolic pressures remain between 90 and 99 mmHg on repeated checking over 3–6 months, non-pharmacological measures are advised; again, drugs will more readily be added in the presence of organ damage or additional risk factors.

In subjects above the age of 60, treatment should be started as readily in women as in men; otherwise all of the above criteria apply.

Moreover, amongst elderly subjects so defined, those with 'isolated systolic' hypertension, in whom the systolic pressure is at least 160 mmHg, but the diastolic below 90 mmHg, should be treated with drugs, as also, by extrapolation, should the rarer younger persons with 'isolated systolic' hypertension.

──────── Objective of treatment ────────

The objective of treatment should be a diastolic pressure of 80–90 mmHg with a systolic of 120–140 mmHg in the absence of unacceptable side-effects.

──── Non-pharmacological measures ────

These have been considered in detail on pages 129–130. Briefly, patients should be advised to moderate their consumption of alcohol; dietary weight reduction should be undertaken if there is a tendency to obesity; and adequate physical exercise should be encouraged. Especially in patients older than around 45–50, restriction of sodium chloride intake to 70–100 mmol/day may help and, if tolerated, is worthy of trial; the small elevation of serum cholesterol consequent upon salt restriction is unlikely to be harmful, especially in the more elderly

subjects. Most importantly, because cigarette smoking compounds the risks of hypertension, all patients should stop smoking.

## Choice of drug therapy
## –(see also Chapter 22 and Appendix 1)–

### Comparative antihypertensive effect

Most trials of antihypertensive therapy undertaken in adequate numbers of patients have found that overall there is little to choose between one form of drug therapy and another in the ability to lower arterial pressure.

$\beta$-Antagonists, however, may be less effective in reducing systolic blood pressure than are alternative agents.[10] This probably relates to their slowing of the heart and little effect on arterial compliance. Nevertheless, atenolol was one of the drugs employed in a trial showing significant benefit in patients with isolated systolic hypertension.[7]

Suggestions that certain classes of drugs possess differential efficacy according to the age of the patient are not, at least so far, well-substantiated.[10] There is no good evidence presently available to support the claims that diuretics and calcium antagonists are more effective, and $\beta$-blockers and ACE inhibitors less so, in older patients. The response of an individual's blood pressure to any particular agent cannot readily be predicted from the age.

### Differential effects on morbidity

While the various antihypertensive drug classes have broadly similar ability to lower blood pressure, it is possible, and a source of much interest, that there could be important differential effects on morbidity. Nevertheless, the evidence, albeit sometimes suggestive, is not accepted by all critics. The large trials of treatment of hypertension have employed a wide range of antihypertensive agents (page 302), and especially $\beta$-blocking drugs, methyldopa, reserpine, hydralazine and thiazide diuretics. These older agents undoubtedly, when compared with placebo or with no therapy, lower cardiovascular morbidity. Newer drug classes, such as calcium antagonists and ACE inhibitors, have not been subjected to similar extended studies of their effect on morbidity, and, however attractive these drugs appear, this aspect remains uncertain. As discussed on page 303, this has led to some hesitancy in recommending their use.[1,2]

### Comparative benefits and demerits of thiazides and β-blockers

Two trials which compared the effects of β-blockers with those of thiazides showed significantly fewer sudden deaths with β-blockade.[11–14] A later analysis[15] of one of these, the British MRC trial, found that when both overt and latent coronary events were assessed, patients allocated to propranolol had significantly lower coronary morbidity than those given either bendrofluazide or placebo (page 105). The second MRC trial, in old subjects, which, as mentioned, might have been confounded,[6] found fewer morbid events with a thiazide/amiloride combination than with atenolol[5] (page 106).

### Side-effect burden of different antihypertensive drugs

Side-effects certainly separate the different groups of drugs and here it is possible for the clinician to select, or more usually to avoid, some agents in individual patients.

β-Antagonists must not be used in an asthmatic subject but they are an obvious choice in one with angina of effort. Tiredness and breathlessness seem less troublesome with the $\beta_1$-selective than with the non-selective β-blockers and are increasingly preferred. Earlier suggestions that ACE inhibitors might carry a lighter burden of side-effects than β-blockers have not been confirmed when newer β-blockers than propranolol were evaluated.[16–18] Nevertheless, those active in aerobic sports find β-blockers unacceptable. One trial indicated that captopril was better accepted than enalapril,[19] although this has not been seen by others.[16]

Thiazide diuretics should usually be avoided in patients with diabetes mellitus.

### Initiation of therapy in patients with mild-to-moderate hypertension

Here, we offer current, albeit perhaps conservative, advice. The recommendations given by the British Hypertension Society, the American Joint National Committee, and the conjoint WHO/ISH Committee, are given in Table 25.2 for comparison (see also Appendix 3).[1–3]

A small dose of a β-antagonist or diuretic is usually chosen as first-step therapy. Typical regimes would start with atenolol 50 mg or bendrofluazide 2.5 mg once daily. Most of the likely effect will be achieved by the end of 1 month, but blood pressure reduction can be more gradual with some agents such as serotonin antagonists. Thus, continuation of therapy for at least 3 months before increasing the dose is advisable unless there are special reasons for haste. The dose of atenolol can be raised to 100 mg or of bendrofluazide to 5 mg. If arterial pressure still remains inadequately controlled, one drug can be exchanged for the other, or indeed, an agent of another class substituted. There is increasing enthusiasm for this approach which may, it is felt, permit sometimes a more relevant correction of the pathophysiological derangements causing hypertension (see also page 20).

Despite persistent conservatism,[1,2] ACE inhibitors and calcium antagonists are gaining acceptance[3] as appropriate alternative first-step drugs (page 303).

### Frequent need for more than one class of drug

Despite the foregoing considerations, a majority of patients require two or more agents given together for adequate control of pressure. Suitable drug combinations have been discussed on page 127 (Table 22.2).

Most often, initially, a diuretic and β-blocker will be combined. There are several alternative two-drug combinations. β-Antagonists or ACE inhibitors are effective in blocking the tachycardia sometimes found, particularly with the initial pressure reduction, when giving a vasodilating drug like nifedipine. Patients with angina and hypertension might benefit from a $\beta$-antagonist/calcium antagonist combination; those with heart failure not related to the hypertension as such might respond to a diuretic with ACE inhibitor.

Any antihypertensive drug, but particularly those that act primarily as vasodilators, may in occasional patients cause unwanted precipitous falls in blood pressure. Such occurrences can be especially hazardous in older patients. Diuretics should be stopped for a few days before introducing an ACE inhibitor to the regime; however, adding a diuretic to an ACE inhibitor is not associated with a severe initial fall in pressure.

Currently, as discussed above, physicians are moving increasingly to extensive exploration of alternative one- or two-drug regimes rather than proceeding to a third agent in a 'stepped care' approach. If a third drug is required, a vasodilating agent is usually added to the $\beta$-blocker/diuretic combination; direct-acting vasodilators like hydralazine, $\alpha_1$-antagonists such as prazosin, or a class II calcium antagonist such as nifedipine are commonly used.

In two studies which addressed the issue directly, captopril, hydralazine or prazosin were found to be particularly suitable additions to a $\beta$-blocker/thiazide combination.[20,21]

## ———— The elderly patient ————

As discussed on page 102, antihypertensive drug therapy has been shown to be especially worthwhile in subjects over 60 years of age. Special problems may, however, also be encountered in elderly patients, and these issues will govern the choice of drug and its dose.[10,22,23] It should be re-emphasized that most claims for age-related differential efficacy and acceptability of different classes of antihypertensive drugs are not well-founded, and require re-evaluation.

Older patients tend to be lighter, and to have progressive impairment of renal and hepatic function. Thus, drug doses should usually be less with advancing years. Sexual interest and function tend to decline with age, and drugs that exacerbate this trend, for example, thiazides, centrally acting agents or $\beta$-blockers, should be employed cautiously. Postural hypotension may be a feature of ageing, and agents that worsen this, such as methyldopa or prazosin, should be used with care. First-dose hypotension with prazosin may be especially hazardous in the elderly. Rarely in old patients, and apparently irrespective of plasma renin level, first-dose hypotension may occur with ACE inhibitors. Diuretics, especially loop diuretics, can provoke urinary retention in older men with prostatic enlargement. By contrast, there is evidence that the use of diuretics can limit osteoporosis, and thus lessen the likelihood of hip fractures. Verapamil may cause or worsen constipation or cardiac conduction defects; it is regarded by some physicians as a drug unsuitable for the old patient. Agents such as methyldopa, clonidine or reserpine, which can cause depression or worsen mental confusion, should also be used with caution in the elderly.

Particularly in old patients, who may have atheromatous changes in the arteries supplying the brain, blood pressure reduction should be gradual, preferably over several weeks, rather than sudden. Ketanserin has been suggested as attractive in this respect.

Occult renal artery stenosis will also be more likely to be present in the elderly. The use of ACE inhibitors can, in these circumstances, lead to a loss or decline of function in the affected kidney by removing the compensatory intrarenal actions of angiotensin II.

Subjects over the age of 60 years comprise a large and rapidly expanding subgroup of the hypertensive population. Treatment requires careful attention to the needs of each individual. Indeed in the old patient especially, the choice of drug, and its deployment, needs particular personal care. Chronological age is an imperfect indicator of biological age; senility and decrepitude cannot be reliably predicted from the birthdate.

## Education of the patient and of relatives

It is most important that the patient, as well as all concerned with the patient's care, such as a responsible relative in the case of an elderly subject, understand fully the purpose of antihypertensive treatment, that it is preventive rather than therapeutic, and lifelong. A common misconception is that drug treatment may be stopped once the blood pressure has been controlled.

## Post-stroke hypertension

As described on pages 55 and 71, blood pressure may increase transiently after an acute stroke. This has been attributed to increased sympathetic discharge, and plasma noradrenaline can rise.[24] Cardiac rhythm can be disturbed. The appropriateness of drug treatment in this situation is unknown. Antihypertensive therapy is usually avoided and pressure allowed to settle. Should antihypertensive therapy be necessary, $\alpha$-adrenergic blockade has logic, but the potential risk of 'first dose' hypotension would for many preclude its use. Carefully monitored parenteral therapy might be considered to avoid lowering pressure too far (see page 151). $\beta$-Adrenergic blockade can be added to control arrhythmias, but should await the establishment of adequate $\alpha$-blockade.

The combined serotonergic type 2 (5-$HT_2$) and $\alpha_1$-antagonist ketanserin has been given intravenously in these circumstances with good blood pressure control and with intracranial pressure maintained steady.[25]

Treatment of post-stroke hypertension should always be cautious.[30]

## Resistant hypertension

Resistant hypertension can be defined arbitrarily as the persistence of a diastolic pressure $> 110$ mmHg despite the prescription of three drugs in com-

bination. Hypertension resistant to therapy may result from poor compliance with therapy, inadequate dosing, fluid retention induced by treatment, a pressor effect of concomitant therapy, undetected secondary hypertension or, rarely, from genuine drug refractoriness.[31]

### Poor compliance

Poor compliance with therapy is frequently found to underlie inability to control the blood pressure. Failure of the pulse rate to slow in a patient ostensibly taking a $\beta$-blocker should, for example, alert the physician. Asking for tablets to be brought to the clinic may help identify some problems. Older patients and alcoholics particularly can be forgetful and thus comply poorly.

Reversion to a simpler, rather than advance to a more complex, therapeutic regime often improves control. The less often patients need to take medication the better; compliance probably tends to diminish when dosing becomes more frequent than twice daily, although clear evidence on this point is elusive. Direct confrontation is sometimes useful; asking if the tablets are 'difficult to take for some reason' or enquiring about specific side-effects may help without endangering the doctor–patient relationship. Only occasional patients are frankly perverse (Plate 25.1). Informing patients of their blood pressure reading and reconfirming the need for therapy sometimes improves control. Overzealous pressure reduction may induce symptoms, and less than satisfactory pressure control may have to be accepted.

Systolic pressure elevation, especially in older patients, may be particularly difficult to control without inducing distressing side-effects; a reasonable aim then is to achieve the best pressure reduction possible without side-effects unacceptable to either patient or doctor.

### Concomitant treatment

Concurrent administration of non-steroidal anti-inflammatory drugs, such as indomethacin, or of oestrogen-containing compounds, can attenuate the effect of hypotensive agents, and is often over-looked (see also pages 158 and 163).

### Alcohol ingestion

Occult alcoholism should always be considered.

### Adequate dosage

It is not rare for a range of drugs to be prescribed together, but in inadequate doses. This should be checked.

### Need for diuretic

Several antihypertensive drugs (for example, nife-dipine, hydralazine or methyldopa) cause sodium and water retention, which then attenuates their effect. Adding, or raising the dose of diuretic can often then be effective.

### Undetected secondary hypertension

Patients resistant to therapy should always be investigated adequately to exclude an underlying cause of secondary hypertension. Thyroid defi-ciency is in this respect especially likely to be over-looked (Chapter 41).

### Treatment of resistant hypertension

Truly resistant essential hypertension can require aggressive therapy. A diuretic should always be included.

The powerful vasodilator minoxidil is particu-larly effective but always needs the conjoint use of a diuretic, and usually a loop-acting diuretic, to pre-vent fluid retention as well as of a drug, typically a $\beta$-blocker, to control tachycardia. Moreover, min-oxidil is not acceptable to a majority of women because of the hypertrichosis it causes.

Alternatively, large doses of loop diuretic com-bined with an ACE inhibitor will often achieve blood pressure control.

## Acute reduction of blood pressure: hypertensive emergencies: parenteral treatment

It is emphasized that the requirement for acute reduction of blood pressure is rare, and should be reserved for genuine hypertensive emergencies such as encephalopathy. Blood pressure should not be lowered acutely simply because it is very high. Moreover, the pressure should not be lowered sud-denly into the 'normal' range, which can take it below the lower limits of autoregulation of cerebral or ocular blood flow (Figure 13.4, page 64) and thus cause ischaemic damage.

Oral atenolol 50 or 100 mg can be rapidly effec-tive and will suffice in many circumstances.

Oral nifedipine, administered as a 5-mg capsule chewed or cut open and ingested is an alternative, although some authorities[26] have advised against its use in this context. Although this mode of dosing is sometimes termed 'sublingual' this is probably erroneous; nifedipine requires to be swal-lowed to be absorbed.[26,27]

### Parenteral antihypertensive treatment

In the rare situations where parenteral therapy is justified we advise sodium nitroprusside, hydralazine, trimetaphan or labetalol. Diazoxide by bolus injection intravenously is no longer recommended; the sudden uncontrolled fall in pressure can readily cause cerebral ischaemia, whilst accompanying tachycardia with increase in cardiac output can provoke myocardial ischaemia or infarction.[28] Parenteral clonidine is also unsuit-able because of an initial $\alpha$-adrenoceptor-mediated rise in pressure preceding the hypotensive effect, and since accompanying sedation hinders neuro-logical assessment.

Labetalol, given as intravenous infusion of 1–2 mg over 10 min, or as repeated intravenous bolus injections of 25 or 50 mg at 10-min intervals, can control crises of hypertension without increasing heart rate (Figure 25.1).[28,29,31]

Intravenous sodium nitroprusside by regulated infusion usually at 0.5–6.0 $\mu$g/kg per min offers an

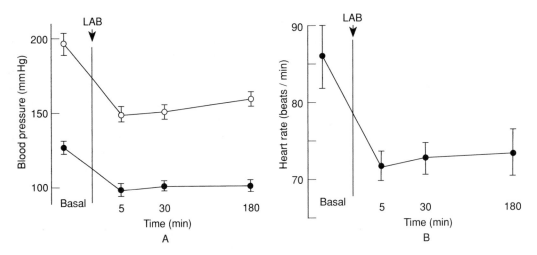

**Figure 25.1.** Effect of labetalol (LAB) intravenously in 20 severely hypertensive patients on (A) systolic and diastolic pressures and (B) heart rate. Mean $\pm$ SE. (Redrawn from Ref. 28, with permission.)

easily controlled way of reducing pressure, but it requires careful monitoring. Tachycardia can be a problem.

Rapid reduction of pressure can alternatively be achieved by intravenous or intramuscular hydralazine, given usually as boluses of 10 mg initially, doubling if necessary at 30-min intervals to a maximum dose of 80 mg.

Trimetaphan by regulated intravenous infusion, usually at 0.5–6.0 mg per min can control blood pressure accurately, with adjustable tilting of the patient providing further refinement if needed. Tachycardia can be troublesome.

Again, it is emphasized that urgent antihypertensive therapy, and especially parenteral therapy, is only rarely needed.

## Follow-up

Once adequate control is achieved with therapy, blood pressure reviews every 3 or 6 months are adequate for many patients. Such visits are useful to reinforce instructions, advice and encouragement, to ensure optimal pressure control and to check on renal function and possible alterations of plasma

potassium. Home blood pressure monitoring is appropriate for some patients, although it is important to avoid the development of an unrealistic and obsessional attitude to the treatment of blood pressure.

The ideal outcome is a subject free of symptoms, side-effects and anxiety, who has a systolic pressure below 140 and a diastolic pressure below 90 mmHg.

## Anaesthesia and surgery in the hypertensive patient

An issue frequently raised concerns the management of a patient with essential hypertension, already under drug therapy, who requires anaesthesia and surgery for some reason.

Almost invariably, it is best to continue therapy unchanged, ensuring that all persons involved with the patient's care are fully consulted throughout. Withdrawal of treatment before operation is more likely to create, rather than alleviate, problems. Although the risk is probably exaggerated, withdrawal of $\beta$-blockade can precipitate myocardial ischaemia; withdrawal of diuretic can predispose to fluid retention; withdrawal of clonidine can cause rebound hypertension, headache and tachycardia; and any pre-operative elevation of blood pressure is undesirable, not least because it may worsen bleeding tendencies at surgery.

Likewise, post-operatively, antihypertensive therapy should be reintroduced as promptly as is feasible, although careful continual supervision is necessary. $\beta$-Adrenergic blockade and, less markedly, ACE inhibition or the giving of centrally acting drugs can inhibit tachycardia and hence mask internal bleeding. Plasma potassium concentration needs to be carefully monitored when there is administration of drugs which cause either loss (thiazides; loop-acting diuretics) or retention (potassium-conserving diuretics; ACE inhibitors; $\beta$-blockers) of potassium.

Also noteworthy is that centrally acting drugs (reserpine; methyldopa; clonidine) can impair alertness and so interfere with clinical assessment.

Several secondary forms of hypertension should always be brought under control with specific drugs before the patient comes to surgery. Details are given in the respective chapters, but can be summarized briefly here.

Patients with renin-secreting tumours should be treated with adequate doses of an ACE inhibitor or an orally active angiotensin II antagonist (Chapter 30).

Cases of renovascular hypertension (Chapter 31) should be treated for 3–4 weeks with an ACE inhibitor before having either surgery or transluminal angioplasty. Some doctors argue contrariwise that such pre-operative therapy carries an undue risk of causing occlusion of the narrowed renal artery; however, our view is that operation is less risky with the blood pressure under control and electrolyte status corrected.

Patients with mineralocorticoid-producing tumours should be fully controlled with adequate doses of potassium-conserving diuretic before surgery (Chapters 35 and 36).

Patients with phaechromocytoma (Chapter 38) must, pre-operatively, have first the blood pressure controlled with $\alpha$-adrenergic blockers, and then a non-selective $\beta$-blocker introduced to prevent arrhythmia and hypokalaemia. During the operation, sodium nitroprusside must be available for intravenous use as necessary in the event of hypertensive crises.

## Case studies

See Case studies 1–4, 9–11, 13, 15 and 23, Appendix 2.

## References

1. Sever P, Beevers G, Bulpitt C *et al*. Management guidelines in essential hypertension: report of the second working party of the British Hypertension Society. *Br. Med. J.*. 1993; **306**: 983–7.

2. Fifth Report of the Joint National Committee on Detection, Evaluation, and Treatment of High Blood Pressure (JNCV). *Arch. Intern. Med.* 1993; **153**: 154–83.

3. Zanchetti A, Chalmers J, Arakawa K *et al*. 1993 Guidelines for the management of mild hypertension: memorandum from a WHO/ISH meeting. *J. Hypertens.* 1993; **11**: 905–18.

4. Robertson JIS. Guidelines for treating hypertension: a critical review. *Cardiovasc. Drugs Ther.* 1994; **8**: 91–8.

5. MRC Working Party. Medical Research Council trial of treatment of hypertension in older adults: principal results. *Br. Med. J.* 1992; **304**: 405–12.

6. Robertson JIS. The case for antihypertensive drug treatment in subjects over the age of 60. *Cardiovasc. Drugs Ther.* 1992; **6**: 579–83.

7. SHEP Cooperative Research Group. Prevention of stroke by antihypertensive drug treatment of older persons with isolated systolic hypertension. *J. Am. Med. Assoc.* 1991; **265**: 3255–64.

8. Dahlöf B, Lindholm L, Hansson L *et al*. Morbidity and mortality in the Swedish Trial in Old Patients with Hypertension (STOP-Hypertension). *Lancet* 1991; **338**: 1281–5.

9. Amery A, Birkenhäger W, Brixko P *et al*. Mortality and morbidity results from the European Working Party on High blood pressure in the Elderly trial. *Lancet* 1985; **i**: 1349–54.

10. Robertson JIS, Doyle AE, Vanhoutte P. (eds) Age-related effects of antihypertensive therapy: the Corsendonk Symposium. *J. Cardiovasc. Pharm.* 1988; **12** (suppl. 8).

11. Medical Research Council Working Party on Mild Hypertension. Coronary heart disease in the Medical Research Council trial of treatment of mild hypertension. *Br. Heart J.* 1988; **59**: 364–78.

12. Wikstrand J, Warnold I, Olsson G *et al.* Primary prevention with metoprolol in patients with hypertension: mortality results from the MAPHY study. *J. Am. Med. Assoc.* 1988; **259**: 1976–82.

13. Wikstrand J. Warnold I. Tuomilehto J *et al.* Metoprolol versus thiazide diuretics in hypertension: morbidity results from the MAPHY study. *Hypertension* 1991; **17**: 579–88.

14. Olsson G, Tuomilehto J, Berglund G *et al.* Primary prevention of sudden cardiovascular death in hypertensive patients: mortality results from the MAPHY study. *Am. J. Hypertens.* 1991. **4**: 151–6.

15. Green KG. British MRC trial of treatment for mild hypertension: a more favorable interpretation. *Am. J. Hypertens.* 1991; **4**: 723–4.

16. Steiner SS, Friedhoff AJ, Wilson BL *et al.* Antihypertensive therapy and quality of life: a comparison of atenolol, captopril, enalapril and propranolol. *J. Human Hypertens.* 1990; **4**: 217–25.

17. Herrick AL, Waller PC, Berkin KE *et al.* Comparison of enalapril and atenolol in mild to moderate hypertension. *Am. J. Med.* 1989; **86**: 421–6.

18. Palmer AJ, Fletcher AE, Rudge PJ *et al.* Quality of life in hypertensives treated with atenolol or captopril: a double-blind crossover trial. *J. Hypertens.* 1992; **10**: 1409–16.

19. Testa MA, Anderson RB, Nackley JF *et al.* Quality of life and antihypertensive therapy in men: a comparison of captopril with enalapril. *N. Engl. J. Med.* 1993; **328**: 907–13.

20. McAreavey D, Ramsay LE, Latham L *et al.* 'Third Drug' trial: comparative study of antihypertensive agents added when blood pressure remains uncontrolled by a beta blocker plus thiazide diuretic. *Br. Med. J.* 1984; **288**: 106–11.

21. Bevan EG, Pringle SD, Waller PC *et al.* Comparison of captopril, hydralazine and nifedipine as third drug in hypertensive patients. *J. Human Hypertens.* 1993; **7**: 83–8.

22. Robertson JIS. Hypertension and its treatment in the elderly. *Clin. Exp. Hypertens.* 1989; A11: 779–805.

23. Tuck M, Golub M. The older hypertensive patient. In *Handbook of Hypertension*, Vol. 15: *Clinical Hypertension* (ed. JIS Robertson). Amsterdam: Elsevier, 1992: 747–77.

24. Myers MG, Norris JW, Hachinski VC. *et al.* Cardiac sequelae of acute stroke. *Stroke* 1982; **13**: 838–42.

25. Kay R, Poon WS, Nicholls MG. Effect of intravenous ketanserin on arterial and intracranial pressures in patients with systemic hypertension following intracerebral haemorrhage. *J. Human Hypertens.* 1993; **7**: 369–71.

26. Spence JD, Arnold JMO, Gilbert JJ. Vascular consequences of hypertension and effects of antihypertensive therapy. In *Handbook of Hypertension*, Vol. 15: *Clinical Hypertension* (ed. JIS Robertson). Amsterdam: Elsevier, 1992: 621–54.

27. Van Harten J, Burggraaf K, Danhof M *et al.* Negligible sublingual absorption of nifedipine. *Lancet* 1987; **ii**: 1363–5.

28. Trust PM, Rosei EA, Brown JJ *et al.* Effect on blood pressure, angiotensin II and aldosterone concentrations during treatment of severe hypertension with intravenous labetalol: comparison with propranolol. *Br. J. Clin. Pharmacol.* 1976; **3** (suppl. 3): 799–803.

29. Cumming AMM, Brown JJ, Lever AF *et al.* Treatment of severe hypertension by repeated bolus injections of labetalol. *Br. J. Clin. Pharmacol* 1979; **8** (suppl. 2): 199–204.

30. Phillips SJ. Pathophysiology and management of hypertension in acute ischemic stroke. *Hypertension* 1994; **23**: 131–6.

31. Mackay A, Isles C, Atkinson AB *et al.* The treatment of resistant hypertension. In *Advanced Medicine*, Vol. 17 (ed. DP Jewell). London: Pitman Medical, 1981: 39–58.

# Section 4
## Secondary forms of hypertension

α

# 26
# Secondary forms of hypertension: Prevalence, variety, nature

Secondary hypertension comprises a variety of disparate conditions, which are uncommon in comparison with primary or essential hypertension. In unselected populations of hypertensive patients, probably no more than 1–5% of cases are secondary,[1] although a much higher proportion of a particular disease may be seen in a specialized centre. Even so, it is in our view appropriate to consider secondary forms of hypertension in some detail, for a variety of reasons.

First, physicians need to be acquainted with syndromes of secondary hypertension, and to have access to guidance on their investigation and treatment. Many forms of secondary hypertension are readily responsive to medical or surgical therapy, whereas mistaken or missed diagnosis can be disastrous.

Second, while some syndromes of secondary hypertension are rare, others, notably that induced by oestrogen–progestogen oral contraceptives, are not uncommon. Moreover, raised blood pressure following ingestion of a wide range of different drugs is becoming increasingly prevalent. Hypertension induced by pregnancy is a special case, dealt with in detail in Chapter 47.

Third, a study of the mechanisms whereby arterial pressure is elevated in these conditions of known pathogenesis is likely to have wider relevance, and to facilitate insight into primary (essential) hypertension and its causation.

Two most interesting aspects of secondary hypertension, first noted by Pickering,[2] are that virtually every form of secondary hypertension can enter the malignant phase, and that the hypertension may persist in a substantial proportion of cases even after the primary cause has been removed or corrected (pregnancy-induced hypertension is an exception to this rule). Persistent hypertension is probably due in part to hypertension-induced changes, including structural thickening in the wall of resistance vessels (Chapter 13), and especially alterations in the arteries of the kidney (Chapter 16). Renal functional impairment in any form of secondary hypertension usually presages a less satisfactory fall in blood pressure after correction of the causal abnormality.

The main forms of secondary hypertension are listed in Table 1.1 on page 5.

## References

1. Gross FH, Robertson JIS (eds). *Arterial Hypertension*. London: Pitman Medical, 1979.
2. Pickering GW. *High Blood Pressure*, 2nd edn. London: Churchill, 1968.

# 27
# Drug-induced hypertension

## Hormonal contraceptives

The most numerous of the drug-induced forms of hypertension and almost certainly the commonest of all the secondary hypertensive syndromes is that caused by hormonal contraceptives.[1]

### Compounds used

Two kinds of oestrogen are generally employed in combined oestrogen–progestogen oral contraceptives,[1] ethinyloestradiol or its 3-methyl ether, mestranol. The progestogens used are various derivatives either of 19-nortestosterone (norethynodrel, norethisterone, ethynodiol diacetate, lynestrol or norgestrel) or of 17-hydroxyprogesterone (megestrol acetate, medroxyprogesterone acetate or chlormadinone acetate). The derivatives of nortestosterone may partly be metabolized to oestrogenic substances.

Early oral contraceptive preparations contained 100 $\mu$g of oestrogen and from 1 to 4 mg of progestogen. Subsequently, and progressively, the dose of oestrogen has been reduced to 50, 35, 30 and 25 $\mu$g; in some preparations, the dose of progestogen also has been lowered, for example, to 150 $\mu$g of norgestrel.

A triphasic low-dose combination tablet containing ethinyloestradiol and laevonorgestrel has been formulated, containing of each, respectively, 30 $\mu$g and 50 $\mu$g for the first 6 days of the menstrual cycle, rising to 40 $\mu$g and 75 $\mu$g for the next 10 days. Progestogen-only preparations are less reliable contraceptives. Examples in use are ethynodiol diacetate 500 $\mu$g, laevonorgestrel 30 $\mu$g, norgestrel 75 $\mu$g and norethisterone 350 $\mu$g.

### Blood pressure changes

The balance of current opinion indicates that the magnitude of any blood pressure increase is in proportion to the dose of oestrogen. There is no good evidence that progestogen-only preparations can influence blood pressure.

Virtually all women who take the combined oestrogen–progestogen pill show a rise in arterial pressure (Figure 27.1). This is usually mild, although it has been estimated that some 5% of pill-takers show blood pressure levels exceeding 140/90 mmHg, which could represent a considerable increase in young women. In one early prospective study (Figure 27.1), average increases of 12 mmHg systolic and 8 mmHg diastolic at 5 years were shown. A few susceptible individuals show a more marked rise in pressure and the malignant phase of hypertension is a well-recorded, albeit rare, complication with oral contraceptives containing 50 or 30 $\mu$g of oestrogen.

Blood pressure usually rises steadily for the first 6 months, then settles to a plateau which is maintained while therapy continues. On stopping the pill, pressures usually, but not always (see below), subside to control values within 3–6 months.

### Predisposing factors

It has been suggested that women with a genetic or environmental predisposition to essential hypertension are more at risk of a severe rise in blood pressure on the pill, although this is not well-substantiated. Women with pre-existing hypertension do not seem to be more susceptible.[2] Black American women have been reported to be less prone to develop hypertension with oral contra-

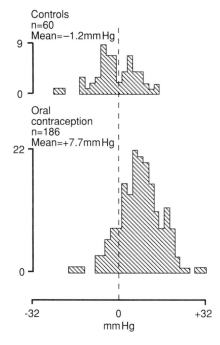

**Figure 27.1.** Changes in systolic blood pressure after 2 years in 186 women aged 21–30 years taking oestrogen–progestogen oral contraceptives, and in 60 matched controls. (Redrawn from Ref. 1, with permission.)

ceptive use. Black women in the UK appear at least as susceptible as others. There is no good evidence of a correlation with pregnancy-induced hypertension, social class or cigarette smoking.

### Complications

Progress into the malignant phase carries the attendant serious consequences of this complication whatever the underlying cause. The risks of the commoner more mild elevations of arterial pressure are less certain, but cannot be regarded with complacency, especially when accompanied by the other sequelae of oral contraception, which include distortion of the plasma lipid pattern, impairment of glucose tolerance, and changes in the blood coagulation system.

There has hence been much concern about the possible long-term vascular consequences of oral contraceptive therapy. There is evidence that cardiovascular mortality is increased fivefold in young women taking oestrogen–progestogen oral contraceptives, and tenfold in those so treated for 5 or more years. Smoking compounds these risks.

Although data are scanty, it is likely that in some women, elevation of blood pressure, at least to an extent, may persist after stopping the pill. If so, this brings pill-induced hypertension into conformity with the general rule that, in secondary hypertension, the blood pressure of many patients fails to return to the levels of age- and sex-matched normal subjects even after the initial cause of the hypertension has been corrected.

### Mechanism of blood pressure rise

Oestrogens cause a rise in the level of plasma renin-substrate (angiotensinogen) concentration. As there is no consistent compensatory fall in the plasma concentration of the active enzyme renin, plasma levels of angiotensin II, a powerful vasoconstrictor, rise. This has been shown to occur in the absence of changes in total body sodium and must therefore in some cases contribute to blood pressure elevation (Table 27.1).[3] However, it is not known how important this mechanism is in the majority of instances.

Although plasma aldosterone would be expected to rise in association with any increase in plasma angiotensin II, and such changes have been reported, there is no good evidence of sodium or water retention that can consistently explain the blood pressure increase, or of expanded extracellular fluid or plasma volume. The changes in pressure do not usually correlate with changes in body weight.

Other suggested pressor mechanisms, not as yet fully explored, are increased sympathetic nerve activity, changes in circulating noradrenaline, and alterations in the proportions or quantities of prostaglandins.

Rarely, oral contraceptives cause intrarenal arteritis (page 180).

**Table 27.1.** Comparison of data in 6 women with oral contraceptive-induced hypertension and those of 6 women with untreated essential hypertension (means shown; * $P < 0.02$)

|  | Oral contraceptive users | Essential hypertensives |
|---|---|---|
| Age (years) | 36.3 | 38.2 |
| BP (mmHg) | 178/101 | 187/108 |
| Angiotensinogen ($\mu$mol/litre) | 1.38 | 0.55* |
| Active renin ($\mu$u/ml) | 27.0 | 27.0 |
| Angiotensin II (pmol/litre) | 38.0 | 20.0* |
| Aldosterone (pmol/litre) | 378.3 | 373.3 |
| Total body Na (% normal) | 100.1 | 94.5 |
| Total body K (% normal) | 97.7 | 104.6 |

*Source:* From Ref. 3.

### Management

All women undertaking oestrogen–progestogen oral contraceptive therapy should have their blood pressure measured before commencing therapy, and at intervals no greater than every 3 months while receiving treatment.

In the event of marked blood pressure elevation, therapy should be changed to a progestogen-only pill, or to an alternative form of contraception. Blood pressure should be monitored carefully to confirm a fall to normal limits; if this has not occurred within 6 months of discontinuation, a search should be made for an additional or alternative form of secondary hypertension. If blood pressure remains high 6 months after stopping the pill and in the absence of evidence of secondary hypertension, the patient should receive drug treatment as for essential hypertension.

A woman who develops malignant hypertension while receiving an oral contraceptive should have this stopped forthwith and should be treated urgently with antihypertensive drugs. After blood pressure has been adequately controlled for 6 months, treatment should be carefully withdrawn and the blood pressure monitored. In the event of sustained blood pressure elevation, long-term antihypertensive treatment will be necessary.

It is not appropriate for a woman to continue to take an oestrogen–progestogen oral contraceptive while remaining hypertensive and thus to require concomitant antihypertensive therapy.

## Post-menopausal oestrogen replacement therapy

### Inadequacy of data

This is a remarkably neglected and poorly studied field, a defect particularly obtrusive given the potential importance of any pressor effects of post-menopausal oestrogen administration. Requiring emphasis is that in contrast to oral contraceptive use, post-menopausal doses of oestrogen are not supraphysiological.[4] The benefits of such long-term post-menopausal oestrogen therapy include diminution of oesteoporosis, whilst amongst the risks are possible enhanced incidences of endometrial cancer and breast cancer,[5] and drug dependence or addiction.[6]

The cardiovascular effects of post-menopausal oestrogens are complex and partly controversial.[34] Data from Framingham indicated that such treatment was accompanied by an increased risk of cardiovascular morbidity.[7] Myocardial infarction was more frequent in post-menopausal oestrogen users who smoked, and stroke in those who did not. Both occurred less often in women who did not take post-menopausal oestrogen.[7] Several other studies have by contrast reported a diminution in the prevalence or prominence of coronary artery disease with post-menopausal oestrogen therapy.[8-13] McDonald and Stewart found, however, that tamoxifen, a non-steroidal anti-oestrogen, given for at least 5 years as adjuvant therapy for breast cancer, significantly reduced the risk of fatal myocardial infarction.[14] The disputed coronary artery benefit has been attributed to oestrogen-induced increases in serum high density lipoprotein cholesterol (HDL) concentrations.[8] Little or no reduction in stroke was observed in these various studies.

In a case-control study of 210 patients with stroke, in the age-group 70–79, in which the largest numbers of strokes occurred, there was an association between stroke risk and oestrogen use.[15] Most of the excess risk seemed to operate through a link between oestrogen use and hypertension.

Despite its obvious relevance, the influence of any oestrogen-induced changes in arterial pressure on the observed patterns of cardiovascular disease has, however, been largely neglected. Several of the papers quoted above deal with large, and necessarily crude, epidemiological surveys, in which blood pressure measurements are either absent or inadequate. For example, although Bush *et al.*[8] report little difference in either systolic or diastolic pressures between users and non-users of oestrogens, their study is severely compromised by lack of information on the type, dose and duration of administration of oestrogen. Oestrogen users and non-users are consistently disparate in various relevant respects, those women taking oestrogen usually being better educated, thinner and smoking less.

As discussed above (page 158), the oestrogenic component of oral contraceptives is responsible for their blood pressure elevating effect.[1] That post-menopausal oestrogen use could be pressor, at least in some women, is plausible, even though the dose is lower, and ostensibly more physiological, than with oral contraceptives.[4] Subjects who become

addicted could well take excessive quantities.[6] In one prospective study, Wren and Routledge[16] reported that post-menopausal women given conjugated oestrogen had a higher rate of rise in blood pressure than others who received piperazine oestrone sulphate together with laevonorgestrel. Occasional patients have been observed to have a distinct rise of blood pressure with post-menopausal oestrogen administration;[1,16,17] this has also been asserted, *ex cathedra*, by the US Joint National Committee.[18] Other workers[19] have stated, by contrast, that they have seen patients whose blood pressure fell in these circumstances.

There is an increasing fashion, most marked in the USA, tending to the broadscale and prolonged use of post-menopausal oestrogens.[5-10,19,20,34] Some other parts of the world remain more cautious.[4,12] There is an obvious and urgent need for properly controlled critical studies of the effects of such treatment on blood pressure. There may be no rise in pressure; or there may, as with oral contraceptives containing oestrogen, be a general, usually modest, rise; or occasional women may be susceptible to a marked pressure increase. Reliable data from focused studies are urgently necessary.

### Management

For the present, as with oral contraceptives, all women being considered for post-menopausal oestrogen treatment should have their blood pressure measured before, and no less often than three times yearly during such therapy.[1,18,21] However, control of blood pressure in post-menopausal women receiving oestrogens and already on antihypertensive drugs does not seem to cause major problems.[35]

## Adrenocorticotrophic hormone (ACTH)

The rare abnormalities of corticosteroid biosynthesis (Chapter 36) demonstrate the ability of increased endogenous adrenocorticotrophic hormone (ACTH) to raise arterial pressure. In those diseases, excessive quantities of endogenous ACTH-dependent mineralocorticoids appear to be principally responsible for the hypertension.

The pressor effect of exogenous ACTH has also been confirmed and extensively studied in experimental animals, notably the sheep.[22] Administration of ACTH to humans likewise raises arterial pressure,[23] an effect dependent on an intact adrenal cortex, because it does not occur in patients with Addison's disease. This potential hazard of long-term therapeutic administration of ACTH should always be borne in mind, and regular checks of arterial pressure made. Cardiovascular morbidity is prominent with iatrogenic Cushing's syndrome.[33]

The development of hypertension in Cushing's syndrome (Chapter 37) similarly suggests the ability also of glucocorticosteroids, such as cortisol, to induce hypertension in humans. This has been demonstrated experimentally, and the similarity in volunteers of the responses to cortisol and ACTH suggests that cortisol could be at least partly responsible for the pressor effects of administered ACTH.[33]

## ———————— Glucocorticoids ————————

As mentioned above, the administration of exogenous glucocorticoids to volunteers can raise arterial pressure.[23] However, several surveys[24,25] have indicated that chronic glucocorticoid therapy in humans has little effect on blood pressure, at least if the daily dose is less than 20 mg of prednisone or its equivalent. By contrast, Whitworth has stated[26] that 20% of patients showing other features of iatrogenic Cushing's syndrome also had hypertension.

It appears prudent, therefore, to monitor blood pressure regularly in all patients on glucocorticoid treatment.

## ———————— Mineralocorticoids ————————

Less controversial is that administration of steroids with a predominant mineralocorticoid action, for example fludrocortisone or fluroprednisolone, can induce hypertension.[25,27] This syndrome has the typical features of mineralocorticoid excess (page 196), as described in detail for aldosterone-secreting adenoma (Chapter 35), except that with exogenous mineralocorticoid administration, aldosterone secretion and plasma aldosterone concentrations are low. Hypokalaemia is prominent.

It is noteworthy that when mineralocorticoids are given as therapy for postural hypotension, hypertension may appear only with the patient recumbent.

Hypertension due to therapeutic administration of mineralocorticoids can sometimes be severe, and malignant phase retinopathy has been reported.

## ———————— Anabolic Steroids ————————

It appears likely, albeit as yet poorly documented, that the administration of excessive amounts of anabolic steroids, often indulged secretly in an attempt to boost athletic performance, can raise blood pressure.[27]

## ———————— Liquorice and carbenoxolone ————————

### Causative compounds

Extracts of liquorice, a substance prepared from the root of the plant *Glycyrrhiza glabra*, contain glycyrrhetinic acid, a compound with mineralocorticoid activity. Carbenoxolone, the semi-synthetic hemisuccinate derivative of glycyrrhetinic acid, is a drug employed to speed the healing of peptic ulcers. It is used little in the U.K.

People who ingest large quantities of liquorice-containing sweets or beverages, and susceptible individuals taking carbenoxolone or liquorice, may develop typical mineralocorticoid hypertension.[27] Some patients may be especially sensitive to the biochemical changes and to the blood pressure increases. More generally, it has been found that 300 mg/day of carbenoxolone regularly induces metabolic and blood pressure changes, whereas 20 mg/day does not.

### Mechanism of pressor effect

The pathogenesis is closely akin to that of congenital deficiency of the enzyme 11-$\beta$-hydroxysteroid dehydrogenase (11-$\beta$-OHSD) (page 204).

11-$\beta$-OHSD is responsible for converting the active steroid cortisol to inactive cortisone. This enzyme is inhibited by liquorice or carbenoxolone. With the consequent deficiency of 11-$\beta$-OHSD, therefore, the renal mineralocorticoid receptor becomes similarly responsive *in vivo* to cortisol as to the usual major physiological mineralocorticoid, aldosterone. Mineralocorticoid hypertension then ensues.

### Clinical and biochemical features

The pattern and biochemical accompaniments of this condition thus closely resemble those of an aldosterone-secreting tumour, except that aldosterone secretion and plasma aldosterone concentration are low. The raised blood pressure is characteristically associated with hypernatraemia, hypokalaemia, increased body sodium and diminished body potassium content, and depression of plasma renin, angiotensin II and aldosterone. The hypokalaemia may be accompanied by muscular weakness, paraesthesiae, polyuria, cardiac arrhythmias and, occasionally, red urine because of the presence of myoglobin.

### Diagnosis and management

Any patient with hypertension, especially if this is associated with hypokalaemia, should be questioned concerning possible ingestion of liquorice or carbenoxolone. If these substances are being taken, they should be discontinued and the patient re-assessed initially after 3–4 weeks. It may sometimes, however, take 6–8 weeks before the biochemical abnormalities and the blood pressure are fully corrected. Even if blood pressure does not return to normal values, its control with antihypertensive drugs should be facilitated.

## Non-steroidal anti-inflammatory drugs

These agents can both induce hypertension and interfere with antihypertensive therapy.[27]

Whilst most information has been obtained with indomethacin, similar, but more limited data are available also on aspirin, diclofenac, ibuprofen, flurbiprofen, naproxen, piroxicam, sulphinpyrazone and sulindac. Possibly aspirin and sulindac are less prone than the other agents to cause these unwanted effects. Although the pressor effect of the non-steroidal anti-inflammatory drugs is usually modest, occasionally severe, life-threatening blood pressure elevation can be caused. Moreover, because many elderly subjects are prescribed non-steroidal anti-inflammatory drugs, and there is increasing use of antihypertensive therapy in this age-group, the problem is of considerable prevalence.

### Mechanism of pressor effect

The mechanism of the pressor effect is uncertain. All possibilities considered relate to a reduction in prostaglandin synthesis; those most favoured include sodium retention, facilitation of sympathetic nervous activity, and enhancement of the effect of vasoconstrictor substances such as angiotensin II.

Furthermore, non-steroidal anti-inflammatory drugs can cause various renal problems, including acute renal failure, worsening of renal impairment in the presence of intrinsic renal diseases, papillary necrosis, nephrotic syndrome and interstitial nephritis.

### Management

It follows that non-steroidal anti-inflammatory drugs should be introduced with reluctance, and then cautiously, in patients with hypertension. Their capacity for causing drug-resistant hypertension must always be borne in mind. The use of these agents in any patient with hypertension or renal disease should invariably be accompanied by especially close monitoring of blood pressure, renal function and urine composition.

## Sympathomimetic agents and monoamine oxidase inhibitors

Occasional examples have been reported of patients developing hypertensive crises following the ingestion of a large dose of a sympathomimetic agent such as phenylpropanolamine, methylphenidate or dextroamphetamine.[27]

Concurrent administration of monoamine oxidase inhibitors, as for the treatment of mental illness, can greatly enhance the risk. Monoamine oxidase inhibitors interfere with the breakdown of endogenous catecholamines such as adrenaline and noradrenaline, as well as of administered amines. The risks are not confined to concurrent abuse of drugs. A number of foods contain large quantities of tyramine, which can accumulate when monoamine oxidase inhibitors are also taken. Thus, patients on these latter drugs should be warned of the dangers of eating ripe cheese, meat extracts, broad beans, ripe grapes and chocolate.

## Erythropoietin

Erythropoietin is a naturally occurring peptide hormone of 166 amino-acid residues. It is available for the treatment of certain anaemias, especially that accompanying chronic renal failure.

Intravenous erythropoietin treatment has, in a regular but uncertain proportion of patients, been followed by the development of hypertension.[27] In some cases hypertension has been severe and complicated by hypertensive encephalopathy.

This property of erythropoietin has, conversely, been exploited in treating postural hypotension.[28]

The pressor mechanism is uncertain, but does not seem to be a result of a direct pressor effect of erythropoietin itself. Favoured is an erythropoietin-induced increase in haematocrit, with a consequent rise in blood viscosity. Additional possibilities are potentiation of other pressor systems or inhibition of vasodilator mechanisms by erythropoietin.

## Cyclosporin

Cyclosporin is an immunosuppressant agent of fungal origin, widely used in the management of patients following renal, hepatic, cardiac or bone marrow transplantation. Cyclosporin can induce or worsen hypertension, although the frequency of the problem is uncertain; it appears to be proportional to the dose and duration of treatment.[27]

Possible pressor mechanisms include renal damage, with resultant sodium and fluid retention, inhibition of endothelial nitric oxide release, sympathetic activation, and renal and/or peripheral arteriolar constriction.[32,36]

## Vasopressin

As mentioned on page 45, physiological variations in circulating vasopressin are below its pressor threshold; moreover, chronic excess of vasopressin, as for example with a vasopressin-secreting bronchial carcinoma, is not usually accompanied by hypertension (see Figure 9.6, page 46).[29] In some extreme situations, however, as in hypotensive haemorrhage, a direct pressor effect of markedly elevated plasma vasopressin may have a crucial acute defensive role.

The therapeutic intra-arterial administration of vasopressin, which has been employed with gastrointestinal haemorrhage, notably when due to portal hypertension and bleeding oesophageal varices, can however sometimes cause hypertension.[27]

## Oxytocin

The combination of oxytocin with another vasoconstrictor, for example a sympathomimetic agent, or ergot, can cause severe hypertension.

## Methylmethacrylate

The use of methylmethacrylate, acrylic bone cement, in orthopaedic surgery has been observed to be occasionally accompanied by an acute rise in blood pressure and plasma cortisol.[27]

## Mitomycin

Mitomycin, used in the treatment of malignancies, has been found to cause microangiopathic haemolytic anaemia, with blood pressure elevation in up to a quarter of patients.[27]

## Cocaine

Cocaine both increases the release, and inhibits neuronal re-uptake, of noradrenaline; thus it can cause hypertension, palpitations and headache, usually within 1 h of its administration. Coronary artery constriction can be added.[30] Stroke or myocardial ischaemia may ensue.[31]

Treatment is based on α-adrenergic blockade, as for phaeochromocytoma (page 218). A non-selective β-blocker can usefully be added later to control arrhythmias; it is crucial to ensure adequate α-blockade first, however.

## Case studies

See Case studies 7 and 14, Appendix 2.

## References

1. Weir RJ, Weinberger MH. Oral contraceptives, hypertension, and cardiovascular disease. In *Handbook of Hypertension*, Vol. 15: *Clinical Hypertension* (ed. JIS Robertson). Amsterdam: Elsevier, 1992: 177–94.

2. Spellacy WN, Birk SA. The effects of mechanical and steroid contraceptive methods on blood pressure in hypertensive women. *Fertil. Steril.* 1974; **25**: 467.

3. McAreavey D, Cumming AMM, Boddy K *et al*. The renin–angiotensin system and total body sodium and potassium in hypertensive women taking oestrogen–progestogen oral contraceptives. *Clin. End.* 1983; **18**: 111–18.

4. Isles CG. Prevention of coronary disease in women. *Scott. Med. J.* 1993; **38**: 103–6.

5. Goldman L, Tosteson ANA. Uncertainty about postmenopausal estrogen. *N. Engl. J. Med.* 1991; **325**: 800–2.

6. Bewley S, Bewley TH. Drug dependence with oestrogen replacement therapy. *Lancet* 1992; **339**: 290–1.

7. Wilson PWF, Garrison RJ, Castelli WP. Postmenopausal estrogen use, cigarette smoking, and cardiovascular morbidity in women over 50. *N. Engl. J. Med.* 1985; **313**: 1038–43.

8. Bush TL, Barrett-Connor E, Cowan LD *et al*. Cardiovascular mortality and non-contraceptive use of estrogen in women: results from the Lipid Research Clinics Program follow-up study. *Circulation* 1987; **75**: 1102–9.

9. Henderson BE, Ross RK, Paganini-Hill A *et al*. Estrogen use and cardiovascular disease. *Am. J. Obstet. Gynecol.* 1986; **154**: 1181–6.

10. Stampfer MJ, Colditz GA, Willett WC *et al*. Postmenopausal estrogen therapy and cardiovascular disease: ten-year follow-up from the Nurses' Health study. *N. Engl. J. Med.* 1991; **325**: 756–62.

11. Sullivan JM, Van der Zwaag R, Hughes JP *et al*. Estrogen replacement and coronary disease: effect on survival in postmenopausal woman. *Arch. Intern. Med.* 1990; **150**: 2557–62.

12. Beaglehole R. Oestrogens and cardiovascular disease. *Br. Med. J.* 1988; **297**: 571–2.

13. Rosano GMC, Sarrel PM, Poole-Wilson PA *et al*. Beneficial effect of oestrogen on exercise-induced myocardial ischaemia in women with coronary artery disease. *Lancet* 1993; **342**: 133–6.

14. McDonald CC, Stewart HJ. Fatal myocardial infarction in the Scottish adjuvant tamoxifen trial. *Br. Med. J.* 1991; **303**: 435–7.

15. Pfeffer RI, van den Noort S. Estrogen use and stroke risk in postmenopausal women. *Am. J. Epidemiol.* 1976; **103**: 445–56.

16. Wren BG, Routledge DA. Blood pressure changes: oestrogens in climacteric women. *Med. J. Aust.* 1981; **2**: 528–31.

17. Robertson JIS. Hypertension in the female. In *The Circulation in the Female: From the Cradle to the Grave* (ed. J Ginsburg). New Jersey: Parthenon, 1989: 51–9.

18. Fifth Report of the Joint National Committee on Detection, Evaluation, and Treatment of High Blood Pressure (JNCV). *Arch. Intern. Med.* 1993; **153**: 154–83.

19. Sarrell P. The effects of ovarian steroids on the cardiovascular system. In *The Circulation in the Female: From the Cradle to the Grave* (ed. J Ginsburg). New Jersey: Parthenon, 1989: 117–40.

20. Editorial: More than hot flushes. *Lancet* 1991; **338**: 917–18.

21. Zanchetti A, Chalmers J, Arakawa K *et al.* 1993 Guidelines for the management of mild hypertension: memorandum from a WHO/ISH meeting. *J. Hypertens.* 1993; **11**: 905–18.

22. Humphrey TJ, Fan JSK, Coghlan JP *et al.* Inter-relationships between sodium and potassium intake and the effects of ACTH in the sheep. *J. Hypertens.* 1983; **1**: 19–29.

23. Connell JMC, Whitworth JA, Davies DL *et al.* Effects of ACTH and cortisol administration on blood pressure, electrolyte metabolism, atrial natriuretic peptide, and renal function in normal man. *J. Hypertens.* 1987; **5**: 425–33.

24. David DS, Grieco MH, Cushman P. Adrenal glucocorticoids after twenty years: a review of their clinically relevant consequences. *J. Chron. Dis.* 1970; **22**: 637–44.

25. Jackson SMD, Beevers DG, Myers K. Does long-term low-dose corticosteroid therapy cause hypertension? *Clin. Sci.* 1981; **61** (suppl.): 381–3.

26. Whitworth JA. Mechanisms of glucocorticoid-induced hypertension. *Kidney Int.* 1987; **31**: 1213–24.

27. Nicholls MG, Richards AM, Lai KN. Drug-induced hypertension. In *Handbook of Hypertension*, Vol. 15: *Clinical Hypertension* (ed. JIS Robertson). Amsterdam: Elsevier, 1992: 195–235.

28. Hoeldtke RD, Streeten DP. Treatment of orthostatic hypotension with erythropoietin. *N. Engl. J. Med.* 1993; **329**: 611–15.

29. Padfield PL, Brown JJ, Lever AF. *et al.* Blood pressure in acute and chronic vasopressin excess: studies of malignant hypertension and the syndrome of inappropriate antidiuretic hormone secretion. *N. Engl. J. Med.* 1981; **304**: 1067–70.

30. Gawin FH, Ellinwood EH. Cocaine and other stimulants: actions, abuse, and treatment. *N. Engl. J. Med.* 1988; **318**: 1173–82.

31. Levine SR, Brust JCM, Futrell N *et al.* Cerebrovascular complications of the use of the 'crack' form of alkaloidal cocaine. *N. Engl. J. Med.* 1990; **323**: 699–704.

32. Sturrock NDC, Struthers AD. Hormonal and other mechanisms involved in the pathogenesis of cyclosporin-induced nephrotoxicity and hypertension in man. *Clin. Sci.* 1994; **86**: 1–9.

33. Whitworth JA. Studies in the mechanisms of glucocorticoid hypertension in humans. *Blood Pressure* 1994; **3**: 24–32.

34. Belchetz PE. Hormonal treatment of postmenopausal women. *N. Engl. J. Med.* 1994; **330**: 1062–71.

35. Lip G, Beevers M, Holmes A *et al.* Hormone replacement therapy and blood pressure in hypertensive women. Medical Research Society, Autumn meeting, Nov. 1993, Abstract 74.

36. Lyson T, McMullan TM, Ermel DL *et al.* Mechanism of cyclosporine-induced sympathetic activation and acute hypertension in rats. *Hypertension* 1994; **23**: 667–75.

# 28
# Coarctation of the aorta

Coarctation of the aorta results from an abnormality of development of the aortic arch system, such that there persists a structural narrowing of the aorta, usually in its descending intrathoracic course.[1,2] An extensive collateral arterial system develops so as to circumvent the coarctation and thus to supply adequate blood to the lower part of the body. Hypertension, readily detected in the upper limbs, is characteristic. If the site of the coarctation is such as to impair the blood flow to the left upper limb, hypertension may not be detectable in the left arm (see later).

## Pathogenesis of hypertension

The cause of the hypertension in coarctation of the aorta is disputed, although several theories have been advanced.

### Mechanical factors

One of the most plausible concepts, albeit unconfirmed, is that mechanical factors predominate. de Leeuw and Birkenhäger[1] have summarized these as follows. Initially, there is marked vascular resistance because of aortic narrowing, thus diverting blood to the upper part of the body, with hypoperfusion of the lower part. A consequent increase in cardiac output then delivers more blood to the lower body, but provides excessive circulation in terms of metabolic requirements to regions above the coarctation. As a result, the excessively perfused tissues increase their vascular resistance ('autoregulation') until a normal blood flow is restored. Thus, more blood then passes via the coarctation and the collaterals to the lower part of the body. Depending on the requirements of these tissues distal to the narrowing, cardiac output may remain elevated or revert to normal. In either event, the increased vascular resistance above the coarctation is responsible for proximal hypertension. As de Leeuw and Birkenhäger point out,[1] however, although this hypothesis is attractive, there are few convincing data either to support or refute it.

### The renin–angiotensin system

An alternative or additional theory proposes that renal ischaemia causes increased release of renin from the kidneys.[1,2] According to this notion, pathogenesis would be similar to that in the Goldblatt one-kidney one-clip or two-kidney two-clip models (page 172). In these models, plasma renin is elevated only transiently, whilst in the established condition there is sustained expansion of body sodium content.

In human coarctation, peripheral plasma levels of renin and renal vein renin values are normal as would be expected (Figure 28.1). There is, however, evidence that renin release in coarctation is hyper-responsive to stimuli such as orthostasis or sodium deprivation.[2] Relevant measurements of body sodium content in clinical aortic coarctation are wanting, although there are reports of expansion of plasma and extracellular fluid volumes.[1]

In experimental aortic constriction with resultant hypertension in animals, the renin system is stimulated transiently, values later declining into the normal range.[2] Transplantation of a kidney

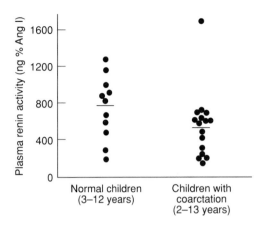

**Figure 28.1.** Peripheral plasma renin activity in children with coarctation of the aorta, compared with control children (all fasted and supine). The differences are not significant. (Redrawn from Ref. 2, with permission, from original data of Ref. 5.)

from below to above the aortic narrowing[2] can correct the hypertension.

For this theory of involvement of the renin–angiotensin system in pathogenesis, there is only slender evidence in favour and little against it. Any such participation is at most partial, and does not fully explain the raised arterial pressure.[1,2,5]

There is, however, clearer evidence of involvement of the renin–angiotensin system in the 'paradoxical' hypertension which can follow surgical repair of coarctation[2,6] (see below).

## Diagnosis

Although diagnosis of aortic coarctation should be made in infancy or childhood, some cases can escape detection until adult life. Thus, coarctation of the aorta, despite its rarity, must be considered in every patient of any age presenting with hypertension.[1]

Detection is usually straightforward. Concurrent palpation of the radical and femoral pulses, which should always be performed, reveals the femoral pulse as feeble although often easily palpable, with

a delayed summit. Once suspected, collateral arteries, with pronounced pulsation, can be felt and seen especially over the back of the thorax. Chest radiography will show, in nearly every patient over the age of 6 years, notching of the lower borders of the ribs resulting from enlarged collateral arteries. There will also probably be evident left ventricular enlargement.

The arterial pressure in the upper limbs is elevated, the systolic to a greater extent than the diastolic. If the aortic constriction lies proximal to the origin of the left subclavian artery, blood pressure will be lower, and the pulse more feeble, in the left arm than the right.

Blood pressure measurement in the leg is performed by auscultation of the popliteal artery in the popliteal fossa, employing an appropriately large cuff to compress the thigh. Systolic pressure always, and diastolic usually, is with coarctation lower in the legs than in the arms. The pulse pressure is diminished below the coarctation.

## Complications

Coarctation of the aorta is the one form of hypertension, primary or secondary, that is rarely complicated by the malignant phase. It is possible that, because the condition is present from birth or earlier, the arteries exposed to the hypertension have adequate time in which to adapt to the raised pressure.[2] However, one very suggestive example has been reported, with the ocular lesions and impaired vision correcting after surgical treatment and relief of the hypertension.[3]

Other complications of aortic coarctation include cardiac failure, aortic rupture, bacterial endocarditis or endaortitis, and cerebral haemorrhage. Associated cardiovascular malformations (especially patent ductus arteriosus and bicuspid aortic valve) are not unusual.[1]

**Treatment**

Coarctation should be treated by surgical reconstruction as early in life as is feasible.

### 'Paradoxical' hypertension

Following surgical repair of coarctation, transient exacerbation of hypertension (so-called 'paradoxical' hypertension) can occur over the next few days (Figure 28.2).[2] There is evidence that plasma renin is raised, and may be largely responsible for this paradoxical hypertension.[2,6] Paradoxical hypertension may be accompanied in up to a quarter of patients by a post-coarctectomy syndrome comprising abdominal pain and tenderness, ileus, fever, melaena, vomiting and leucocytosis. Necrotizing fibrinoid necrosis is found in mesenteric arteries, and bowel necrosis can occur.

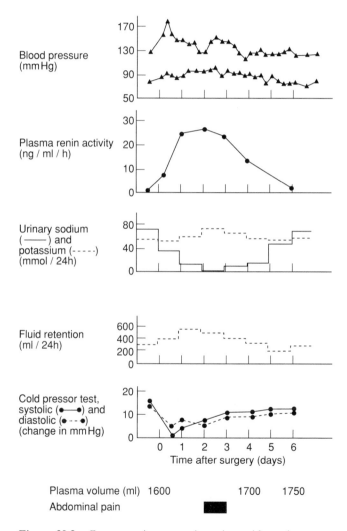

**Figure 28.2.** Post-operative events in patient with aortic coarctation. Plasma renin activity increases markedly after surgery, reaches a maximum at days 2–4, and is accompanied by retention of sodium and water and by abdominal pain. (Redrawn from Ref. 2, with permission, from original data of Ref. 6.)

It appears that change to a more pulsatile blood flow after repair of coarctation leads to these arterial lesions, probably because the mesenteric arteries, having been exposed to subnormal pulse pressure previously, are unduly fragile.[2]

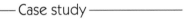

## Prognosis of hypertension

Coarctation of the aorta conforms to the general rule that after correction of the causal abnormality in secondary hypertension, blood pressure remains elevated in a substantial proportion of cases.[2,4] These may then require drug treatment as for essential hypertension.

## Case study

See Case study 8, Appendix 2.

## References

1. de Leeuw PW, Birkenhäger WH. Coarctation of the aorta. In: *Handbook of Hypertension*, Vol. 15: *Clinical Hypertension* (ed. JIS Robertson). Amsterdam: Elsevier, 1992: 236–65.
2. Robertson JIS. Renin and aortic coarctation. In *The Renin–Angiotensin System* (eds JIS Robertson and MG Nicholls). London: Gower Medical, 1993: chapter 59.
3. Cleland WP, Counihan TB, Goodwin JF, Steiner RE. Coarctation of the aorta. *Br. Med. J.* 1956; **2**: 379–90.
4. Pickering GW. *High Blood Pressure*, 2nd edn. London: Churchill, 1968.
5. Amsterdam EA, Albers WH, Chistlieb AR *et al.* Plasma renin activity in children with coarctation of the aorta. *Am. J. Cardiol.* 1969; **23**: 396–9.
6. Rocchini AP, Rosenthal A, Barger AC *et al.* Pathogenesis of paradoxical hypertension after coarctation resection. *Circulation* 1976; **54**: 382–7.

# 29
# Hypertension of renal origin: The Goldblatt models

A wide range of renal disorders can cause hypertension[1-8] (Table 29.1). Amongst the secondary forms of hypertension, these diverse renal conditions are outnumbered only by pre-eclampsia (page 243), and the various syndromes of drug-induced hypertension (Chapter 27).

## —Unilateral and bilateral renal disease—

Renal hypertension can usefully be considered under two main headings: that due to unilateral renal disease,[2] and that which is associated with bilateral renal abnormalities.[3] In unilateral renal

**Table 29.1.** Hypertension of renal origin

*Unilateral renal disease:*
  Renal artery stenosis or occlusion
  Renin-secreting tumour
  Other renal tumour
  Renal cyst or cysts
  Hypertensive small vessel damage[a]
  Arteritis following oral contraceptive use[a]
  Arteritis with collagenosis (systemic lupus erythematosus, scleroderma, or polyarteritis)[a]
  Renal arteriovenous fistula
  Intrarenal vascular malformation
  Chronic pyelonephritis
  Reflux nephropathy
  Hydronephrosis
  Tuberculosis
  Radiation nephritis
  Ask-Upmark kidney
  Page kidney
  [a] (often bilateral: see below)

*Bilateral renal disease:*
  Renal artery stenosis
  Primary or secondary glomerulonephritis
  Interstitial nephritis
  Hypertensive small vessel damage
  Arteritis following oral contraceptive use
  Arteritis with collagenosis (systemic lupus erythematosus, scleroderma, or polyarteritis)
  Chronic pyelonephritis
  Polycystic disease

disease, it is suggested that the pathogenesis of hypertension, in virtually all forms, shares a common path, namely stimulation, by whatever mechanism, of hypersecretion of renin by the afflicted kidney. In bilateral renal disease, overall impairment of kidney function provides the principal mechanism of the raised arterial pressure, although in some cases hypersecretion of renin may be an additional factor. It has, for example, been suggested, but not proved, that with adult polycystic disease, hypertension occurring before the onset of renal impairment may be due to bilateral sources of excessive renin secretion because of arterial constriction from cyst compression (see later).[6] In some patients with malignant phase hypertension likewise,[1] multiple intrarenal arterial lesions may sometimes stimulate renin secretion and so exacerbate hypertension independently of the supervention of renal impairment. Similar hypersecretion of renin with hypertension can be seen with acute glomerulonephritis. Moreover, raised arterial pressure as such can lead to intrarenal vascular damage, with consequent acceleration of renal functional decline.[1–3,7]

It will therefore be apparent that the renin–angiotensin system is either perceived or suspected as being involved in a range of forms of renal hypertension. Because much of the evaluation of the renin–angiotensin system in pathogenesis has been studied in terms of the various Goldblatt models of experimental hypertension, and their supposed clinical counterparts, these are described briefly below.

## The Goldblatt models of experimental hypertension[7]

### The two-kidney one-clip model

Goldblatt two-kidney one-clip hypertension comprises one kidney bearing a main renal artery constriction ('clipped'), with the other kidney and renal artery intact. The initiation of hypertension is due to increased renin release from the clipped kidney and thus to the immediate direct pressor effect of the consequently elevated peripheral plasma angiotensin II (Figure 29.1).

Continued exposure to raised plasma angiotensin II, even if the increase is only modest, results in an upward shift of the angiotensin II/pressor dose–response curve; thus in this second phase, blood pressure is disproportionately elevated in relation to the circulating concentration of angiotensin II, as compared with phase one. In both phases one and two, hypertension can be corrected either by removal of the renal artery constriction or by excision of the kidney distal to the stenosis. Hypertension in this model can be prevented by prolonged administration of inhibitors of the renin–angiotensin system, and can be corrected, even in the second phase, by extended treatment with such agents.

This form of hypertension can develop in the absence of changes in sodium balance and is not prevented by sodium restriction. Indeed, with severe unilateral renal artery stenosis or occlusion, frank and progressive sodium depletion can develop, with consequent ever-higher plasma renin and angiotensin II concentrations, and worsening, often malignant phase, hypertension. This is the hyponatraemic hypertensive syndrome, which is described from the clinical aspect on page 182. Sodium repletion can be therapeutically useful when this complication has supervened.

In a much later third phase with this model, removal of the clip, or of the kidney beyond the clip, no longer corrects the hypertension. However, excision of the contralateral, initially uninvolved, kidney can lower blood pressure, which is believed then to be dependent on hypertension-induced arterial lesions in that kidney.

The clinical counterparts of the two-kidney one-clip model are found in most cases of renovascular hypertension, and in many forms of hypertension due to unilateral renal disease.

### The one-kidney one-clip and two-kidney two-clip models

Goldblatt one-kidney one-clip hypertension is due to the application of a constriction to the artery

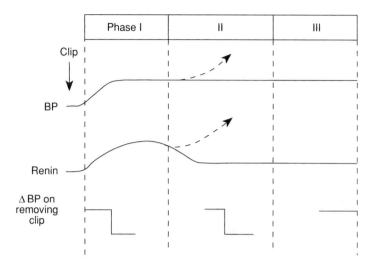

Arrows show course in hyponatraemic syndrome

**Figure 29.1.** Diagram illustrating the three phases of Goldblatt two-kidney one-clip hypertension. The arrows in phase II indicate the course in the hyponatraemic hypertensive syndrome. (Redrawn from Ref. 7, with permission.)

supplying a sole remaining kidney; pathogenesis in the two-kidney two-clip model is closely similar.

Application of the clip in the one-kidney one-clip model is followed by an immediate, though transient, rise in peripheral plasma renin and angiotensin II. In this brief phase, the hypertension is directly attributable to the immediate pressor action of the elevated plasma angiotensin II. Thereafter, plasma renin and angiotensin II return to normal and usually remain so, even though arterial pressure can continue to rise. Antagonism of the renin–angiotensin system during the initial brief phase of its stimulation prevents the early rise of blood pressure. However, prolonged antagonism of the renin–angiotensin system does not hinder the later appearance of sustained hypertension, which does not therefore in this model require the initial transient rise in plasma angiotensin II.

One-kidney one-clip hypertension throughout its stable phase is accompanied by modest, constant expansion of body sodium, even though the hyper-tension can be progressive. Relief of the renal artery constriction promptly returns body sodium and blood pressure to normal, whilst plasma renin is unaltered. Combined sodium restriction and antagonism of the renin–angiotensin system will also usually correct hypertension, although renal function may well then be worsened.

With severe renal artery constriction in this model, there can be progression to a terminal phase of severe hypertension and uraemia, with a secondary rise in plasma renin and angiotensin II. Administration of an antagonist of the renin–angiotensin system at this late phase will usually cause profound hypotension, worsening uraemia, and early death.

The one-kidney one-clip and two-kidney two-clip experimental models have their obvious clinical counterparts in patients with renal vascular disease. There may be further parallels with some diseases in which multiple intrarenal arterial lesions occur. Although not agreed by all, the pathogenesis of hypertension in coarctation of the aorta may likewise be akin to that in the two-kidney two-clip model[7] (page 167).

──────────── Case studies ────────────

See Case studies 15 and 16, Appendix 2.

──────────── References ────────────

1. Robertson JIS. Renin and malignant hypertension. In *The Renin–Angiotensin System* (eds JIS Robertson and MG Nicholls). London: Gower Medical, 1993: chapter 60.
2. Robertson JIS. Unilateral renal disease in hypertension. In *Handbook of Hypertension*, Vol. 15: *Clinical Hypertension* (ed. JIS Robertson). Amsterdam: Elsevier, 1992: 266–325.
3. Whitworth JA. Renal parenchymal disease and hypertension. In *Handbook of Hypertension*, Vol. 15: *Clinical Hypertension* (ed. JIS Robertson). Amsterdam: Elsevier, 1992: 326–56.
4. Lindop GBM, Leckie BJ, Mimran A. Renin-secreting tumours. In *The Renin–Angiotensin System* (eds JIS Robertson and MG Nicholls). London: Gower Medical, 1993: chapter 54.
5. Bakris GL, Gavras H. Renin in acute and chronic renal failure: implications for treatment. In *The Renin–Angiotensin System* (eds JIS Robertson and MG Nicholls). London: Gower Medical, 1993: chapter 56.
6. Robertson JIS. Polycystic kidney disease and the renin system. In *The Renin–Angiotensin System* (eds JIS Robertson and MG Nicholls). London: Gower Medical, 1993: chapter 57.
7. Robertson JIS. Renin and the pathophysiology of renovascular hypertension. In *The Renin–Angiotensin System* (eds JIS Robertson and MG Nicholls). London: Gower Medical, 1993: chapter 55.
8. Robertson JIS. Angiotensin-converting enzyme inhibitors in clinical renovascular hypertension. In *The Renin–Angiotensin System* (eds JIS Robertson and MG Nicholls). London: Gower Medical, 1993: chapter 88.

# 30
# Renin-secreting tumour

This rare condition[1-3] has excited interest disproportionate to its frequency because it offers insight into the pathophysiology of hypertension resulting solely from hypersecretion of renin. As it is proposed that the common pathogenetic route of most, if not all, forms of hypertension resulting from unilateral renal disease is overproduction of renin, excessive secretion of which has been stimulated in one way or another by the lesion, close study of patients with renin-secreting tumour is merited. Moreover, the condition is eminently treatable in its own right.

## Pathology

The classic and commonest form of the disease is a benign tumour of the renin-producing cells of the juxtaglomerular apparatus (juxtaglomerular cell tumour) (Figures 30.1 and 30.2). However, more rarely, renin hypersecretion with hypertension has been observed with a variety of other neoplasms, arising both within and outside the kidney, including Wilms' tumour, renal carcinoma, pulmonary carcinoma, pancreatic adenocarcinoma, parovarian tumour, fallopian tube adenocarcinoma, orbital haemangiopericytoma, epithelial liver hamartoma, angiolymphoid hyperplasia with eosinophilia, retroperitoneal leiomyosarcoma, and epithelioid sarcoma. A feature of many of these atypical, and especially of the malignant, renin-secreting tumours, is that they can produce substantial pro-

portions, often predominantly, of inactive renin; this can hinder diagnosis.

## Pathophysiology

The principal features of the condition are the consequences of excessive secretion of renin from the tumour. The resulting syndrome is characterized by hypertension with elevated peripheral plasma levels of renin and of its product the peptide angiotensin II, with secondary aldosterone excess and thus low plasma potassium concentrations.

Renin-secreting tumour, particularly the classic juxtaglomerular cell tumour, provides critical evidence of the relationship between chronic elevation of renin, and hence of angiotensin II, and hypertension. The analysis of such cases strongly indicates that, with prolonged exposure to high peripheral plasma concentrations of angiotensin II, much higher levels of arterial pressure are achieved than by the short-term elevation of angiotensin II to similar values. Thus, herein is clinical evidence of the slow, as well as of the fast, pressor effect of angiotensin II, now well-established both in experimental animals and man.[3] This phenomenon is compatible with the often slow return of blood pressure to normal values when patients or animals with hypertension due to excess of circulating angiotensin II are treated long term with angiotensin II antagonists or ACE inhibitors.

These observations also have important implications for the much commoner clinical hypertensive syndromes resulting from hypersecretion of renin, notably renovascular hypertension.

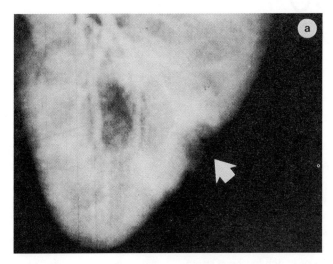

**Figure 30.1.**    Renin-secreting tumour at selective left renal angiography. (Reproduced from Ref. 1, with permission.)

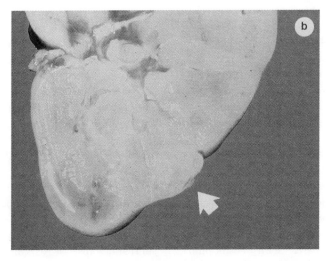

**Figure 30.2.**    Renin-secreting tumour shown in Figure 30.1 after nephrectomy. (Reproduced from Ref. 1, with permission.)

## Clinical features

The classic benign juxtaglomerular cell tumour is seen most often in children or young adults, which can be an important diagnostic clue.

In many patients, the history and physical findings are unremarkable, the condition being revealed often following the discovery of hypertension with hypokalaemia at routine examination. However, some of the rarer malignant renin-secreting neoplasms may manifest evidence of the primary or secondary carcinoma, with the renin excess and hypertension being noted subsequently. As mentioned earlier, if mainly inactive renin is secreted, diagnosis can be elusive.

## Diagnosis

In a patient with hypertension and hypokalaemia, and with concurrent elevation of plasma renin and aldosterone, once the more common forms of aldosterone excess, such as that induced by diuretic therapy or resulting from renal artery stenosis or the malignant phase, have been excluded, the possibility of renin-secreting tumour should be considered, especially in a young patient. Untreated, the raised arterial pressure may lead to the various sequelae of that condition, including progression to the malignant phase.

Estimation of renin in renal venous blood is critical, but it should be emphasized that, in contrast to renal artery stenosis, renal blood flow on the affected side is not usually reduced, and thus a high rate of renin secretion in a patient with renin-secreting tumour can be reflected in only a modest differential in renin values between the two renal veins. This is an important point because in several instances the difference, albeit genuine, has been close to the limit of discrimination of the relevant assay method. In rare instances, and especially with malignancy, the diagnosis may be missed unless both inactive and active renin are assayed in plasma.

The tumour may be localized definitively by selective angiography or tomographic scanning.

## Treatment

Local excision, if possible, or unilateral nephrectomy, are usually curative in the case of the most common form, renal juxtaglomerular cell tumour. With the more varied and rarer malignant neoplasms causing this condition, outcome is less certain.

Medical treatment can be useful pre-operatively or as definitive therapy in a patient with an inoperable or metastasizing renin-secreting neoplasm. An orally active ACE inhibitor will prevent the excessive formation of angiotensin II from the secreted renin, and should limit or correct the hypertension, aldosterone excess and hypokalaemia.

## Case study

See Case study 21, Appendix 2.

## References

1. Robertson JIS. Unilateral renal disease in hypertension. In *Handbook of Hypertension*, Vol. 15: *Clinical Hypertension* (ed. JIS Robertson). Amsterdam: Elsevier, 1992: 266–325.
2. Lindop GBM, Leckie BJ, Mimran A. Renin-secreting tumors. In *The Renin–Angiotensin System* (eds JIS Robertson and MG Nicholls). London: Gower Medical, 1993: chapter 54.
3. Robertson JIS. Renin and the pathophysiology of renovascular hypertension. In *The Renin–Angiotensin System* (eds JIS Robertson and MG Nicholls). London: Gower Medical, 1993: chapter 55.

# 31
# Renovascular hypertension

## Definition of renovascular hypertension

By definition, renovascular hypertension is hypertension resulting from narrowing of one or both renal arteries. Full confirmation of this condition clinically requires restoration of blood pressure to normal following either surgical relief of the renal artery constriction or removal of the afflicted kidney.[1] However, in some patients with a unilateral renal artery lesion, correction of the stenosis may not return blood pressure to normal, particularly if the hypertension has persisted over a long time. This is the result, at least in certain instances, of hypertension-induced lesions in the contralateral kidney, as has also been described in relation to experimental renovascular hypertension which has progressed to phase three (page 173). Thus occasional patients have been reported in whom, following correction of a unilateral renal artery stenosis, blood pressure fell only when the contralateral kidney was excised – a rare and best avoided clinical scenario.

It must be emphasized, therefore, that the co-existence of hypertension with renal artery stenosis does not establish that there exists genuine renovascular hypertension. In addition to the relationships mentioned above, there is the possible development of renal artery stenosis superimposed upon, and in part consequent on, pre-existent hypertension with its accompanying disturbances of blood flow (Chapter 13). Further, a patient with essential hypertension can develop significant renal artery stenosis with further elevation of blood pressure; a conjunction of a common condition with a rare one. Last, it should be pointed out that

the findings of clinical and post-mortem studies have shown anatomical renal artery stenosis in up to 46% of normotensive subjects. Evidently, the coexistence of a renal artery lesion with high blood pressure is not always easily interpreted.

## Prevalence of renovascular hypertension

Accurate estimation of the frequency of renal artery stenosis as a cause of hypertension is difficult; patients tend to be selected and referred preferentially to a centre where clinicians have an interest in the condition, and this distorts the apparent prevalence. In retrospective surveys of hypertensive populations, frequency rates from 2 to 30% have variously been quoted; a prevalence of 6% was found in a prospective study of an unselected hypertensive population. Speculative estimates have suggested that up to 920 000 people in the USA and 200 000 in the UK could have potentially curable hypertension associated with a renal artery stenosis. A further reason for identifying these subjects is that relief of a renal arterial lesion can improve renal function.

## Causes of renal artery stenosis

Clinical renal artery stenosis may result from various pathological lesions.

### Atheroma (atherosclerosis)

The commonest clinical cause of renal artery stenosis, accounting overall for about two-thirds

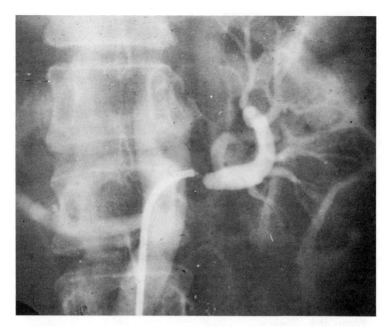

**Figure 31.1.**   Selective left renal arteriogram in a hypertensive man with left renal artery stenosis, showing atheromatous stenosis at origin of the left renal artery. The right renal artery is normal.

of cases, is atheroma (atherosclerosis) or a combination of atheroma with thrombus formation, usually found either at the origin of the main renal artery (Figure 31.1), along the proximal third of the renal artery, or at the first bifurcation of the main renal artery. Dilatation of the artery immediately distal to the stenosis is frequent. A collateral circulation may often develop via the inferior adrenal, peri-ureteric or other vessels.

Atheromatous renal artery disease occurs predominantly in older men who are cigarette smokers and who often show atheromatous disease at other sites. It is also not unusual in the artery to a transplanted kidney.

### Fibromuscular dysplasia

About one-third of cases of renal artery stenosis in hospital populations are due to fibromuscular dys-

plasia. This lesion predominantly affects women. The pathogenesis is disputed. On average, patients with fibromuscular dysplasia present some 10 years earlier in life than do patients with atheromatous lesions. An association with cigarette smoking is seen, as with atheromatous renal artery stenosis.

The middle and distal thirds of the main renal artery are principally involved, the right side more often than the left. There is with fibromuscular dysplasia less frequent involvement of arteries at other sites than in the case of atheroma. Other arteries that may nevertheless be implicated in fibromuscular dysplasia are the iliacs, mesenterics, carotids and coronaries, in that order.

Although the classic arteriographic appearance of this lesion mimics a 'string of beads' affecting an appreciable length of artery (Figure 31.2), fibromuscular dysplasia can present as a single discrete

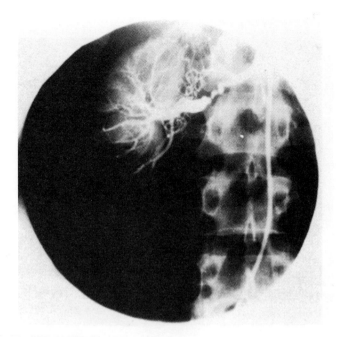

**Figure 31.2.** Right selective renal arteriogram in a 46-year-old woman showing appearances of fibromuscular dysplasia. Collateral circulation is evident via the inferior adrenal and periureteric vessels. (Reproduced from Ref. 1, with permission.)

renal artery stenosis with post-stenotic dilatation (Figure 31.3).

### Other causative lesions

A variety of other conditions has been reported as occasionally causing renal artery stenosis. These include external compression, as from various tumours, such as phaeochromocytoma (Figure 31.4) or neurofibroma; haematoma; encroaching diaphragmatic crura and sympathetic chains; accidental trauma; nephroptosis; arterial dissection; and various forms of renal arteritis as from systemic connective tissue diseases (page 66), oral contraceptive use (page 159), or Takayasu disease.

### Clinical Pathophysiology

The pathophysiology of hypertension resulting from renal artery stenosis is, as was outlined in Chapter 29 from the experimental aspect, complex.[2] There are two distinct varieties of the condition. The commoner clinical version shows a unilateral renal artery stenosis, the opposite kidney and its artery remaining intact; this has as its experimental counterpart the 'two-kidney one-clip' model. The second, and rarer, variety has either bilateral renal artery stenosis or stenosis of the artery to a sole remaining kidney; experimentally these are represented by the 'two-kidney two-clip' and 'one-kidney one-clip' models respectively. In patients with anatomical bilateral lesions only one of the lesions may be sufficiently severe to be of functional relevance and these patients are akin to unilateral

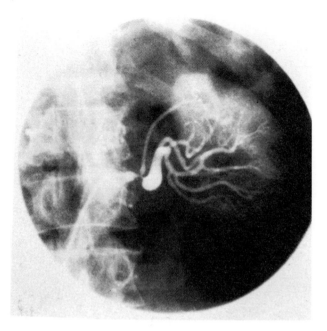

**Figure 31.3.** Left selective renal arteriogram showing tight stenosis of renal artery with poststenotic dilatation. Smaller artery to upper pole is also involved and also has post-stenotic dilatation. (Reproduced from Ref. 1, with permission.)

renal artery stenosis and the two-kidney one-clip model. Elucidation of pathogenetic mechanisms has been easier in the various experimental models than in patients. Many aspects remain uncertain.

These pathophysiological processes were summarized in Chapter 29.

## Unilateral renal artery stenosis, with contralateral side normal

The pathogenesis of 'two-kidney one-clip' hypertension has been divided into three phases that merge into one another (page 173, Figure 29.1). The initial phase is rarely seen clinically. In this first phase, lasting for a few days at most, plasma renin, plasma angiotensin II and blood pressure rise together. There is good evidence that at this stage the blood pressure is elevated by the immediate direct pressor effect of the raised circulating angio-

tensin II. Relief of the stenosis, or removal of the affected kidney, promptly returns the plasma concentrations of renin and angiotensin II and the blood pressure to normal.

### Phase two clinical renovascular hypertension

Within days or weeks, phase one is succeeded by phase two, in which, although blood pressure remains high, there is, proportionately, less marked elevation of plasma renin and of angiotensin II than in phase one. In many patients in this second phase of renovascular hypertension, circulating levels of renin and angiotensin II may be only marginally elevated, or even in the upper part of the normal range. There is little disturbance of plasma electrolytes, and body sodium content is normal. Nevertheless, correction of the stenosis, excision of the afflicted kidney or the administration of antagonists of the renin–angiotensin system can, in phase

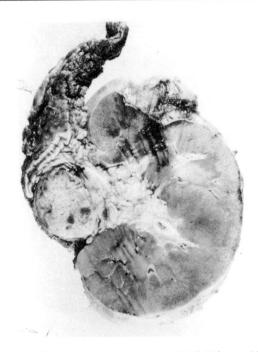

**Figure 31.4.** Operation specimen of left kidney with spherical phaeochromocytoma lying in the hilum. The tumour involved the renal arteries; note scarring of the upper pole of the kidney. Normal left adrenal lies above the phaeochromocytoma. (Reproduced from Ref. 1, with permission.)

two, alleviate the hypertension. Evidently, slow, as well as fast, components of the pressor action of angiotensin II are involved.

### Presentation with nephrotic syndrome

Occasionally in phase two, severe unilateral renal artery stenosis can cause plasma renin and angiotensin II to rise sufficiently high that, combined with systemic hypertension, marked proteinuria is provoked mainly via the contralateral kidney, and the nephrotic syndrome can ensue.[4]

### The hyponatraemic hypertensive syndrome

If, in phase two, there is a very severe unilateral renal artery stenosis or unilateral renal artery occlusion, intense stimulation of renin release, with consequent very marked elevation of plasma angio-

tensin II concentration and severe hypertension can occur (Figures 29.1 and 31.5). However, because of the severity of the renal artery lesion, systemic blood pressure cannot rise sufficiently to eliminate the intrarenal signal to renin secretion. The hypertension causes loss of sodium by pressure natriuresis from the contralateral kidney (Figure 31.6), and the consequent sodium deficiency provides a reinforcing stimulus to the already excessive renin secretion. Even so, the sodium loss, while undoubtedly moderating the pressor effect of angiotensin II, is insufficient to abrogate it. Secondary aldosterone excess follows, with resulting potassium deficiency, which provides yet another stimulus to renin secretion. Potassium loss may well moderate the pressor effect of angiotensin II, although in this context, evidently not markedly. The elevated angiotensin II can cause thirst and

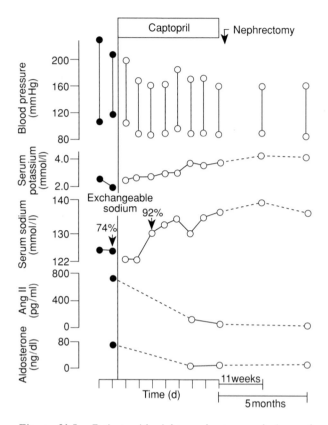

**Figure 31.5.** Patient with right renal artery occlusion and acute onset of the hyponatraemic hypertensive syndrome with malignant hypertension. Shows effect of 1 week of treatment with captopril (450 mg daily) – such high doses of captopril would no longer be considered appropriate – followed by unilateral nephrectomy, when all treatment was stopped. Note correction of hypertension, hyponatraemia, hypokalaemia and deficiency of exchangeable body sodium on captopril. Unilateral nephrectomy was curative. Normal upper limit of plasma angiotensin II (Ang II) is 35 pg/ml. (Redrawn from Ref. 3, with permission.)

increased vasopressin secretion. The hyponatraemia thus has multiple causes; these include direct renal actions of angiotensin II, together with angiotensin II-stimulated thirst and elevation of vasopressin.

The abnormalities can be corrected by relief of the renal artery constriction, by removal of the kidney distal to the renal arterial lesion, or by lowering plasma angiotensin II by the administration of an ACE inhibitor. Indeed, because of the marked sodium deficit, the introduction of ACE inhibition will lower blood pressure often precipitously. Correction of the sodium deficit can also be therapeutically beneficial.

A very similar hyponatraemic syndrome can occur in malignant-phase essential hypertension, where presumably multiple intrarenal hypertension-induced arterial lesions cause scattered renal

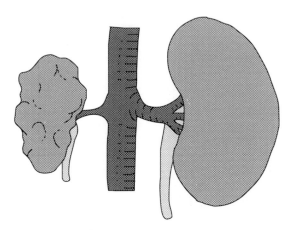

- Unilateral renal artery stenosis or occlusion–intense
  stimulus to renin secretion
- Rise in Ang II and blood pressure–natriuresis from
  opposite kidney
- Sodium loss–further renin stimulation

**Figure 31.6.** The essential features in the pathogenesis of the hyponatraemic hypertensive syndrome. Severe unilateral renal artery stenosis or occlusion causes intense stimulation of renin secretion, with hypertension and consequent pressure natriuresis from the contralateral kidney. (Redrawn from Ref. 3, with permission.)

artery stenoses. The hyponatraemic syndrome is also encountered in some patients in end-stage renal failure undergoing haemodialysis, and occasionally with intensive diuretic therapy.

### Late (phase three) clinical renovascular hypertension

Months or years later, phase two of renovascular hypertension is succeeded by phase three, in which it appears that hypertension-induced lesions in the contralateral kidney are responsible for perpetuating the hypertension. Much evidence suggests that the renin–angiotensin system is not relevant to the hypertension in phase three, although some authorities disagree. In phase three, surgical relief of the renal arterial lesion or removal of the affected kidney does not correct the hypertension (Figure 29.1), although, as previously mentioned, subsequent excision of the contralateral kidney may be effective. Clinical recognition of phase three is important, in order to avoid unnecessary or inappropriate surgical intervention.

### Renal artery stenosis with a single kidney —— and bilateral renal artery stenosis ——

The 'one-kidney one-clip' variety of hypertension (page 172) is clinically rarer.

The established clinical condition shows, as does the experimental form, normal or near-normal plasma renin and angiotensin II values. There is, however, generally stable expansion of body sodium content, which presumably is a main, but not the sole, mechanism responsible for the hypertension.

Bilateral renal artery stenosis has closely similar pathophysiology.

------------ Clinical features ------------

Renovascular hypertension is largely devoid of specific symptoms. However, in up to 20% of patients, the malignant phase may have supervened and given rise to visual disturbance, other neurological features such as fits or clouding of consciousness, hypertensive heart failure, headache or nocturia.

As described on page 182, a few patients with a severe unilateral renal artery stenosis or thrombosis develop a characteristic and striking constellation of features including polyuria, polydipsia, weight loss and rapidly advancing sodium and potassium depletion. Malignant-phase hypertension is usually also present. Plasma renin, angiotensin II, aldosterone and vasopressin values are high or very high, and plasma sodium and potassium low. This is the 'hyponatraemic hypertensive syndrome', which will advance rapidly to a fatal conclusion unless the stenosis is relieved, the affected kidney is removed, or the gross excess of circulating angiotensin II is corrected or antagonized, as by the administration of an ACE inhibitor. The use of orally active angiotensin II antagonists (page 123) in this syndrome has yet to be described.

Another rare mode of presentation with unilateral renal artery stenosis is as sudden onset of the nephrotic syndrome[4] (page 182).

Patients with occlusion of a renal artery or one of its main branches may develop infarction of renal tissue, with consequent loin pain and haematuria. Such a lesion may supervene on a previously occult renal artery stenosis. Alternatively, the infarct may be the consequence of abdominal trauma or a deceleration injury, or there may be evidence of a source of embolus, such as cardiac arrhythmia or endocarditis.

Physical signs are often lacking in renovascular hypertension. An abdominal or loin bruit may arise from turbulent blood flow across a renal artery stenosis, and a bruit audible in both systole and diastole is held to be particularly suggestive. Abdominal bruits have been reported in up to 58% of patients with demonstrable renal artery stenosis but can also occur frequently in subjects with aortic atheroma and no renal arterial lesion. An abdominal bruit must therefore be regarded as an unreliable sign of renal artery stenosis.

A suspicion of either bilateral renal artery stenosis or of stenosis of the artery to a single kidney is raised, first, on features suggestive of renal artery stenosis set out above. Second, hypertension resistant to drug therapy should suggest this possibility. Third, if the overall renal function is already compromised and/or if renal function deteriorates as systemic blood pressure is lowered with drugs, especially with ACE inhibitors, the possibility of either bilateral renal artery stenosis or of stenosis of the artery supplying a single kidney should be seriously considered. Renal artery stenosis can develop not unusually in the artery to a transplanted kidney.

It is mandatory that no patient should be subjected to regular haemodialysis for renal failure unless the possibility of correctable bilateral renal artery stenoses (or of renal artery stenosis in a single kidney), with potential restoration of renal function, has been excluded. This is important not least because the kidney distal to a renal artery stenosis is largely protected from damage due to hypertension, and may therefore function well once its blood supply is restored.

------------ Screening tests ------------

### Intravenous urography

In unselected hypertensive patients, intravenous urography yields few abnormalities, and its value has been questioned. Nevertheless, it is a frequent first indicator of renal artery stenosis.

The characteristic features of this disease on pyelography are usually fourfold. The affected kidney is usually smaller, although the right kidney can normally be as much as 1.5 cm shorter than the left. On the affected side, there is delayed appearance of contrast in the first minutes after injection, with later hyperconcentration. There is usually visibly reduced urine volume, despite the hyperconcentration of dye, on the affected side

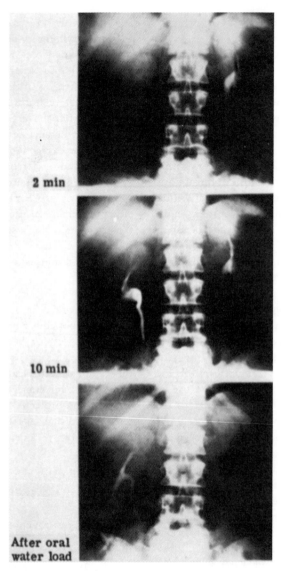

**Figure 31.7.** Intravenous urogram in a 46-year-old woman with right-sided renal arterial fibromuscular dysplasia (same case as Figure 31.2). (A) Two minutes after injection of dye a delay in appearance of dye on the affected right side can be seen. (B) At 10 min, hyperconcentration can be seen on the right. (C) After water load only the affected right side can be seen. (Reproduced from Ref. 1, with permission.)

(Figure 31.7). On the normal, but not on the affected, side, there may be disappearance or fading of contrast after the administration of a water load. It is important that these last three features are appreciated; because of them, suspicion can easily focus on the good kidney, which can then be inappropriately attacked surgically. More rarely, in the presence of a very severe stenosis or occlusion, dye may fail to appear at all stages on the affected side.

The value of intravenous pyelography as a screening test may be lost in those patients with bilateral renal artery stenosis.

### Ultrasound

Abdominal ultrasound can demonstrate disproportionate kidney size. Again, it should be remembered that the right kidney can normally be up to 1.5 cm shorter than the left.

### Intravenous renal arteriography

The advent of intravenous renal arteriography,[9] combined with digital subtraction methods, has greatly facilitated screening for renal artery stenosis, permitting in many cases not only the detection but also the localization and definition of the lesion.

### Isotope renography

In the past, this procedure enjoyed a transient vogue as a screening test, despite the occurrence of a substantial proportion of both false-negative and false-positive results. It has also been combined with intravenous urography.

It was later noted that the administration at renography of an ACE inhibitor such as captopril would often depress the function of the affected kidney. The use of isotope renography was enthusiastically espoused as a screening test by some, assessed more critically by others, and sometimes rejected outright. The value of captopril provocation with isotope renography as a screening test for renal artery stenosis likewise remains controversial. The role of renography in this disease nowadays is more appropriately directed to assessing the severity of a renal artery stenosis.

### Plasma renin estimation

An elevated value for plasma renin in peripheral blood has long been regarded as indicative of renovascular hypertension. However, many patients with this condition have circulating concentrations of both renin and angiotensin II that are only marginally elevated, or in the upper part of the overall normal range (page 181). Therefore, this should be regarded as only a tenuous lead.

More recently, this approach has been expanded and refined, by measuring plasma renin following the administration of the fast-acting ACE inhibitor captopril. It has been reported that, following captopril, patients with renal artery stenosis show a more marked rise in plasma renin than do those with essential hypertension, with virtually complete separation of the two groups. Other workers, however, have not been able to confirm these findings, and have queried the reliability of the procedure.

## Diagnosis of renovascular hypertension

### Radiological tests

Of the screening procedures enumerated above, intravenous angiography may permit diagnosis of anatomical renal artery stenosis, but not necessarily of renovascular hypertension. However, intra-arterial angiography will usually be required to provide the detail needed to guide the surgeon (Figures 31.1–31.3). Excretion urography can indicate functional renal artery stenosis (Figure 31.7).

Isotope renography has progressed in recent years so that a quantitative assessment of both the extent of reduction of renal plasma flow and the glomerular filtration rate may be made non-invasively.

### Bilateral ureteric catheter studies

Bilateral ureteric catheterization provides the most detailed functional and diagnostic information in unilateral renal artery stenosis. The procedure is no longer popular because it is time-consuming and expensive, requires expert urological skills, calls for saddle-block anaesthesia, is uncomfortable for the patient and may be complicated by loin or bladder pain, haematuria or urinary infection.

Typical features of unilateral renal artery stenosis are, on the affected side, reduction in urine flow and urinary sodium concentration, enhanced concentrations of creatinine and, if administered, inulin and *para*-aminohippurate (PAH), with reduced clearances of creatinine, inulin and PAH.

There remain few, if any, patients in whom the precise details provided by this procedure are needed.

### Renal vein renin estimation

Comparison of the values of renin (less commonly of angiotensin II) in the two renal veins is a widely employed confirmatory procedure.

Increased values of renin on the affected side are the combined result of increased renin secretion and diminution of renal plasma flow; renin secretion is usually suppressed on the contralateral normal side, with renin values in renal venous plasma being closely similar to those in the aorta.

In the steady state, increased renin secretion alone cannot in unilateral renal artery stenosis raise the renal vein renin ratio to more than 1.5:1. Values higher than this reflect also reduction of renal blood flow on the affected side, and the procedure has thus been used to estimate changes in blood flow.

The ratio of renin in renal venous plasma on the affected side to that on the unaffected side can be raised transiently by stimulating renin secretion acutely; this has been performed as an aid to diagnosis employing various procedures such as orthostasis or the administration of vasodilators or ACE inhibitors. ACE inhibitors will enhance this ratio not only by stimulating renin secretion on the affected side; there are contributions also from ipsilateral further reduction of renal blood flow, with contralateral increased blood flow and extraction of renin.

## Diagnostic pathways

There are several alternative pathways through the foregoing screening and diagnostic procedures. Much will depend on local facilities, preferences and expertise. Two possible alternative routes are suggested in Table 31.1.

## Prognostic indicators

Many procedures, some of dubious value, have been employed to attempt the prediction of blood pressure reduction after successful relief of the stenosis.

### Clinical features

A poor outcome in terms of blood pressure reduction is more likely with older age, long-standing

**Table 31.1.** Two possible pathways for the screening and subsequent diagnosis of renal artery stenosis and renovascular hypertension

| | | |
|---|---|---|
| I | 1) | History of suggestive features (see text). |
| | 2) | Abdominal ultrasound for disparity of renal size. |
| | 3) | Intravenous renal arteriogram with attention to accompanying excretion urogram. |
| | 4) | Renal vein renin (with captopril stimulation). |
| | 5) | Selective renal arteriogram. |
| II | 1) | History of suggestive features (see text). |
| | 2) | Abdominal ultrasound for disparity of renal size. |
| | 3) | Intravenous urogram. |
| | 4) | Renal vein renin (with captopril stimulation). |
| | 5) | Selective renal arteriogram. |

Preferences and especially sensitivity and specificity will depend on local facilities, and particular interest or expertise.

An alternative early test is peripheral venous renin sampling with captopril stimulation; this could be incorporated in Step 4 in either of the two schemes.

Not all workers agree on the value of captopril enhancement either on isotope renography or renal vein sampling.

There are also fears that the large dose of contrast needed for intravenous renal arteriography may provoke renal impairment occasionally.

hypertension, cigarette smoking, atheroma, vascular disease at other sites, renal functional impairment and male sex. Conversely, a better result may be expected with youth, fibromuscular dysplasia, good renal function and female sex.

### Renin estimation

High levels of renin in peripheral blood and a high renal vein renin ratio have been claimed to herald a good prognostic outcome. Suppression of renin release by the unaffected kidney has also been deemed an encouraging feature. However, none of these has been reliably consistent.

### Ureteric catheterization studies

The information provided by ureteric catheterization studies has not proved reliable in prediction of surgical success.

### Antagonists of the renin–angiotensin system

The extent of the immediate blood pressure fall following acute administration of antagonists of angiotensin II, such as saralasin, or of ACE inhibitors, such as captopril, has been widely employed as an indicator of prognosis with unilateral renal artery stenosis. However, our experience and that of other workers has demonstrated the fallibility of this approach, with the acute blood pressure fall in such circumstances variously over- and underestimating the long-term outcome following relief of the stenosis. This is not surprising in view of the pathophysiological considerations discussed already.

However, it has been reported that the long-term blood pressure response (i.e. over several weeks) to orally active ACE inhibitors predicts well, in absolute terms, both for systolic and diastolic pressures, the long-term outcome following either surgical intervention or transluminal angioplasty. This observation is in accord with pathophysiological notions, and, although the findings have not been universally accepted, they deserve further critical evaluation.

## Treatment of renovascular hypertension

### Surgical intervention

The two main reasons for surgical relief of renal artery stenosis are to lower arterial pressure or to improve renal function. To these may be added a much rarer indication, where the cause of the renal artery narrowing requires excision in its own right, e.g. phaechromocytoma involving the renal hilum (Figure 31.4).

As the kidney distal to the stenosis is protected from the effects of systemic hypertension, in most cases this kidney has potentially excellent function. Such considerations make a strong case for operative relief of a renal artery constriction as the treatment of choice with unilateral renal artery stenosis. Although both unilateral nephrectomy or reconstruction can relieve high blood pressure, the former consistently diminishes, whereas the latter enhances, overall renal function. Reconstructive arterial surgery is almost always necessary with bilateral renal artery stenosis, or with stenosis to the artery of a single kidney.

The foregoing comments emphasize that nephrectomy should be avoided if at all possible. However, there are circumstances in which with unilateral disease, nephrectomy or heminephrectomy is indicated, such as an obviously shrunken kidney or part of the kidney, or in which there exist severe technical problems such as aberrant or friable renal arteries, multiple intrarenal branch lesions or renal artery aneurysm. There are also rare cases in which successful reconstruction of a renal artery stenosis fails to relieve hypertension, which is then corrected only after the contralateral kidney, the seat of hypertension-induced renal changes, has been removed.

Conservative surgical procedures include endarterectomy with or without patch angioplasty; splenorenal, hepatorenal, iliac-renal or superior mesenteric-renal arterial anastomosis; aortorenal bypass grafting employing Dacron velour, saphenous, ovarian or testicular vein or splenic or hypogastric artery; and autotransplantation, usually to the internal iliac artery.

**Table 31.2.**   Results of surgery for renal artery stenosis: a review of
26 reports

| No. of patients | Blood pressure | | |
|---|---|---|---|
| | Normal | Improved | Unchanged |
| 3347 | 1686 (50%) | 1026 (31%) | 635 (19%) |

*Source:* From Ref. 1.

The introduction of extracorporeal methods for reconstructing extensive renal and intrarenal vascular disease has in recent years greatly enhanced the scope and success of these procedures, notably bypass grafting and autotransplantation. At one time, revascularization techniques carried an anatomical failure rate of 18–45%. However, better surgical expertise and especially the use of extracorporeal reconstruction methods have considerably improved these figures, at least in centres where there is extensive experience.

### Evaluation of outcome: blood pressure

Comparison of the results of surgical 'successes' and 'failures' among centres is difficult because of differing criteria adopted by various authors. Most reviewers include a category of 'partial' success, in which, although blood pressure has not been lowered to normal, control with drugs has been easier, and/or the burden of side-effects of medical therapy has been lightened. We have defined a successful outcome, in terms of blood pressure reduction, as the lowering of pressure to within one standard deviation of age- and sex-adjusted values observed in the general population.

Despite the differences of definition, some worthwhile comparisons of outcome among various centres can be made. In a review of 26 series in which 3347 patients were operated upon between 1961 and 1989, 50% of patients were regarded as having had a successful outcome in terms of blood pressure reduction, 31% were regarded as improved, and 19% of the operations were judged as failures (Table 31.2). Diverse other forms of secondary hypertension managed surgically yielded overall success rates that are not dissimilar from those of operated renal artery stenosis, ranging from 40 to 65%.

### Evaluation of outcome: renal function

The assessment of the success or otherwise of operation to improve renal function is more readily achieved. However, no large series in which patients were operated upon specifically for this reason appear to have been reported. It deserves emphasis that normal renal function can be restored even after several weeks of main renal arterial occlusion, especially if an extensive collateral blood supply has developed. Nevertheless, acute renal artery occlusion, if diagnosed, is a surgical emergency.

A chronically shrunken kidney is unlikely, however, to benefit from restoration of its arterial supply.

### Transluminal angioplasty

Percutaneous transluminal balloon angioplasty has steadily gained in popularity in recent years as an alternative to surgical intervention for renal artery stenosis. The procedure is usually performed under local anaesthesia.

Anticoagulants are usually administered subsequently. Improved outcome can in future be expected, with the more enlightened use of antiplatelet agents across the procedure. Thus far, any supportive medical therapy has been largely arbitrary and unassessed.

Not all renal arterial lesions are amenable to angioplasty. Those most suitable are proximal, accessible, discrete, concentric non-calcified lesions.

**Table 31.3.** Results of angioplasty for renal artery stenosis: a review of 10 reports

| No. of patients | Excluded because blood pressure not followed | Technical failure | Blood pressure | | |
|---|---|---|---|---|---|
| | | | Normal | Improved | Unchanged |
| 691 | 21 | 84 (12%) | 163 (24%) | 286 (43%) | 221 (33%) |

*Source:* From Ref. 5.

In general, fibromuscular dysplastic stenoses do better than atheromatous lesions. The use of intra-arterial stents has extended the applicability of angioplasty.

Complications include pain, segmental or total renal infarction, renal failure, intimal dissection leading to worsening of the stenosis, retroperitoneal bleeding, balloon rupture with embolization of the fragments, and inability to remove the balloon with consequent need for surgery.

Facilities for open surgery must therefore always be available when practising balloon angioplasty.

A summary of the outcome after angioplasty for renal artery stenosis in ten published series of hypertensive patients is given in Table 31.3.

### Medical treatment

Stimulation of the renin–angiotensin system is, as described earlier, almost certainly responsible for the initiation and, in both phase one and phase two of 'two-kidney, one-clip' renovascular hypertension, the maintenance, of the raised blood pressure. The role of the renin–angiotensin system in phase three is less certain.

Thus, it is to be expected that in phase two, that most often encountered clinically, the administration of agents that neutralize the effects of the renin–angiotensin system will alleviate the hypertension.

The orally active ACE inhibitors are suitable for long-term treatment, and the fall in blood pressure after several weeks of pre-operative therapy with such agents has, as discussed above (page 188), been taken by some workers as a good index of the likely blood pressure response following operation or transluminal angioplasty. The efficacy of ACE inhibitors can sometimes be enhanced by adding a diuretic. However, diuretic therapy is often super-

fluous; an ACE inhibitor given alone has been shown to lower total exchangeable body sodium in hypertensive patients with unilateral renal artery stenosis (Figure 31.8).

While the response of systemic hypertension to ACE inhibition in patients with renovascular disease is frequently gratifying, it is not established beyond doubt that these drugs are in this disease superior to other classes of antihypertensive agent. There are, nevertheless, some strongly suggestive comparative trials.

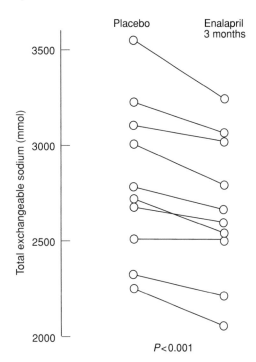

**Figure 31.8.** Total exchangeable sodium in mmol per patient in 10 subjects with hypertension and renal artery stenosis before and at the third month of enalapril monotherapy. (Redrawn from Ref. 3, with permission.)

However, as well as being responsible probably for the maintenance of systemic hypertension in this disease, important intrarenal compensatory actions of angiotensin II occur in the kidney beyond the stenosis, helping that kidney, despite the reduction in perfusion, to an extent to sustain glomerular filtration rate, the capacity to excrete urea, and the pressure in the main renal artery distal to the stenosis. These compensatory effects will be diminished or lost with ACE inhibition; moreover, there are fears that with such medical treatment there may be not only reversible diminution of unilateral renal function, but also a predisposition to occlusion of the afflicted renal artery.

For these reasons, many physicians are reluctant to employ ACE inhibitors, other than briefly, in patients with hypertension accompanied by renal artery stenosis. There is particular concern that their use in patients with bilateral renal artery stenosis may regularly induce renal failure. The conjoint administration of diuretics almost certainly enhances the risks in patients with both unilateral and bilateral renal artery narrowing. For contrasting opinions on these contentious issues, the reader is referred to the reviews by Ménard et al.[6] and by Hollenberg.[7]

Fears have been expressed concerning the possible dangers also of $\beta$-adrenoceptor blockers in this condition, because these agents again in part work via the renin–angiotensin system, inhibiting renin secretion. However, $\beta$-blockers less potently interfere with the renin system, and the risk is probably less than that associated with ACE inhibitors.

The above considerations do not preclude the use of either ACE inhibitors or $\beta$-blockers, alone or in combination, in the long-term treatment of renovascular hypertension in patients unsuitable or unwilling to undergo operation. However, it has to be recognized that treatment using antagonists of the renin–angiotensin system cannot improve, and will almost certainly worsen, the already compromised function of the diseased kidney. Moreover, with bilateral renal artery stenosis, or with a solitary kidney having renal artery disease, especially if diuretics are also administered, renal failure can readily be provoked.

## Case studies

See Case studies 15 and 16, Appendix 2.

## References

1. Robertson JIS. Unilateral renal disease in hypertension. In *Handbook of Hypertension*, Vol. 15: *Clinical Hypertension* (ed. JIS Robertson). Amsterdam: Elsevier, 1992: 266–325.

2. Robertson JIS. Renin and the pathophysiology of renovascular hypertension. In *The Renin–Angiotensin System* (eds JIS Robertson and MG Nicholls). London: Gower Medical, 1993: chapter 55.

3. Robertson JIS. Angiotensin-converting enzyme inhibitors in clinical renovascular hypertension. In *The Renin–Angiotensin System* (eds JIS Robertson and MG Nicholls). London: Gower Medical, 1993: chapter 88.

4. Robertson JIS. Renin and the nephrotic syndrome. In *The Renin–Angiotensin System* (eds JIS Robertson and MG Nicholls). London: Gower Medical, 1993: chapter 58.

5. Ramsay LE, Waller PC. Blood pressure response to transluminal angioplasty for atheromatous renal artery stenosis: an overview of published series. *Br. Med. J.* 1990; **300**: 569–72.

6. Ménard J, Michel JB, Plouin P-F. A cautious view of the value of angiotensin-converting enzyme inhibition in renovascular disease. In *The Renin–Angiotensin System* (eds JIS Robertson and MG Nicholls). London: Gower Medical, 1993: chapter 89.

7. Hollenberg NK. A buoyant view of the value of angiotensin-converting enzyme inhibition in renovascular disease. In *The Renin–Angiotensin System* (eds JIS Robertson and MG Nicholls). London: Gower Medical, 1993: chapter 90.

8. Robertson JIS, Ball SG. Hypertension. In *Diseases of the Heart*, 1st edn (eds DG Julian, AJ Camm, KM Fox et al.). London: Baillière Tindall, 1989: 1227–92.

9. Fournier A, Cecile JP, Remond A et al. Value of combined intravenous renal arteriography and pyelography in the diagnosis of renovascular hypertension. *Clin. Sci.* 1980; **59** (suppl. 6): 423–5.

# 32
# Other forms of unilateral renal disease with hypertension

A wide variety of unilateral parenchymal renal lesions may occur with hypertension (see Table 29.1) and, at least in some instances, blood pressure may be lowered following removal of the affected kidney.[1] It has been proposed that the common pathogenetic pathway is stimulation of renin secretion by the lesion. If this is so, these patients should show, as in renal artery stenosis or renal renin-secreting tumour, differential renin values in renal venous blood, and also probably a fall in blood pressure with pre-operative administration of ACE inhibitors.

The number and variety of conditions listed in Table 29.1 give an idea of the protean modes of presentation. Many of these conditions require nephrectomy irrespective of hypertension; consequently, any fall in blood pressure resulting from surgical intervention may often be regarded as a bonus.

The reader is referred to specialist texts for a detailed account of these lesions. Two require brief elucidation here.

## Ask–Upmark kidney

This rarity consists of apparently congenital unilateral renal lobular hypoplasia, with small blind-ending recesses in the renal pelvis.[2] Pyelonephritis may complicate the pathology. The condition is found predominantly in young females and often progresses to the malignant phase.

## Page kidney

Page described experimental cellophane wrapping of the kidney, with consequent perinephritis, capsular fibrosis and subcapsular ischaemia with hypertension. Clinically, the term 'Page kidney' has been applied to capsular fibrosis and hypertension resulting from a perirenal haematoma.[3]

## Reference

1. Robertson JIS. Unilateral renal disease in hypertension. In *Handbook of Hypertension*, Vol. 15: *Clinical Hypertension* (ed. JIS Robertson). Amsterdam: Elsevier, 1992: 266–325.
2. Zezulka A, Arkell DG, Beevers DG. The association of hypertension, the Ask–Upmark kidney and other congenital abnormalities. *J. Urol.* 1986; **135**: 1000–1.
3. Weinberger MH, Grim CE, Donohue JP. A rare but curable form of hypertension: the 'Page kidney'. In *Juvenile Hypertension* (eds MI New and LS Levine). New York: Raven, 1977: 133.

# 33
# Hypertension with bilateral renal disease

Hypertension can be seen, as has been discussed in detail in Chapters 29 and 31, in association with bilateral renal artery stenosis.

As indicated in Table 29.1, hypertension can also complicate a range of bilateral renal parenchymal disorders, particularly if overall renal functional impairment supervenes.[1-3]

It has further been proposed that in bilateral polycystic kidney disease, compression by the enlarging cysts can attenuate renal arteries and stimulate renin secretion, thereby provoking hypertension before the onset of renal impairment.[3] Despite much suggestive evidence, this concept remains controversial.

Hypersecretion of renin and hypertension can occur in acute glomerulonephritis, sometimes with only modest azotaemia.[2]

## Bilateral parenchymatous renal disease

### Pathology

As shown in Table 29.1, a diverse range of bilateral intrinsic renal diseases can be associated with hypertension; detailed description of these is beyond the scope of this present chapter. Diagnoses include bilateral polycystic disease, which is inherited as a Mendelian dominant disorder; acute and chronic glomerulonephritis; interstitial nephritis; pyelonephritis; radiation nephritis; intrarenal arteritis caused by oral contraceptives; analgesic nephropathy; diabetic nephropathy; and the con-

nective tissue diseases systemic lupus erythematosus, progressive systemic sclerosis (scleroderma), and polyarteritis nodosa. All of these can cause elevation of arterial pressure. Moreover, hypertension-dependent nephrosclerosis may add to renal damage and accelerate the rate of deterioration of renal function and the rise of blood pressure.[5] These concepts emphasize the need for prompt recognition and treatment of hypertension. Terminally, when both kidneys are shrunken and scarred, it may be almost impossible to differentiate the initial abnormality from lesions resulting from hypertension.[5]

Systemic lupus erythematosus and polyarteritis nodosa can pose especial problems because retinal haemorrhages and exudates reflecting the underlying vascular disease mimic the retinopathy of malignant hypertension (pages 65–66 and 69).

### Pathophysiology

In some instances, the pathophysiological mechanism underlying the hypertension is hypersecretion of renin caused by the renal lesions, and these are likely to have affinities with the Goldblatt two-kidney two-clip experimental model (page 172). In these circumstances, the blood pressure can be raised in the absence of azotaemia. Conditions in which this may or does occur include acute glomerulonephritis[2] and polycystic disease.[3]

More often, however, hypertension with bilateral renal disease is accompanied by, and dependent upon, renal impairment.[2] In these latter circumstances, fluid and sodium retention are almost certainly important influences in the causation of raised arterial pressure. Significant correlations have been described between the severity of hypertension and total exchangeable sodium in series of patients with chronic renal failure. The renin–angiotensin system then can provide an additional or alternative factor in some cases.

Other pressor mechanisms that have been proposed, but which are less clearly defined, are increases in plasma noradrenaline and deficiencies of vasodepressor prostaglandins and of kinins.

## Treatment

The underlying disorder may well require appropriate therapy in its own right; this is notably so with the systemic connective tissue diseases. In patients who have hypertension accompanying bilateral renal disease, but who do not require regular dialysis for renal impairment, drug therapy may suffice to control the blood pressure. Care should be taken that overzealous blood pressure reduction does not provoke renal failure. ACE inhibitors in particular may effectively control the blood pressure, especially if there is evidence of hypersecretion of renin; however, these drugs are also prone to cause renal failure, notably if given together with aggressive diuretic therapy.

As stated earlier, no patient should proceed to long-term dialysis without the possibility of bilateral renal artery stenosis being excluded.

In patients who are hypertensive and require regular dialysis, blood pressure can usually be controlled by the removal of water and sodium at dialysis, with the addition of antihypertensive drugs as necessary.

Rarely, patients are encountered in whom the intrinsic renal lesion responds to the removal of sodium at dialysis with gross hypersecretion of renin. There is then a resulting marked excess of circulating angiotensin II, with severe and worsening hypertension, raised plasma aldosterone and often intolerable thirst.[4] Formerly, bilateral nephrectomy was required in such patients in order to control the hypertension and other features. Plasma angiotensin II can now be lowered with the use of ACE inhibitors. Care must be taken in introducing these agents, however, because, with a very high plasma angiotensin II concentration, its sudden reduction may lead to severe hypotension.

## Case study

See Case study 13, Appendix 2.

## References

1. Whitworth JA. Renal parenchymal disease and hypertension. In *Handbook of Hypertension*, Vol. 15: *Clinical Hypertension* (ed. JIS Robertson). Amsterdam: Elsevier, 1992: 326–56.
2. Bakris GL, Gavras H. Renin in acute and chronic renal failure: implications for treatment. In *The Renin–Angiotensin System* (eds JIS Robertson and MG Nicholls). London: Gower Medical, 1993: chapter 56.
3. Robertson JIS. Polycystic kidney disease and the renin system. In *The Renin–Angiotensin System* (eds JIS Robertson and MG Nicholls). London: Gower Medical, 1993: chapter 57.
4. Fitzsimons JT. Renin in thirst and sodium appetite. In *The Renin–Angiotensin System* (eds JIS Robertson and MG Nicholls). London: Gower Medical, 1993: chapter 32.
5. Epstein M. Hypertension as a risk factor for progression of chronic renal disease. *Blood Pressure* 1994; **3** (suppl. 1): 23–8.

# 34
# Mineralocorticoid-induced hypertension: The 'escape' phenomenon

Exposure of the organism to excessive quantities or effects of compounds with a mineralocorticoid action consistently produces hypertension (see also Chapters 35 and 36). The accompanying pathophysiology has been studied in detail, and much is known of the mechanisms underlying the raised arterial pressure.[1-3] Even so, several aspects remain uncertain.

## Metabolic effects of mineralocorticoid excess: the 'escape' phenomenon

The critical action of a mineralocorticoid such as aldosterone is to promote, at distal renal tubules, sodium reabsorption in exchange for potassium, magnesium and hydrogen ions. Thus, sodium is retained, while potassium, magnesium and hydrogen are lost. When there is a physiologically inappropriate excess of such a mineralocorticoid (as for example with an aldosterone-secreting tumour), there is consequent elevation of arterial pressure accompanied by sodium retention, hypernatraemia, potassium deficiency, hypokalaemia and extracellular alkalosis.

With such long-term mineralocorticoid excess there is chronic stable expansion of body sodium content (assessed either as total exchangeable or total body sodium), of plasma volume, of extracellular fluid volume, and of total body water, while body potassium content (assessed as total exchangeable or total body potassium) is deficient.

It is emphasized that these alterations in body composition and related hormones are stable; after an initial period of sodium and water retention when the organism is first exposed to mineralocorticoid excess, equilibrium is re-established and the excretion rates of sodium, potassium and water return so as to balance intake. The physiological events that enable the re-establishment of metabolic equilibrium ('mineralocorticoid escape'), have attracted considerable attention and investigation. It seems likely that the interplay of several influences, prominent amongst which are rises in arterial pressure and in plasma atrial natriuretic peptide (ANP), is responsible for the renal escape from mineralocorticoid excess (Figure 34.1). The renin–angiotensin system is markedly suppressed.

Various mechanisms have been invoked to explain the increase of arterial pressure in mineralocorticoid hypertension: a direct vasoconstrictor effect of hypokalaemia, increased plasma vasopressin, a direct action of the mineralocorticoid on vascular smooth muscle, and sodium retention acting either though whole-body autoregulation or by its stimulant effect on a sodium transport inhibitor (pages 28 and 48). These mechanisms are not mutually exclusive. Some of them could be different steps in a sequence linking excess mineralocorticoid and hypertension. It is fairly clear that abnormal sodium retention is one of the necessary components and that hypokalaemia, vasopressin and the direct vascular action of mineralocorticoid are relatively unimportant.

Some of the main varieties of mineralocorticoid-induced hypertension are listed in Table 35.1. Of these, hypertension caused by ingestion of liquorice or carbenoxolone is discussed on page 162.

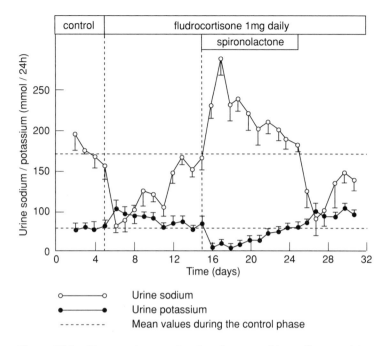

**Figure 34.1.**   Data on six normal male volunteers taking a diet containing constant amounts of sodium and potassium daily for each individual. No treatment for 5 days (control) was followed by oral fludrocortisone 1 mg daily for 27 days. Spironolactone 50–200 mg daily was added on days 16–25. The data are presented as mean $\pm$ SEM for 24-h urinary excretion of sodium and potassium. (Redrawn from Ref. 4, with permission.)

─────────── References ───────────

1. Ferriss JB. Primary hyperaldosteronism: Conn's syndrome and similar disorders. In *Handbook of Hypertension*, Vol. 15: *Clinical Hypertension* (ed. JIS Robertson). Amsterdam: Elsevier, 1992: 357–89.

2. Fraser R. Inborn errors of corticosteroid biosynthesis and metabolism: their effects on electrolyte metabolism. In *Handbook of Hypertension*, Vol. 15: *Clinical Hypertension* (ed. JIS Robertson). Amsterdam: Elsevier, 1992: 420–60.

3. Padfield PL, Edwards CRW. Mineralocorticoid-induced hypertension and the renin-angiotensin system. In: *The Renin–Angiotensin System* (eds JIS Robertson and MG Nicholls). London: Gower Medical, 1993; chapter 63.

4. Nicholls MG, Ramsay LE, Boddy K *et al*. Mineralocorticoid-induced blood pressure, electrolyte, and hormone changes, and reversal with spironolactone, in healthy men. *Metabolism* 1979; **28**: 584–93.

# 35
# Primary aldosterone excess: Conn's syndrome and related disorders

The classic form of mineralocorticoid excess with hypertension is true Conn's syndrome, due to an aldosterone-secreting adenoma of the adrenal cortex. The syndrome can be mimicked by several other conditions which have similarities, affinities and also important differences.[1-3]

## Pathology

A classification of the conditions that will be considered in this section is presented in Table 35.1.

All are characterized by aldosterone excess and low plasma renin.

## Pathophysiology

Aldosterone is a powerful mineralocorticoid secreted by the zona glomerulosa of the adrenal cortex. Its main action is on distal nephrons to promote sodium reabsorption in exchange for potassium and hydrogen ions. Aldosterone secretion is normally regulated principally by the renin–

**Table 35.1.** Classification of mineralocorticoid-induced hypertension

|   |   |
|---|---|
| i) | Conn's syndrome and related disorders: primary aldosterone excess |
|  | True primary hyperaldosteronism |
|  |    Aldosterone-secreting adenoma (Conn's syndrome proper) |
|  |    Aldosterone-secreting carcinoma |
|  |    ?Primary adrenocortical hyperplasia |
|  | Glucocorticoid-remediable hyperaldosteronism |
|  | Idiopathic ('non-tumorous'; 'pseudoprimary') hyperaldosteronism. This is now considered to be part of the continuum of essential hypertension |
| ii) | Ingestion of liquorice, carbenoxolone, or mineralocorticoids |
| iii) | 17-$\alpha$-hydroxylase deficiency |
| iv) | 11-$\beta$-hydroxylase deficiency |
| v) | Idiopathic deoxycorticosterone excess |
| vi) | Carcinoma secreting corticosterone or deoxycorticosterone |
| vii) | 11-$\beta$-hydroxysteroid dehydrogenase deficiency |
| viii) | Liddle's syndrome |

angiotensin system and, therefore, in most physiological and pathophysiological circumstances, plasma renin, angiotensin II and aldosterone levels move in conjunction. By contrast, in the syndromes described herein, largely autonomous aldosterone excess is accompanied by depression of the renin–angiotensin system.

## Conn's syndrome: aldosterone-secreting adrenocortical adenoma

Aldosterone-secreting adrenocortical adenoma is an interesting rarity, probably representing no more than 0.1% of the hypertensive population according to most surveys. By contrast, Gordon and his colleagues have claimed[4] that Conn's syndrome is one of the most prevalent forms of secondary hypertension. This claim, which revives an earlier notion of Conn et al.,[5] remains unsubstantiated. The disease can present at any age, more often in women than in men. Adrenocortical adenoma can be associated with the multiple endocrine neoplasia syndrome type 1 (MEN 1), which characteristically features tumours of the pituitary, parathyroid and pancreas. More often, but still rarely, there has been seen an accompaniment just with parathyroid adenoma. Several patients with both acromegaly and Conn's syndrome have been described.

### Pathology

Most aldosterone-secreting tumours are roughly spherical, of 2 cm or less in diameter (Plate 35.1). They usually project from the adrenal cortex but can be wholly intraglandular. The cut surface is typically golden yellow. The left gland is affected more often than the right. Bilateral tumours are sometimes found. The hypertension is accompanied by hypokalaemia, contraction of body potassium content, extracellular alkalosis, hypernatraemia and expansion of body sodium. If diuretics have been given, muscle weakness, polyuria, nocturia and polydipsia may be present. Most patients, however, are devoid of symptoms.

### Diagnosis

Although low plasma (or serum) potassium concentration usually provides the initial clue, it must be recognized that on occasions this feature may be masked by a low dietary sodium intake, or by the use of fist clenching to aid venepuncture.[6]

Despite the low prevailing plasma renin concentrations, and hence angiotensin II concentrations, aldosterone is typically unresponsive to administered angiotensin II or by stimulating an increase in endogenous angiotensin II by the assumption of the upright posture. These tests have been used as an aid to diagnosis. For example, in a patient with Conn's syndrome a blood sample taken after overnight recumbency will reveal low renin and angiotensin II with high aldosterone. A further sample taken at midday, after the patient has been upright and ambulant, will show little change in renin and angiotensin II, but the plasma aldosterone falls; this contrasts with the rise in renin and angiotensin II and rise (or lack of fall) in aldosterone in those without 'autonomous' aldosterone secretion. Aldosterone in Conn's syndrome appears to track the diurnal fall in ACTH secretion. However, a rare angiotensin II responsive variety has been described (see below).[7]

Once suspected, diagnosis can be further pursued by locating an adrenocortical tumour on computed tomography, adrenal ultrasonography or adrenal scintillation scanning, of which computed tomography is the most sensitive and precise.

Confirmation by bilateral adrenal vein sampling may be undertaken. This will reveal high plasma aldosterone values on the suspect side; at the same procedure, adrenal venography can confirm the presence and location of the adenoma. This test has been largely superseded in recent times by computed tomography; however, it may still be useful in, for example, the presence of bilateral lesions with only one functional tumour.

### Treatment

Pre-operative treatment with a potassium-conserving diuretic (spironolactone up to 300 mg/day or amiloride up to 75 mg/day) will correct the various biochemical abnormalities (apart from aldosterone excess), the distortions of body spaces and lower the raised arterial pressure. The magnitude of blood pressure reduction during 4–6 weeks of treatment with these agents has been taken to predict the subsequent response to surgical removal of the adenoma.

Definitive therapy is surgical excision, best performed via a posterior (loin) approach. Blood pressure returns, after removal of the tumour, to strictly normal age- and sex-matched values in only about 50% of cases, even though operation has corrected the aldosterone excess. Blood pressure reduction tends to be less adequate in patients with renal functional impairment. In the event of persistent elevation of arterial pressure after operation, treatment is as for essential hypertension.

## Angiotensin-responsive adrenocortical adenoma

This variant[7] may be distinguished from true Conn's syndrome by showing a rapid rise in plasma aldosterone in response to either infused angiotensin II or orthostasis, which latter raises plasma renin and angiotensin II. The pathways of aldosterone biosynthesis are believed to be distinct from those of classic Conn's syndrome. As blood pressure may be adequately lowered by excision of the adenoma, it is important to distinguish this variety from non-tumorous aldosterone excess (see later), which does not respond well to adrenal surgery.

## Aldosterone-secreting carcinoma

### Pathology

An aldosterone-secreting carcinoma is most often of adrenocortical origin, but it can also arise in the ovary.

### Clinical features

Aspects additional to those of the more usual Conn's syndrome should raise the possibility of carcinoma. Fever, muscle weakness and a large abdominal or pelvic mass may be alerting features. Excessive secretion of corticosteroids in addition to aldosterone is common, and occasionally the predominant mineralocorticoid may be 11-deoxy-corticosterone or corticosterone (page 204). Prompt surgical excision is indicated.

## Glucocorticoid-remediable hyperaldosteronism

Glucocorticoid-suppressible (-remediable) aldosterone excess, a rare variant of primary aldosterone excess, was first described by Sutherland et al.[8]

In this usually evidently familial form of hyperaldosteronism, the administration of glucocorticoids, such as dexamethasone (2 mg/day), produces a reversal of the abnormalities, usually within 2 weeks. However, as with other secondary forms of hypertension, blood pressure may not fall adequately and the use of higher doses of dexamethasone can lead to problems of steroid excess. Amiloride is considered by some as a more appropriate long term approach to treatment for many patients.

There is evidence of a genetic defect in this condition involving a mutation whereby the 5′ regulatory region of 11-$\beta$-hydroxylase is fused to the coding sequences of aldosterone synthetase on chromosome 8. This unequal crossing over allows the expression of aldosterone synthetase in the zona fasciculata so that aldosterone can then be produced under continuing adrenocorticotrophic hormone (ACTH) control.[3]

As the disease is inherited in an autosomal dominant fashion, other members of the family are likely to be affected. The adrenal cortices usually show bilateral nodular hyperplasia.

The diagnosis is based on the usual criteria for primary hyperaldosteronism, that is, high plasma aldosterone concentration or aldosterone secretion rate, low plasma renin and hypokalaemia, as well as the special criterion for this disease—sustained correction of blood pressure and of biochemical abnormalities by administration of the synthetic glucocorticoid dexamethasone. Dexamethasone suppresses ACTH secretion; aldosterone secretion, which is particularly sensitive to ACTH infusion in this condition, also then falls. The difficulty of assessing the response to dexamethasone makes identification of the abnormal genotype a simpler and more certain means of diagnosis.

## Idiopathic aldosteronism (sometimes termed 'pseudo-primary' aldosterone excess or 'non-tumorous hyperaldosteronism')

This condition, once confused with Conn's syndrome, is now recognized as distinct from it, and is instead believed to be part of the same continuum as essential hypertension. The confusion arose because, in essential hypertension, plasma renin falls progressively with the course of the disease, whereas the aldosterone response to angiotensin II becomes more pronounced. Thus, some patients with essential hypertension, with low renin and rather high aldosterone levels, come increasingly to resemble, at least superficially, true Conn's syndrome. Hypokalaemia, contraction of body potassium, hypernatraemia and expansion of body sodium are all less marked, however, than in patients with aldosterone-secreting adenoma. These quantitative differences have formed the basis of multifactorial statistical tests to differentiate idiopathic aldosteronism from Conn's syndrome. The greatest danger of diagnostic confusion is likely to be with the more recently recognized angiotensin-responsive adrenocortical adenoma.

In patients with idiopathic aldosteronism, specific adrenocortical lesions are wanting, although nodular changes, or widening, of the zona glomerulosa can be found, as in essential hypertension, and may add to the confusion. The response to surgery is usually poor. These cases should be treated medically, including, if appropriate, potassium-conserving diuretics.

## Case study

See Case study 20, Appendix 2.

## References

1. Ferriss JB. Primary hyperaldosteronism: Conn's syndrome and similar disorders. In *Handbook of Hypertension*, Vol. 15: *Clinical Hypertension* (ed. JIS Robertson). Amsterdam: Elsevier, 1992: 357–89.
2. Fraser R. Inborn errors of corticosteroid biosynthesis and metabolism: their effects on electrolyte metabolism. In *Handbook of Hypertension*, Vol. 15: *Clinical Hypertension* (ed. JIS Robertson). Amsterdam: Elsevier, 1992: 420–60.
3. Padfield PL, Edwards CRW. Mineralocorticoid-induced hypertension and the renin-angiotensin system. In: *The Renin–Angiotensin System* (eds JIS Robertson and MG Nicholls). London: Gower Medical, 1993; chapter 63.
4. Gordon RD, Klemm S, Stowasser M *et al.* How common is primary aldosteronism? Is it the most frequent cause of curable hypertension? *Sixth European Meeting on Hypertension*, Milan, 1993; Abstract no. 278.
5. Conn JW, Rovner DR, Cohen EL *et al.* Normokalaemic primary aldosteronism: its masquerade as 'essential' hypertension. *J. Am. Med. Assoc.* 1966; **195**: 21–6.
6. Singh BN, Hollenberg NK, Poole-Wilson PA, Robertson JIS. Diuretic-induced potassium and magnesium deficiency: relation to drug-induced QT prolongation, cardiac arrhythmias and sudden death. *J. Hypertens.* 1992; **10**: 301–16.
7. Gordon RD, Gomez-Sanchez CE, Hamlet SM *et al.* Angiotensin-responsive aldosterone-producing adenoma masquerades as idiopathic hyperaldosteronism (IHA: adrenal hyperplasia) or low-renin essential hypertension. *J. Hypertens.* 1987; **5** (suppl. 5): 103–6.
8. Sutherland DJA, Ruse JL, Laidlaw JC. Hypertension, increased aldosterone secretion and low plasma renin activity relieved by dexamethasone. *Can. Med. Assoc. J.* 1966; **95**: 1109–120.
9. Robertson JIS, Ball SG. Hypertension. In *Diseases of the Heart*, 1st edn (eds DG Julian, AJ Camm, KM Fox *et al.*). London: Baillière Tindall, 1989: 1227–92.

# 36
# Hypertension due to excess of mineralocorticoids other than aldosterone. Liddle's syndrome

In a variety of conditions, hypertension, with suppression of the renin–angiotensin system, results from excess of endogenous or exogenous mineralocorticoids other than aldosterone.[1,2] Nearly always, in this range of conditions, plasma aldosterone concentration is subnormal. In most other respects, the patterns of changes in body spaces, and their relation to the renin–angiotensin system, are closely similar to those described earlier for patients with aldosterone-secreting adenoma. However, in several of these disorders, some of which are rare, the detailed changes are much less fully elucidated than they are in Conn's syndrome.

Hypertension due to exogenous ACTH or corticosteroids, and to ingested liquorice or carbenoxolone, is discussed in Chapter 27.

## 17-α-Hydroxylase deficiency

This very rare hypertensive syndrome is of considerable interest, in particular because of the light it sheds on the role of ACTH in the pathogenesis of hypertension.[2,6]

The basic defect is lack of the enzyme 17-α-hydroxylase, which results in deficiencies of adrenal steroid synthesis. Both androgens and oestrogens are subnormal; thus, genetic males present as pseudohermaphrodites, and females fail to develop secondary sexual characteristics.

Central to the pathogenesis of the hypertension is a deficiency also of cortisol biosynthesis, leading to excess secretion of ACTH and hence to an overproduction of ACTH-dependent mineralocorticoids, notably deoxycorticosterone, 11-hydroxydeoxycorticosterone, corticosterone and 11-hydroxycorticosterone (Figure 36.1, Table 36.1). Sodium is retained and potassium lost; total exchangeable sodium is expanded and exchangeable potassium contracted. Plasma potassium is reduced, plasma sodium tends to be raised, and there is extracellular alkalosis. Plasma renin and angiotensin II fall, and consequently aldosterone levels also are low.

Treatment with dexamethasone lowers the excessive ACTH secretion, the ACTH-dependent mineralocorticoids drop to normal values and blood pressure falls, while renin, angiotensin II and aldosterone rise into the normal range. The sodium and potassium balance is restored, and plasma sodium, potassium and bicarbonate concentrations are corrected.

## 11-β-Hydroxylase deficiency

This congenital defect of the enzyme 11-β-hydroxylase also leads to deficient biosynthesis of cortisol and hence to overproduction of ACTH. Androgen secretion is unimpaired, thus male patients show precocious sexual development, whereas females are virilized. The site of the en-

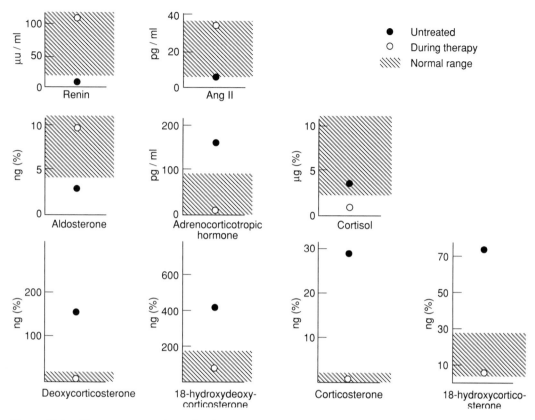

**Figure 36.1.**    Plasma concentrations of renin, angiotensin II (Ang II), adrenocorticotrophic hormone (ACTH), cortisol, deoxycorticosterone, 18-hydroxycorticosterone, corticosterone and 18-hydroxydeoxycorticosterone untreated and during therapy with dexamethasone 0.5 mg twice daily in a patient with 17-α-hydroxylase deficiency (same patient as in Table 36.1). (Redrawn from Ref. 2, with permission, from original data of Ref. 6.)

zymic defect means that secretion rates of both corticosterone and aldosterone are low. Deoxycorticosterone, however, is produced in excess, leading to sodium retention, potassium depletion, hypokalaemia and hypernatraemia, lowering of plasma renin and angiotensin II levels, and hypertension.

In this disease, treatment with dexamethasone corrects the excess of ACTH, lowers the secretion of deoxycorticosterone, restores sodium and potassium balance, returns the suppressed plasma renin and angiotensin II levels into the normal range, and alleviates the hypertension.

## Apparently idiopathic deoxycorticosterone excess

Occasional patients with hypertension and low plasma renin values have been described in whom high circulating levels of the mineralocorticoid deoxycorticosterone were present. Other stigmata of mineralocorticoid excess such as hypokalaemia were usually lacking.

Demonstrable excess of a mineralocorticoid hormone is otherwise unusual in low-renin essential hypertension (page 42).

**Table 36.1.** Plasma sodium, potassium and bicarbonate, exchangeable body sodium and potassium, and blood pressure in a 29-year-old genetic female with 17-$\alpha$-hydroxylase deficiency, untreated and during treatment with dexamethasone 0.5 mg twice daily

|  | Untreated | On dexamethasone (0.5 mg/b.i.d.) |
|---|---|---|
| Sodium (mmol/litre) | 146 | 136 |
| Potassium (mmol/litre) | 2.8 | 4.4 |
| Bicarbonate (mmol/litre) | 32 | 28 |
| Exchangeable sodium |  |  |
| (mmol) | 2801 | 2258 |
| (per kg) | 43.6 | 34.3 |
| Exchangeable potassium |  |  |
| (mmol) | 2110 | 2489 |
| (per kg) | 32.8 | 37.8 |
| Blood pressure (mmHg) | 250/165 | 136/94 |

*Source:* From Ref. 2, from original data of Ref. 6.

## Carcinoma secreting deoxycorticosterone or corticosterone

Rare cases have been reported of patients with carcinoma secreting excessive quantities of deoxycorticosterone or of corticosterone. These patients can show the typical features of mineralocorticoid excess, including hypertension, hypokalaemia, and suppression of the renin–angiotensin system.

## 11-$\beta$-Hydroxysteroid dehydrogenase deficiency (the 'apparent mineralocorticoid excess' syndrome)

With the extremely rare condition of congenital deficiency of the enzyme 11-$\beta$-hydroxysteroid dehydrogenase (11-$\beta$-OHSD) severe hypertension, with the features of mineralocorticoid excess, including suppression of the renin–angiotensin system and low levels of aldosterone, is found.

The enzyme 11-$\beta$-OHSD regulates the conversion of cortisol to cortisone.[2,3] It is known that mineralocorticoids and glucocorticoids have remarkable structural homology and also similar patterns of steroid binding *in vitro*. As the levels of circulating free cortisol are approximately 100-fold higher than those of aldosterone, it is evident that some mechanism is required to prevent the activation of the mineralocorticoid receptor by cortisol. This protection is effected via the local action of 11-$\beta$-OHSD, which converts cortisol to cortisone and thus limits access of active mineralocorticoid to the renal receptor.

Treatment with a glucocorticoid such as dexamethasone, which is not subject to metabolism by renal 11-$\beta$-OHSD, is effective therapy.

The enzyme 11-$\beta$-OHSD is inhibited by glycyrrhetinic acid, a constituent of liquorice and of carbenoxolone. Thus the pathogenesis of the mineralocorticoid hypertension caused by ingestion of these compounds is closely akin to that of congenital 11-$\beta$-OHSD deficiency. Hypertension caused by liquorice or carbenoxolone is discussed further on page 162, Chapter 27.

## Liddle's syndrome

Liddle's syndrome[3,4] has all the clinical and biochemical features of mineralocorticoid hypertension, including sodium retention and hypokalaemia, although no responsible mineralo-corticoid has been identified.

Hypertension does not, in this disorder, respond to treatment with spironolactone but it does to amiloride, implying that there is a tubular transport abnormality in the kidney which is susceptible to amiloride, rather than an excess of a circulating mineralocorticoid substance.[5]

## References

1. Fraser R. Inborn errors of corticosteroid biosynthesis and metabolism: their effects on electrolyte metabolism. In *Handbook of Hypertension*, Vol. 15: *Clinical Hypertension* (ed. JIS Robertson). Amsterdam: Elsevier, 1992: 420–60.

2. Padfield PL, Edwards CRW. Mineralocorticoid-induced hypertension and the renin-angiotensin system. In *The Renin–Angiotensin System* (eds JIS Robertson and MG Nicholls). London: Gower Medical, 1993: chapter 63.

3. Gordon RD, Klemm SA, Tunny TJ. Renin in Liddle's syndrome and in the syndrome of apparent mineralocorticoid excess. In *The Renin–Angiotensin System* (eds JIS Robertson and MG Nicholls). London: Gower Medical, 1993: chapter 66.

4. Gordon RD, Klemm SA, Tunny TJ. Gordon's syndrome and Liddle's syndrome. In *Handbook of Hypertension*, Vol. 15: *Clinical Hypertension* (ed. JIS Robertson). Amsterdam: Elsevier, 1992: 461–93.

5. Botero-Velez M, Curtis JJ, Warnock DG. Brief report: Liddle's syndrome revisited – a disorder of sodium reabsorption in the distal tubule. *N. Engl. J. Med.* 1994; **330**: 178–81.

6. Fraser R, Brown JJ, Mason PA *et al.* Severe hypertension with absent secondary sex characteristics due to partial deficiency of steroid 17α-hydroxylase activity. *J. Hum. Hypertens.* 1987; **1**: 53–8.

# 37
# Cushing's syndrome

Cushing's syndrome results from a prolonged excess of glucocorticoids, notably cortisol. Hypertension, occurring in about 75–85% of patients,[1,2] is a frequent accompaniment of this rather uncommon disease. Untreated, Cushing's syndrome carries a high mortality; thus early diagnosis is important.

## Pathology

The various causes of Cushing's syndrome[2,3] are listed in Table 37.1.

Cushing's disease proper is where the syndrome is caused by an abnormality of the anterior pituitary gland. Such primary pituitary disease or dysfunction of the hypothalamic–pituitary axis accounts for some 70% of all cases.

Excess ACTH or corticotrophin-releasing hormone produced by various other tumours account for about 12% of instances. The most frequent causes of ectopic ACTH secretion are neoplasms, usually malignant, of bronchus, pancreas or thymus. Corticotrophin-releasing hormones can arise in prostate, lung, pancreas or thyroid.

Adrenal tumours occur in about 12% of cases.

Very rare variants include the Carney complex, in which there can be various associated endocrine tumours, myomata, pigmented skin lesions and tumours of peripheral nerves, and where adrenocortical-stimulating immunoglobulins circulate in peripheral blood; the McCune–Albright syndrome, a genetically determined disease in which nodular hyperfunction can occur in various endocrine glands, including the adrenal cortex; and food-dependent stimulation of gastric inhibitory polypeptide (GIP), which then provokes excessive secretion of cortisol from unduly sensitive adrenal cortices.

Iatrogenic Cushing's syndrome, due to the therapeutic administration of ACTH or glucocorticoids, is described on pages 161–162, Chapter 27.

**Table 37.1.** Varieties of Cushing's syndrome

Pituitary-dependent Cushing's syndrome (Cushing's disease proper)
Adrenocortical adenoma
Adrenocortical carcinoma
Ectopic adrenocorticotrophic hormone excess
Exogenous adrenocorticotrophic hormone administration
Carney complex
McCune–Albright syndrome
Food-dependent gastric inhibitory polypeptide stimulation
Exogenous glucocorticoid administration
Ectopic corticotrophin-releasing factor excess
Alcohol-associated pseudo-Cushing's syndrome

Excessive ingestion of alcohol can be associated with a syndrome of Cushingoid appearance with central obesity, plethora, striae and hypertension. The syndrome is said to disappear with abstinence and is of uncertain pathophysiology. It is usually regarded as separate from Cushing's syndrome and has been termed 'alcohol-induced pseudo-Cushing's syndrome' (see pages 31–33). In a detailed review of this topic, Jeffcoate[4] concluded that whilst acute drunkenness and its sequelae could be accompanied by transient excess of corticosteroids, there is little evidence that long-term exposure to alcohol activates the hypothalamic–pituitary–adrenocortical axis or causes cortisol release. In Jeffcoate's view, ethanol rather than cortisol can in these patients be responsible for central adiposity, hypertension, conjunctival injection, myopathy, osteoporosis, thin skin, depression and psychosis.

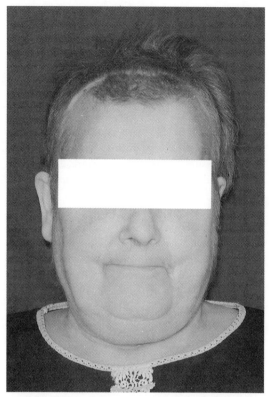

**Figure 37.1.** Patient with Cushing's syndrome showing typical facies. The responsible lesion was an anterior pituitary adenoma which had been removed surgically shortly before this photograph. The craniotomy scar is evident. (Reproduced from Ref. 5, with permission.)

## Clinical features

Hypertension is present in up to 85% of patients with Cushing's syndrome.

Cushing's syndrome may be suspected because of the appearance of the patient (Figure 37.1). There is characteristically a 'moon face', a 'buffalo hump' over the thoracic spine, wasting of muscles and skin, with livid striae in the latter, frequent bruises, and abdominal obesity. Diabetes mellitus is a common complication. There can be osteoporosis with spontaneous fractures. Psychiatric disturbances occur in some 40% of patients. Subjects with ACTH excess secreted from a malignant neoplasm are especially likely to show hypokalaemic alkalosis.

Other frequent features include hirsutism, amenorrhoea or oligomenorrhoea, impotence, proneness to infections, poor wound healing, ankle oedema, headache, polyuria and polydipsia. Virilism and exophthalmos are more rarely found.

Cyclical Cushing's syndrome is considered by some authorities[2] to be more common than was believed earlier; it can cause especial diagnostic problems.

## Pathophysiology of hypertension in Cushing's syndrome

The pathogenesis of hypertension in Cushing's syndrome is not fully elucidated. Various possibilities have been proposed. It is likely that in different forms of the syndrome, and between patients exhibiting the same basic pathology, the several possible pressor mechanisms are variably emphasized, with consequent diversity of pathophysiological and clinical expression.

## Mineralocorticoid effects

Cortisol is a weak mineralocorticoid, and three characteristic features of mineralocorticoid-induced hypertension, expansion of exchangeable body sodium, renin suppression and hypokalaemia, are usually lacking in Cushing's syndrome. Nevertheless, the administration of cortisol, or of ACTH with consequent elevation of plasma cortisol, to normal volunteers raises blood pressure, causes antinatriuresis, expands plasma and extracellular fluid volumes, while depressing renin and elevating atrial natriuretic peptide, at least in the short term.

Potent mineralocorticoids, such as deoxycorticosterone or aldosterone, may also be secreted to excess if Cushing's syndrome is due to an adrenocortical tumour. Alternatively, if the primary pathological lesion produces a long-term surfeit of ACTH, various ACTH-sensitive mineralocorticoids, including deoxycorticosterone and corticosterone (but not aldosterone) can be secreted in large quantities. In these latter circumstances, typical features of mineralocorticoid excess, including expansion of body sodium, suppression of the renin–angiotensin system, hypernatraemia and hypokalaemia, may then be added (see also Chapters 34–36).

## Increased renin substrate (angiotensinogen)

Plasma renin substrate (angiotensinogen) levels rise with cortisol administration and thus can be high in Cushing's syndrome. In the absence of corresponding suppression of plasma renin concentration, plasma angiotensin II will increase and could raise arterial pressure.

However, measurements of plasma renin activity, which should express the net effect of any simultaneous changes in the levels of renin substrate and the enzyme renin, have usually been reported as normal in Cushing's syndrome, although they are sometimes low, and more rarely raised. Thus, elevation of plasma angiotensinogen, although usual, appears not to be a common source of hypertension in Cushing's syndrome.

The therapeutic use of antagonists of the renin–angiotensin system has likewise been accompanied by very varied results.

Given that there will be different patterns of steroid excess in the various forms of Cushing's syndrome, and diverse emphasis on glucocorticoid and mineralocorticoid activity from patient to patient and even from time to time in the same patient, the inconsistency of these findings is hardly unexpected.

## Direct glucocorticoid effects

Various glucocorticoid hormones can have a direct pressor effect without altering sodium metabolism.[6,7] The precise nature of this acute action is unknown but the evidence does not support the theory that the pressor actions of glucocorticoids are a consequence of internal fluid redistribution with plasma volume expansion.

## Increased vascular response to various vasoconstrictors, such as angiotensin II and catecholamines

The possibility that hypertension in Cushing's syndrome is a consequence, at least partly, of increased vascular responsiveness to angiotensin II[8] or catecholamines has been raised, but so far remains inadequately explored.

The variable results of giving inhibitors of the renin–angiotensin system do not indicate that increased response to angiotensin II is a consistent mechanism, if indeed it obtains in occasional cases.

However, some authorities regard the evidence of an enhanced vascular reaction to catecholamines in Cushing's syndrome to be fairly strong.

## Inhibition of prostaglandins

It has been proposed that glucocorticoids could produce hypertension by inhibiting the generation or the effects of prostaglandins and so promoting arterial constriction. Any such mechanism would also imply enhancement of vasoconstriction by agents such as catecholamines or angiotensin II, as discussed earlier.

## Diagnosis

The diagnosis of Cushing's syndrome depends essentially on the demonstration of excessive secretion of cortisol.[2]

The diagnostic difficulties imposed by the not infrequent cyclical variability in the severity of Cushing's syndrome need always to be borne in mind.

### Plasma cortisol assay

The large diurnal and physiological variations in plasma cortisol concentrations make single estimations of limited value. Samples obtained after 2300 h are usually of most diagnostic import.

### Urinary free cortisol

Measurement of urinary free cortisol in a reliable 24-h urine collection can be of considerable value, even though there is some overlap between values found in Cushing's syndrome and the range in normal persons.

### Low-dose dexamethasone suppression test

Suppression of cortisol secretion with the administration of dexamethasone at low dose (0.5 mg 6-hourly for 2 days) is generally more marked in normal subjects than in patients with Cushing's syndrome.

This test can therefore refine the measurement of plasma or of urinary free cortisol described above. Even so, occasional ambiguous cases are still encountered.

### Single-dose dexamethasone suppression test

This is a simplified (and hence less reliable) version of the low-dose dexamethasone suppression test. It consists of the demonstration, in Cushing's syndrome, of a failure of plasma cortisol to fall overnight following a single dose of dexamethasone.

However, up to 25% of control subjects, especially if obese, can show similar failure of cortisol suppression.

### Intravenous dexamethasone test

In cases in which oral dexamethasone testing gives equivocal results, estimation of plasma cortisol concentrations during and after weight-related intravenous dexamethasone infusion can discriminate patients with genuine Cushing's syndrome.

## Determination of the cause of Cushing's syndrome

Once the diagnosis of Cushing's syndrome has been established, the site and nature of the responsible lesion require to be determined, in order that appropriate therapy can be applied.

### Plasma ACTH assay

The availability of a reliable assay for plasma ACTH can greatly facilitate differential diagnosis. Plasma ACTH values are raised if the cause of the disease is hypersecretion of ACTH from a pituitary or ectopic lesion or from administration of exogenous ACTH. A very high ACTH level is particularly suggestive of ectopic, rather than of pituitary, origin. By contrast, plasma ACTH values are low if the causative lesion is an adrenocortical tumour producing an excess of glucocorticoids.

As the demonstration of an undetectable level of ACTH is often clinically important, meticulous attention to detail is needed. Blood should be sampled in the morning, when plasma ACTH is normally high. Later in the day, ACTH is often undetectable in normal subjects because of limitations of current assay methods.

### High-dose dexamethasone suppression test

Dexamethasone 2.0 mg is administered every 6 h for 2 days, and 24-h urinary 17-hydroxycorticosteroids or free cortisol are assayed. Some 40% of patients with ACTH excess of either pituitary or ectopic origin may then show suppression of urinary corticoid excretion, whilst this rarely occurs if the causative lesion lies in the adrenal cortex. This test is less specific than plasma ACTH assay, and it is now obsolescent.

### Metyrapone test

Most patients with pituitary-dependent Cushing's disease will respond with a rise in ACTH if cortisol synthesis is inhibited. Metyrapone inhibits 11-$\beta$-hydroxylase and thus causes a fall in plasma cortisol. Patients with ectopic tumours or primary adrenal lesions show no response. Metyrapone can be given orally or intravenously and the ACTH response measured either directly or by collecting urine over 24 h for assessing excretion rates of precursors of 11-deoxycortisol or 17-oxogenic steroids.

### Corticotrophin-releasing hormone (CRH) test

It has been claimed that the administration of ovine corticotrophin-releasing hormone (CRH) can distinguish true Cushing's disease, that is, originating in an anterior pituitary lesion, from other forms of ACTH excess. According to this view, patients with an anterior pituitary lesion respond to CRH with a further rise in ACTH and cortisol, while other Cushingoid cases do not. However, some workers have emphasized limitations of this test.

## — Anatomical localization of the lesion —

### Computer-assisted tomography

Computer-assisted tomography (CT scanning) can detect lesions as small as 1 cm in diameter, is now well-established in the identification and delineation of pituitary and adrenal tumours, and has substantially replaced arteriography and pneumoencephalography. It is current practice to perform CT scans of pituitary, chest and abdomen in all ACTH-dependent cases of Cushing's syndrome.

Close attention to the possible existence of small neoplasms in lung or pancreas is mandatory. It should also be noted that small lucent pituitary defects are not rare in endocrinologically normal subjects, whilst conversely ACTH-secreting adenomata are often also small.

### Magnetic resonance imaging

This approach has so far had limited application in Cushing's syndrome, but offers obvious promise.

### Scintigraphy

Adrenocortical scintigraphy with radiolabelled cholesterol compounds can identify an adrenocortical tumour and also partly quantify the extent of adrenal dysfunction.

### Ultrasound

Adrenocortical lesions may be identified non-invasively by ultrasound. The limit of resolution is about 3 cm.

### Regional venous sampling

Sampling from veins at various sites, with plasma ACTH assay, has been used to help localize a source of ectopic ACTH secretion.

### Bilateral inferior petrosal sinus sampling

A particular development of regional venous sampling is the use of selective catheterization of the inferior petrosal sinus for the determination of ACTH concentration in diagnosis.[2] The need for sampling higher than the level of the jugular bulb is crucial, since blood taken from the jugular bulb is mixed with blood drained from various other regions of the brain.

In experienced hands this method can reliably detect the presence of pituitary lesions responsible for excessive ACTH secretion. The requirement always for bilateral petrosal sampling has been emphasized.[2]

## Treatment

Successful therapy should ideally relieve all the features of Cushing's syndrome, leaving the hypothalamic–pituitary axis intact, and without the need for steroid replacement or other drug treatment.

Inevitably, these therapeutic ideals are not always achieved.

## Pituitary Cushing's syndrome (Cushing's disease proper)

### Surgery of pituitary gland

Pituitary tumours responsible for Cushing's syndrome may be resected surgically, via either a trans-sphenoidal or trans-frontal (Figure 37.1) approach. With the advent of the dissecting microscope, trans-sphenoidal microsurgery has become the favoured method. In the absence of a large or invasive tumour necessitating near total hypophysectomy, the objective is to correct hyperfunction without causing local damage or a long-term endocrine defect. In occasional patients with Cushing's disease proper (Cushing's syndrome of pituitary origin), cure has been achieved by hypophysectomy even when no pituitary tumour has been found.

### Irradiation

Pituitary tumours may be irradiated externally, usually with conventional external cobalt. α-Particle and proton beam irradiation have also been employed. External irradiation is less effective in adults than in children.

An alternative approach is radiation by implantation, for example with yttrium-90 or gold-198. This method is decreasing in popularity because of a slow onset of action and a low cure rate.

Irradiation, which can be combined with drug treatment (see below), is now largely reserved for patients with recurrent pituitary tumour following pituitary surgery.

### Drug therapy

The administration of either bromocriptine or cyproheptadine may suppress excessive pituitary ACTH secretion, but the effect of these drugs is usually only temporary. Alternatively, agents suppressing adrenocortical steroid synthesis, such as mitotane, metyrapone, aminoglutethimide, keto-conazole or trilostane have been employed, often in conjunction with external irradiation.

### Adrenal surgery

Although bilateral adrenalectomy can relieve the features of Cushing's syndrome of pituitary origin, the subsequent appearance or the progressive enlargement of a pituitary tumour, with grossly excessive ACTH output in some 40% of patients and frequent skin pigmentation (Nelson's syndrome), makes this an unattractive procedure. Life-long steroid replacement therapy is also needed.

## Adrenal Cushing's syndrome

### Surgery

When the primary pathology, be it adenoma or carcinoma, arises in the adrenal gland, surgical excision is required.

### Drug treatment

Agents that interfere with corticosteroid biosynthesis (such as mitotane, metyrapone, aminoglutethimide, ketoconazole and trilostane mentioned above) can be employed as supportive therapy.

## Ectopic ACTH secretion

Cushing's syndrome resulting from ectopic ACTH secretion is often the result of a carcinoma arising in some distant tissue, most often bronchus, pancreas or thymus. Excision or irradiation of the primary lesion, which usually requires therapy in its own right, is necessary.

Such measures are often inadequate, and adrenal surgery, or the administration of drugs inhibiting corticosteroid biosynthesis, may then be also needed to alleviate the accompanying features of Cushing's syndrome.

―――――――――― Prognosis ――――――――――

It will be evident from the diversity of abnormalities that can cause Cushing's syndrome that the efficacy of therapy in correcting glucocorticoid excess and its consequences will vary widely.

Even when the biochemical abnormalities are fully corrected, Cushing's syndrome conforms to the general rule that, in secondary hypertension, removal or correction of the primary lesion restores blood pressure to age- and sex-adjusted normal values in only a proportion of cases. The approach to treatment of residual hypertension is as that for essential hypertension.

## Glucocorticoid resistance and hypertension

A very rare abnormality has been described in which hypertension is associated with glucocorticoid resistance.[1] In the original account, a father and son were found to have hypertension with low plasma renin, low aldosterone and hypokalaemia. There were no clinical features of Cushing's syndrome, although cortisol secretion rate and plasma cortisol were high.

This appears to be an ACTH-driven phenomenon, with consequent high levels of deoxycorticosterone and corticosterone causing mineralocorticoid hypertension. High-dose dexamethasone (3 mg daily) is an effective therapy.

## References

1. Padfield PL, Edwards CRW. Mineralocorticoid-induced hypertension and the renin-angiotensin system. In: *The Renin–Angiotensin System*, (eds JIS Robertson and MG Nicholls). London: Gower Medical, 1993; chapter 63.
2. Atkinson AB. Cushing's syndrome. In *Handbook of Hypertension*, Vol. 15: *Clinical Hypertension* (ed. JIS Robertson). Amsterdam: Elsevier, 1992: 390–419.
3. Bertagna X. New causes of Cushing's syndrome. *N. Engl. J. Med.* 1992; **327**: 1024–5.
4. Jeffcoate W. Alcohol-induced pseudo-Cushing's syndrome. *Lancet* 1993; **341**: 676–7.
5. Robertson JIS, Ball SG. Hypertension. In *Diseases of the Heart*, 1st edn (eds DG Julian, AJ Camm, KM Fox *et al.*). London: Baillière Tindall, 1989: 1227–92.
6. Whitworth JA. Mechanisms of glucocorticoid-induced hypertension. *Kidney Int.* 1987; **31**: 1213–4.
7. Whitworth JA. Studies on the mechanisms of glucocorticoid hypertension in humans. *Blood Pressure* 1994; **3**: 24–32.
8. Sato A, Suzuki H, Murakami M *et al.* Glucocorticoid increases angiotensin II type 1 receptor and its gene expression. *Hypertension* 1994; **23**: 25–30.

# 38
# Adrenal medullary disorders: Phaeochromocytoma

Phaeochromocytoma[1,2] is a rare cause of hypertension.

## Pathology

### Non-malignant phaeochromocytoma

The term phaeochromocytoma denotes, strictly, a tumour of neural crest ectodermal origin with an affinity for chromium salts. Chromaffin cells form the adrenal medulla. They are also distributed adjacent to sympathetic ganglia and nerves, especially in association with nerve plexuses, and are found in the organ of Zuckerkandl, a fetal structure lying anterior to the abdominal aorta near the origin of the inferior mesenteric artery.

Phaeochromocytomas are tumours of the chromaffin cells, and although the majority lie in the adrenal medulla, they may also be widely distributed at other sites where chromaffin cells occur, such as the organ of Zuckerkandl, adjacent to sympathetic ganglia and, less often, in apposition to sympathetic nerve plexuses in the neck, chest, urinary bladder, rectum, testes or ovaries.

More than 97% of all phaeochromocytomas lie within the abdomen. Over 90% arise in the adrenal glands, the right being affected more than the left; 10% of these adrenal tumours are bilateral.

### Malignant phaeochromocytoma

Malignant phaeochromocytomas are rare, and difficult to identify as such histologically, even though some ultrastructural and microscopic findings may provide supportive evidence of malignancy. The diagnosis therefore depends on the discovery of metastases. The occurrence of multiple tumours and local invasion by benign phaeochromocytoma further confounds confirmation of malignancy.

Increased plasma levels of neurone-specific enolase (NSE) have been reported in the presence of malignancy.

### Familial phaeochromocytoma

In some 10% of all cases, phaeochromocytoma is familial, inherited as a dominant trait with a high degree of penetrance. Diagnosis is often made earlier than in sporadic cases, usually before the age of 40 years. Bilateral adrenal tumours are found in 10% of these patients.

More than half of the cases of familial phaeochromocytomas are not associated with evidence of other endocrine gland involvement. In the remainder, there are concomitant tumours that may afflict the parathyroid and thyroid (multiple endocrine neoplasia, 'MEN', type 2). The medullary thyroid carcinoma characteristic of 'MEN' type 2 can be highly malignant, invading locally as well as metastasizing.

The MEN-2 syndrome may occur sporadically. The MEN-2 gene has been localized to chromosome 10 though the precise genetic mechanism is not known. The phaeochromocytomas are usually bilateral though this may not be apparent at presentation.

### Catecholamine-induced cardiomyopathy

Excessive secretion of catecholamines can cause multiple necroses of ventricular myocardial cells and thus lead to cardiac failure or arrhythmias.

A diagnostic label of 'idiopathic cardiomyopathy' should therefore not be given without excluding the rare possibility of phaeochromocytoma. The condition is reversible in some patients.

### Other associations

Five per cent of phaeochromocytomas are associated with neurofibromatosis, although 1% of patients with neurofibromatosis have phaeochromocytoma. Familial phaeochromocytoma is not especially associated with neurofibromatosis. There is a rare association of phaeochromocytoma with von Hippel–Lindau disease.

### Adrenal medullary hyperplasia

Catecholamine excess can sometimes be due to adrenal medullary hyperplasia in the absence of a phaeochromocytoma.

--------------- Pathophysiology ---------------

### Secretion of catecholamines

Phaeochromocytomas can secrete excessive quantities of noradrenaline and adrenaline, together with the catecholamine precursors dopamine and dopa. Noradrenaline is the hormone predominantly released, and seems to be ubiquitous in non-familial phaeochromocytomas. Adrenaline is secreted by a smaller proportion of cases and rarely, if ever, alone; adrenaline-secreting tumours occur only occasionally outside the adrenal gland.

### Secretion of other hormones

Primitive cells of neural crest origin may populate a range of endocrine and other tissues, and can elaborate various hormones and hormone precursors. Thus, neuroendocrine tumours can secrete

adrenocorticotrophic hormone (ACTH), melanin-stimulating hormone, encephalin, calcitonin, somatostatin, vasoactive intestinal peptide, neuropeptide-Y or serotonin in conjunction with catecholamines.

--------------- Clinical features ---------------

The clinical features of phaeochromocytoma result principally from the release of catecholamines, either continuously or paroxysmally, into the circulation. Hypertension is the aspect most likely, but by no means exclusively, to bring the patient to investigation. The elevation of arterial pressure can be intermittent or sustained, or episodes of severe hypertension may be superimposed on a background of continuously elevated blood pressure. The pattern of circulatory disturbance varies with the type of underlying catecholamine excess.

Noradrenaline causes peripheral vasoconstriction, elevation of both systolic and diastolic pressures, and reflex bradycardia; adrenaline raises systolic pressure, lowers the diastolic pressure and increases heart rate. Postural hypotension is a feature in some patients. Hypotension can also occasionally follow a paroxysm in which noradrenaline has been predominantly released.

Other clinical manifestations are protean, especially given the range of hormones additional to catecholamines that may be secreted, and thus a wide variety of conditions can simulate phaeochromocytoma (Table 38.1). The diagnosis is held to be particularly likely in a thin hypertensive patient who experiences paroxysmal severe throbbing headache, marked sweating, palpitations and a sense of impending doom. Any such subject should be referred to a physician promptly.

--------------- Diagnosis ---------------

### Hormone assay

Diagnosis is furthered by demonstrating an excess of catecholamines and/or catecholamine metabo-

**Table 38.1.** Manifestations of phaeochromocytoma and conditions simulating or associated with the disease

*Manifestations:*
  Headache
  Palpitation
  Anxiety
  Sweating
  Tremor
  Weight loss
  Nausea
  Abdominal/chest pain
  Vomiting
  Constipation
  Polyuria/polydipsia
  Heat intolerance
  Thyroid swelling
  Cold extremities
  Raynaud's phenomenon
  Hypertension (sustained ± paroxysms or intermittent)
  Orthostatic hypotension
  Paradoxical response of blood pressure to $\beta$-blockers
  Tachycardia
  Bradycardia
  Arrhythmias
  Pallor
  Flushing
  Ashen cyanosis
  Glycosuria
  Fever
  Retinopathy and other complications of hypertension, e.g. stroke, cardiac failure, renal failure

*Conditions simulating:*
  Anxiety
  Hypoglycaemia
  Diabetes
  Migraine
  Thyrotoxicosis
  Bacterial endocarditis
  Menopause
  Eclampsia
  Carcinoid syndrome
  Porphyria

*Important associations:*
  Multiple endocrine neoplasia
  von Hippel–Lindau disease
  Cardiomyopathy
  Neurofibromatosis

lites in the urine, or of catecholamines in plasma. The methods available, and the relevant normal ranges, will obviously vary considerably among centres.

Valuable, but not infallible, guidance is obtained by finding an excess of urinary noradrenaline, adrenaline, and of the metabolites vanilmandelic acid (VMA) and normetanephrine. It is important to recognize that drugs such as methyldopa, L-dopa, labetalol and phenothiazines can interfere with some methods used for assaying urinary normetanephrine. Moreover, various phenolic acids in addition to VMA appear in the urine, often derived from dietary components such as coffee, tea, bananas, chocolate, vanilla and citrus fruits, and also from aspirin.

The development of improved assays for plasma and urinary catecholamines in recent years has increasingly displaced measurements of urinary metabolites. Impressive diagnostic information has been obtained via assay of plasma or urine noradrenaline and, less often, of adrenaline. The concentrations of catecholamines or of metabolites in urine reflect those in the circulation in most circumstances, an exception being a phaeochromocytoma situated in the bladder.

## Clonidine suppression test

Refinement has come with the clonidine suppression test. In this, the $\alpha$-adrenergic agonist clonidine (300 $\mu$g) is administered, and blood samples are drawn 1, 2 and 3 h later for catecholamine assay. Clonidine suppresses sympathetic activity, and so reduces plasma levels of noradrenaline in normal subjects and in patients with essential hypertension. However, no such lowering of plasma noradrenaline is observed after clonidine administration in patients with phaeochromocytoma (interestingly, clonidine can suppress catecholamine release associated with autonomic epilepsy; page 219). This test has been further improved by giving clonidine before retiring at night and making an overnight urine collection for adrenaline and noradrenaline assay. As sympathetic activity is normally low during the night, this allows excellent separation of catecholamine secretion from a tumour from that of normal production. There is the additional advantage that methods for measuring the usually high amounts in urine are easier than plasma assays.

### Provocative tests

Modern biochemical methods have largely eliminated the use of earlier pharmacological tests based on either the response to a catecholamine-releasing agent, such as histamine, tyramine or glucagon, or the hypertensive reaction to phentolamine. Such procedures are not consistently reliable and can be dangerous.

## ——— Localization of the tumour ———

### Computer-assisted tomography

Once phaeochromocytoma is diagnosed, it is necessary to localize the tumour as a prelude to surgery. The advent of computer-assisted tomography (CT) has greatly facilitated detection. This method can reliably identify lesions as small as 1 cm in diameter, and probably less (Figure 38.1). Computer tomography is best suited to the detailed scanning of a selected region under suspicion; it is less practicable to apply the technique, with its high resolution, to a wide area. However, as 97% of phaeochromocytomas lie within the abdomen and 90% in the adrenal glands, a scan is likely to find most tumours.

### Ultrasound

Ultrasound is a simple and safe method capable of detecting tumours as small as 3 cm in diameter (Figure 38.2). However, a negative scan is unhelpful. Further, most clinicians would like reassurance that, despite the certain presence of a tumour in one adrenal gland, there is not also a second, smaller, lesion on the opposite side.

### Magnetic resonance imaging

This technique allows good tissue contrast and may enable distinction from adrenocortical neoplasms and of metastases.

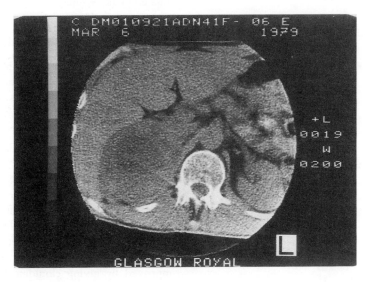

**Figure 38.1.** Computed tomography showing an 8.1 × 9.1 cm mass in the region of the right adrenal gland and indenting the liver. (Reproduced from Ref. 1, with permission.)

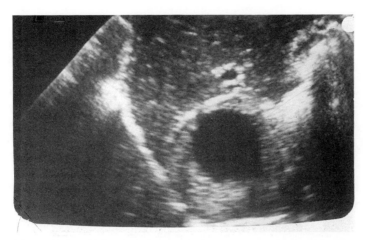

**Figure 38.2.** Abdominal ultrasound showing a mass 8 cm in diameter thought to be a phaeochromocytoma with central necrosis lying above the right kidney. (Reproduced from Ref. 1, with permission.)

In pregnant women suspected of harbouring a phaeochromocytoma this method can offer an attractive alternative to computer tomographic scanning.

### Regional venous sampling

Sampling of blood at various sites in the vena cava, with catecholamine measurement, may be especially useful in identifying the territory in which a phaeochromocytoma lies, if outwith the adrenal glands.

### Scintigraphy

Scintigraphic images using [$^{133}$I]metaiodobenzylguanidine have been obtained with both intra- and extra-adrenal lesions.

Few centres use this technique routinely, though it may help when tumours are multiple and when lesions are outside the adrenal gland.

### Arteriography

Arteriography is a sensitive method for the localization of phaeochromocytoma (Figures 38.3 and 38.4), but its value even in difficult cases has been largely supplanted by computer tomography.

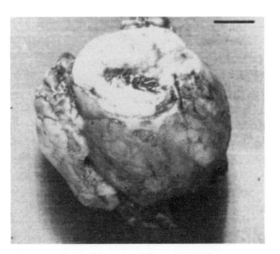

**Figure 38.3.** A spherical phaeochromocytoma removed at operation. Bar = 1 cm. (Reproduced from Ref. 1, with permission.)

Moreover, the injection of contrast material can provoke catecholamine release and a hypertensive crisis. This approach should not therefore be made until the patient is fully controlled medically with both $\alpha$- and $\beta$-antagonists. Even so, marked rises in blood pressure can still occur, and nitroprusside for infusion should be available.

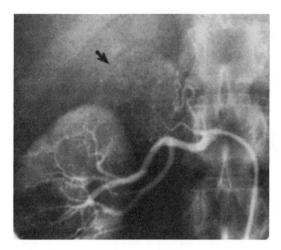

**Figure 38.4.**   Tumour of Figure 38.3 seen on arteriography pre-operatively, lying above right kidney. (Reproduced from Ref. 1, with permission.)

--------- Treatment ---------

The great majority of phaeochromocytomas are amenable to resection. Nevertheless, full medical control is a mandatory prelude to surgery, and it is also required in patients who have metastasizing, inoperable or recurrent tumours.

### Medical treatment

Medical therapy is based on the administration of both $\alpha$- and $\beta$-adrenergic-blocking drugs in order to antagonize the effects of excess catecholamines at various sites. Full $\alpha$-adrenergic blockade is advisable before $\beta$-blockers are administered, so as to limit the risk of hypertensive crises that might otherwise occur.

The non-competitive ('insurmountable') $\alpha$-antagonist phenoxybenzamine is traditionally given, once the diagnosis is seriously entertained, because its use will be unlikely to compromise modern diagnostic biochemical procedures. Phenoxybenzamine should be administered orally, starting at 10 mg/day, and proceeding to the maximum tolerated dose, which usually lies between 20 and

40 mg/day. The drug is best given in divided doses with food, because various gastrointestinal disturbances are common side-effects, and in this way they may be lessened.

The non-selective $\alpha$-antagonist phentolamine has a shorter duration of action than phenoxybenzamine; it can also cause gastrointestinal upsets. Phentolamine, either by mouth or intravenously, has been given as supportive therapy to phenoxybenzamine.

The competitive $\alpha$-antagonists, such as prazosin or indoramin have also been used. Large doses may be needed and first-dose hypotension can be a problem.

Once $\alpha$-adrenergic antagonism is fully established, a non-selective $\beta$-blocker, such as propranolol, is given to control tachycardia and to minimize the risk of arrhythmias. Patients with cardiac failure not consequent upon hypertension may respond adversely to $\beta$-blockade, and caution is needed in these circumstances.

The combined $\alpha$- and $\beta$-antagonist labetalol has been successfully used in the pre-operative control of patients with phaeochromocytoma. However, the $\beta$-adrenergic antagonism of this drug predominates over its $\alpha$-antagonism, which is not the most appropriate balance.

In some patients, the maximum tolerated doses of $\alpha$- and $\beta$-adrenergic antagonists may be inadequate to control hypertension and/or cardiac arrhythmias, especially if massive quantities of catecholamines are released paroxysmally. In such patients, the drug $\alpha$-methylparatyrosine, an inhibitor of the enzyme tyrosine hydroxylase and thus an agent limiting catecholamine biosynthesis at the stage of conversion of tyrosine to dopa, has successfully been employed.

### Operation for phaeochromocytoma

Patients coming to surgery should be fully controlled with medical therapy as outlined. However, further gross release of catecholamines with hypertension can still occur at operation. Intra-arterial pressure monitoring is mandatory, and the anaesthetist should be prepared to manage hypertensive crises by the intravenous administration as necessary of sodium nitroprusside (page 151), which, although a non-specific agent, has been successfully used to control hypertension at operation.

Blood pressure may fall precipitously at the time the tumour is isolated from the circulation.

## Prognosis

Sustained hypertension following removal of a phaeochromocytoma may occur. Provided excision of all tumorous tissue has been achieved and catecholamine output has returned to normal, treatment thereafter is as that for essential hypertension.

Because of the difficulties of determining which tumours are malignant, with metastases dormant for years, long-term follow-up is recommended.

## Phaeochromocytoma in Pregnancy

The presence of phaeochromocytoma complicating pregnancy poses severe problems of diagnosis and management (see also page 255). In the first two trimesters, medical preparation and surgery are generally favoured, whereas in the third trimester medical treatment with combined Caesarian section and tumour removal may be appropriate. Individual circumstances vary widely. The safety of the mother has to be weighed against the viability of the fetus. The combined $\alpha$- and $\beta$-blocker labetalol and a range of other $\beta$-blockers have been extensively used in hypertensive pregnant patients without detectable adverse fetal effects and therefore they are suitable drugs to be used in the treatment of a pregnant woman with phaeochromocytoma. Experience with phenoxybenzamine is more limited. Concerns about adverse drug effects and irradiation accompanying diagnostic procedures recede after the early developmental phase.

## Autonomic epilepsy

Autonomic epilepsy has been described as occasionally accompanied by paroxysmal rises of plasma catecholamines, with hypertension and tachycardia.[3] Clonidine therapy was partially effective.

## Case study

See Case study 19, Appendix 2.

## References

1. Hall AS, Ball SG. Pheochromocytoma. In *Handbook of Hypertension*, Vol. 15: *Clinical Hypertension* (ed. JIS Robertson). Amsterdam: Elsevier, 1992: 494–544.
2. Robertson JIS. Pheochromocytoma and the renin system. In *The Renin–Angiotensin System* (eds JIS Robertson and MG Nicholls). London: Gower Medical, 1993: chapter 67.
3. Metz SA, Halter JB, Porte D *et al*. Autonomic epilepsy: clonidine blockade of paroxysmal catecholamine release and flushing. *Ann. Intern. Med.* 1978; **88**: 189–93.

# 39
# Acromegaly

Acromegaly is the result of excessive production of growth hormone in an adult subject.[1]

## Pathology

The usual cause of acromegaly is a tumour of the anterior pituitary gland producing an excess of the peptide growth hormone. Additionally, ectopic production of growth hormone can occur with tumours of the bronchus, breast or ovary. Acromegaly may comprise part of the multiple endocrine neoplasia ('MEN') type 1 syndrome, in which there are tumours afflicting the pituitary, parathyroid glands and pancreatic islets.

## Pathophysiology

Growth hormone has direct effects on target tissues, and indirect effects mediated by the generation of various low molecular weight growth factors, the somatomedins.

Long-term exposure to excess of circulating growth hormone leads to a series of mainly anabolic reactions and to diabetogenic effects.

Growth hormone has been implicated in the cardiac and vascular hypertrophy of hypertension. The marked excess of pituitary growth hormone characteristic of acromegaly has been thought to be responsible for the high prevalence of cardiovascular complications in this disease (see below).

## Clinical features

Acromegalic subjects have a distinctive facial appearance, with broadening of the nose, protrusion of the lower jaw, prominent lips, and thickened, coarse skin (Figure 39.1). The hands and feet

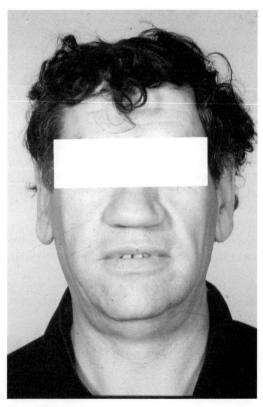

**Figure 39.1.** Patient with acromegaly showing typical facies. (Reproduced from Ref. 3, with permission.)

are enlarged, with an excess of soft tissue. Patients often report an increase in their required size of gloves and shoes, and that rings are difficult to put on or remove. These features result from bony enlargement together with an increase in interstitial oedema fluid rich in hyaluronates. Awareness of a change in appearance by the patient or relatives, or recognition of the characteristic features when seeking advice for other problems often lead to diagnosis.

Additional symptoms include excessive sweating, headache, lethargy, weakness, paraesthesiae, impotence or menstrual irregularities. Arthritis can develop in an unusual site because of degenerative changes in the hyperplastic articular cartilage.

Radiology can reveal a lower jaw prominence, big paranasal sinuses, tufting of terminal phalanges, and enlargement of the heart and abdominal viscera.

In addition to these consequences of growth hormone excess, there can be features directly consequent on the physical presence of an expanding pituitary tumour. These include headache, contraction of visual fields and diplopia. Compression of normal pituitary tissue can produce hypopituitarism.

––––––––––––– Hypertension –––––––––––––

Accurate estimates of the prevalence of hypertension in acromegaly are difficult to make because of varied definitions of 'hypertension' and of methods of blood pressure measurement. However, raised arterial pressure is certainly frequent in association with acromegaly, and possibly affects between 20 and 50% of patients; Davies et al., in a detailed review,[1] give an average figure of 35%.

An important pathogenic influence could be growth hormone-stimulated hypertrophy of arterial smooth muscle and hence elevated peripheral resistance and rapid worsening of hypertension (see also Chapter 19). Moreover, cardiomegaly, cardiac failure and arterial disease are probably disproportionately prominent, even

allowing for the increased prevalence of hypertension, in part because of associated acromegalic myocardial hypertrophy, cardiomyopathy or diabetes mellitus.

Various renal effects of growth hormone have been reported and could contribute to the elevation of arterial pressure, although many of the studies are imperfectly controlled; they have been reviewed in detail by Davies et al.[1] Administration of growth hormone can cause sodium and water retention variously in normal, adrenalectomized, and hypophysectomized animals and man. Acromegalics show, consistently, marked elevation of body sodium, nitrogen, chloride, phosphorus and calcium.[1] Body potassium content is also, it should be emphasized, increased, in contrast to classical forms of mineralocorticoid excess where it is low (Chapters 34–36). Plasma and extracellular fluid volumes and plasma ouabain (page 48) are consistently raised in acromegaly. These changes correlate with growth hormone levels and are corrected when treatment reduces growth hormone secretion.

Such an abnormal sodium-fluid status should have predictable effects both on the basal activity of the renin–angiotensin system and on its sensitivity to various stimuli. Thus, plasma renin might be expected to be severely suppressed, and the response to upright posture or to moderate sodium depletion might be expected to be blunted, compared with normal. Similarly, plasma aldosterone concentration or aldosterone secretion rate should be subnormal in acromegaly, since aldosterone biosynthesis is largely controlled by the renin–angiotensin system and responses to agonists such as angiotensin II or ACTH should be attenuated.[2]

In fact, the situation in acromegaly is less clear-cut, in part because of the inadequacies of control series. The heterogeneity of patient groups in respect of age, stage of disease and treatment make interpretation and comparison between reports difficult. However, it is probably valid to conclude that, although basal plasma renin levels are usually low or low–normal in acromegaly, they are not as suppressed as would be expected from the concurrent sodium and potassium status, nor is there any obvious relationship between the degree of suppression of the renin–angiotensin system and the severity of hypertension.[1,2]

Aldosterone levels are normal or slightly suppressed, but show subnormal responses to dietary sodium restriction, diuretic use, upright posture and ACTH administration. In a few cases, high plasma aldosterone concentrations in acromegaly have been due to a coexisting aldosterone-secreting adenoma (Chapter 35).

A surprising, and probably very relevant, finding is that plasma atrial natriuretic peptide (ANP) concentrations are, despite the sodium retention, normal in acromegaly. The renal and hypotensive responses to exogenous ANP are greater in active acromegaly. Davies et al.[1] have speculated on likely reasons for the lack of rise in plasma ANP in acromegaly despite the sodium and water retention. Among possible explanations are that acromegalic atrial hypertrophy may modify atrial compliance, with consequent alterations in the effects of transmural pressure or atrial stretch, or that growth hormone may modify parasympathetic and sympathetic tone, all with consequent impairment of ANP release. The lack of the expected rise of ANP in acromegaly could well be one factor mediating hypertension (see also page 44).

In summary, the long-term pressor mechanisms in acromegaly are complex and imperfectly elucidated. Acromegaly does not conform to the classic pattern of mineralocorticoid-induced hypertension.[1,2]

--------------------- Diagnosis ---------------------

The diagnosis of acromegaly can be made by observation of the clinical and radiological features described above. Confirmation is by demonstrating an excess of plasma growth hormone which is not diminished by a glucose load; during a standard glucose tolerance test, growth hormone should normally fall to a plasma concentration below 4 milliunits/litre (2 ng/ml).

High-resolution computed tomography identifies the pituitary tumour and reveals its extent.

--------------------- Treatment ---------------------

The pituitary tumour may be removed surgically or irradiated. The drug bromocriptine has also been given to suppress growth hormone secretion, and it can sometimes reduce tumour size. However, values of plasma growth hormone during bromocriptine treatment, although lowered, remain generally higher than after surgery or irradiation. Long-acting analogues of somatostatin can also be used.

--------------------- Prognosis ---------------------

The general tenet that following correction of a condition responsible for secondary hypertension, blood pressure returns to age- and sex-matched normal values in only a proportion of cases, is well-illustrated by acromegaly, in which blood pressure frequently remains high following therapy to the pituitary tumour, even though there is subsequent correction of plasma growth hormone concentrations and of body sodium content.

Treatment of hypertension thereafter is with antihypertensive drugs as in essential hypertension, and should be particularly thorough in view of the high prevalence of hypertension-associated cardiomegaly, cardiac failure and arterial atheroma in this condition.

--------------------- References ---------------------

1. Davies DL, Connell JMC, Reid R et al. Acromegaly: the effects of growth hormone on blood vessels, sodium homeostasis and blood pressure. In Handbook of Hypertension, Vol. 15: Clinical Hypertension (ed. JIS Robertson). Amsterdam: Elsevier, 1992: 545–75.

2. Padfield PL, Edwards CRW. Mineralocorticoid-induced hypertension and the renin-angiotensin system. In: *The Renin–Angiotensin System* (eds JIS Robertson and MG Nicholls). London: Gower Medical, 1993; chapter 63.

3. Robertson JIS, Ball SG. Hypertension. In *Diseases of the Heart*, 1st edn (eds DG Julian, AJ Camm, KM Fox *et al.*). London: Baillière Tindall, 1989: 1227–92.

# 40
# Gordon's syndrome

Gordon's syndrome is a rare condition characterized by hypertension, hyperkalaemia and acidosis in the absence of renal failure.[1,2] Glomerular filtration rate is normal, an unusual feature of syndromes of hyperkalaemia. It has been proposed that the basic defect is a congenital abnormality of renal tubular function leading to sodium retention and hypervolaemia. An alternative suggestion is that atrial natriuretic peptide (ANP) (page 44) is insufficiently responsive and hence subnormal; and/or that there may be resistance to ANP. Plasma concentrations of renin and angiotensin II are depressed in Gordon's syndrome, although aldosterone levels may be normal. Associated, albeit inconsistent, features can include short stature, hypoplastic upper lateral incisor teeth, cardiac valve lesions and intellectual impairment. The condition may be familial, although any genetic basis is not elucidated.

Recognition of this rarity is clinically important because the hypertension and biochemical abnormalities can readily be corrected by treatment with a thiazide diuretic, or by dietary sodium restriction, or by a combination of the two.

## References

1. Gordon RD, Klemm SA, Tunny TJ. Renin in Gordon's syndrome. In *The Renin–Angiotensin System* (eds JIS Robertson and MG Nicholls). London: Gower Medical, 1993: chapter 65.
2. Gordon RD, Klemm SA, Tunny TJ. Gordon's syndrome and Liddle's syndrome. In *Handbook of Hypertension*, Vol. 15: *Clinical Hypertension* (ed. JIS Robertson). Amsterdam: Elsevier, 1992: 461–93.

# 41
# Thyroid disease and hypertension

## Hypothyroidism

High blood pressure is roughly twice as prevalent in patients with thyroid deficiency as in the general population.[1] In the majority of these hypothyroid and hypertensive subjects blood pressure returns to the age- and sex-adjusted normal range with thyroid replacement therapy (Figure 41.1). Thus hypertension could be at least a partial explanation for the high frequency of coronary arterial disease in patients with hypothyroidism. Thyroid deficiency can also evidently be responsible for some drug-resistant hypertension.

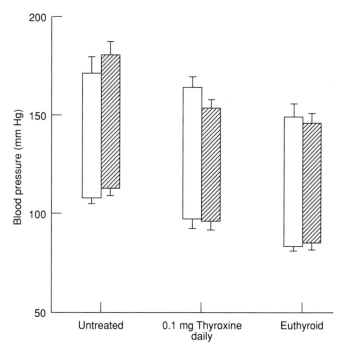

**Figure 41.1.** Blood pressure response in seven hypertensive hypothyroid patients to treatment with thyroxine alone. Means and SEM shown; open columns recumbent, shaded standing. (Redrawn from Ref. 1, with permission.)

### Pathophysiology

In untreated thyroid deficiency, exchangeable body sodium is expanded, and plasma renin low, although the expansion of body sodium content does not seem to explain fully the depression of plasma renin.[1] Diminished $\beta$-adrenergic activity may be a further partial reason for the low renin values. Aldosterone secretion also is diminished, in part reflecting suppression of the renin–angiotensin system, but also in large measure representing a general diminution of adrenocortical activity with hypothyroidism.[1]

Peripheral resistance is elevated, a consequence of reduced tissue perfusion secondary to diminished metabolic activity, together with relatively enhanced peripheral $\alpha$-adrenergic activity.[1] Increased sodium and water content of the walls of resistance arteries could also contribute. Cardiac output and blood volume are reduced.

### Effect of treatment

These various abnormalities are largely reversible with correction of the hypothyroidism. Thus treatment of hypertension in hypothyroid patients should therefore usually await rectification of the thyroid deficiency (see page 295). Careful attention should be given to the well described lipid disturbance in this condition.

## Thyrotoxicosis

Elevation of the systolic pressure ($> 150$ mmHg) occurs in at least 50% of patients with thyrotoxicosis, returning to age- and sex-matched normal values with treatment. A raised diastolic pressure, by contrast, is unusual. Untreated thyrotoxicosis is characterized by a raised cardiac output, tachycardia, decreased peripheral resistance and an expanded blood volume.[1]

## Case study

See Case study 22, Appendix 2.

## Reference

1. Bing RF. Thyroid disease and hypertension. In *Handbook of Hypertension*, Vol. 15: *Clinical Hypertension* (ed. JIS Robertson). Amsterdam: Elsevier, 1992: 576–93.

# 42
# Angiotensinogen-producing tumour

In 1984 a group of Japanese workers reported the case of a 36-year-old man with hypertension (170/96 mmHg), mild hypokalaemia (serum potassium 3.6 mM/litre), and very high serum levels of α-feto-protein (AFP); he was found to have a trabecular hepatocellular carcinoma.[1] There were very high plasma concentrations of renin and of aldosterone; plasma renin activity was also elevated (see page 41). Plasma concentrations of angiotensinogen (renin substrate) were some 5 times higher than normal. Hepatic tissue was obtained post-mortem; the tumour contained extremely high quantities of angiotensinogen as compared with the surrounding normal liver tissue.

The authors proposed[1] that the hypertension was due to excessive quantities of angiotensinogen produced by the hepatocellular carcinoma and released into the blood. The interaction of these high plasma concentrations of angiotensinogen with plasma renin (which was found, at first inexplicably, to be present in high concentrations) had led to elevation of plasma renin activity, also presumably to increased plasma concentrations of angiotensin II, to hypertension, and secondary aldosterone excess.

Subsequently Kew et al.[2] described three South African black patients also with hepatocellular carcinoma and hypertension. Plasma concentrations of angiotensinogen (renin substrate) were increased by 8- to 10-fold in the two patients in whom these measurements were made. One of these two subjects also showed a marked rise in plasma active, inactive and total renin concentrations; inactive renin comprised 90% of the total renin concentration. This subject was shown additionally to have high plasma renin activity. Two of the three patients had elevated plasma levels of aldosterone.

As described in Chapter 30, high plasma concentrations of inactive renin have been reported in association with, and almost certainly secreted by, malignant tumours both of renal and extrarenal[3] origin. Possibly, therefore, the hypertension that sometimes complicates hepatocellular carcinoma may be caused by a combination of eutopic synthesis of excessive quantities of angiotensinogen plus ectopic production and secretion of renin (much of which may be in an inactive form). Alternatively there could be eutopic production of angiotensinogen alone. The former circumstances would explain why, despite very high plasma concentrations of angiotensinogen, plasma renin concentration is not correspondingly lowered, but may conversely be increased.[1,2]

Much needs yet to be learned of this interesting syndrome.[4] It appears that some patients with hepatocellular carcinoma of the liver, the organ which normally is responsible for secretion of the major quantity of angiotensinogen, can develop excessive plasma concentrations of angiotensinogen. Concurrently there can also be increased plasma concentrations of renin. Although much of the renin can be in an inactive form, concentrations of active renin can be sufficiently high that, reacting with the elevated angiotensinogen, increased angiotensin II is generated, resulting in hypertension with secondary aldosterone excess and hypokalaemia.

## References

1. Ueno N, Yoshida K, Hirose S *et al*. Angiotensinogen-producing hepatocellular carcinoma. *Hypertension* 1984; **6**: 931–3.
2. Kew MC, Leckie BJ, Greef MC. Arterial hypertension as a paraneoplastic phenomenon in hepatocellular carcinoma. *Arch. Intern. Med.* 1989; **149**: 2111–13.
3. Lindop GBM, Leckie BJ, Mimran A. Renin-secreting tumors. In *The Renin–Angiotensin System* (eds JIS Robertson and MG Nicholls). London: Gower Medical, 1993: chapter 54.
4. Robertson JIS. Angiotensinogen-producing tumour and hypertension. In: *Handbook of Hypertension*, Vol. 15: *Clinical Hypertension* (ed. JIS Robertson). Amsterdam: Elsevier, 1992: 617–18.

# 43
# Endothelin-secreting tumour

Endothelin is a vasoconstrictor oligopeptide produced by vascular endothelium in response to a variety of stimuli (page 41).

Yokokawa et al.[1] reported on two elderly women with scalp nodules which were found, after excision, to be malignant haemangioendotheliomas. Both patients had high peripheral plasma endothelin concentrations, which fell following surgical excision of the tumours. Recurrence of tumour in one case was accompanied by re-elevation of plasma endothelin concentration.

Both patients had modestly raised blood pressures and the recorded values were lower after operation. In one patient, with recurrence of the neoplasm, blood pressure values then rose again slightly.

It was concluded that these malignant tumours secreted an excess of endothelin and that the latter contributed to the accompanying hypertension.

A more detailed study of further cases, and more objective and controlled arterial pressure measurement, are necessary for an appropriate evaluation and understanding of this potentially interesting syndrome.[2]

## References

1. Yokokawa K, Tahara H, Kohno M. et al. Hypertension associated with endothelin-secreting malignant hemangioendothelioma. Ann. Intern Med. 1991; **114**: 213–15.
2. Robertson JIS. Endothelin-secreting tumor. In Handbook of Hypertension, Vol. 15: Clinical Hypertension (ed. JIS Robertson). Amsterdam: Elsevier, 1992: 619–20.

# 44
# Guillain-Barré neuropathy

The Guillain–Barré syndrome comprises acute polyneuritis with elevated cerebrospinal fluid protein concentration. In many cases the cause is uncertain. Complete recovery usually occurs spontaneously within weeks, although more rarely a chronic, sometimes relapsing, variety is encountered.

Occasionally, the Guillain–Barré syndrome is complicated by acute hypertension,[1,2] which has been attributed to neuropathy affecting the baroreflex arc (see also page 55). Other possibilities are hypersecretion of catecholamines[2,3] and raised haematocrit with increased blood viscosity.[1] Clinical assessment can be complicated, because the Guillain–Barré syndrome can, irrespective of systemic arterial hypertension, be associated with raised cerebrospinal fluid pressure and papilloedema.

Rare cases have been reported of Guillain–Barré syndrome precipitated by the use of the angiotensin-converting enzyme inhibitors captopril[4,5] or enalapril[6] (see also page 125).

## References

1. Richards AM, Nicholls MG, Beard MEJ *et al*. Severe hypertension and raised haematocrit: unusual presentation of Guillain–Barré syndrome. *Postgrad. Med. J.* 1985; **61**: 53–5.
2. Ventura HD, Messerli FH, Barron RE. Norepinephrine-induced hypertension in Guillain–Barré syndrome. *J. Hypertens.* 1986; **4**: 265–7.
3. McInnes GT, Moore MR, McCall KEL. Porphyria and hypertension. In *Handbook of Hypertension*, Vol. 15: *Clinical Hypertension* (ed. JIS Robertson). Amsterdam: Elsevier, 1992: 594–603.
4. Atkinson AB, Brown JJ, Lever AF *et al*. Neurological dysfunction in two patients receiving captopril and cimetidine. *Lancet* 1980; **ii**: 36–7.
5. Chakraborty TK, Ruddell WSJ. Guillain–Barré neuropathy during treatment with captopril. *Postgrad. Med. J.* 1987; **63**: 221–2.
6. Hormigo A, Alvers M. Peripheral neuropathy in a patient receiving enalapril. *Br. Med. J.* 1992; **305**: 1332.

# 45
# Intracranial tumour

An acute rise in blood pressure together with slowing of the heart rate may result from sudden expansion of an intracranial lesion and is termed the Cushing reflex (see also pages 55, 71 and 150).

More rarely, hypertension may be caused by a slowly growing intracranial tumour, usually situated in the posterior fossa.[1] Several reported cases of this kind have shown evidence of hypersecretion of catecholamines, and the distinction from phaeochromocytoma is difficult (see also page 214).

The presence of papilloedema with only a few or no retinal haemorrhages or exudates, the converse of that characteristic of the malignant phase (page 69), can alert physicians to this important rarity.

## Reference

1. Bell GM. Hypertension and intracranial tumor. In *Handbook of Hypertension*, Vol. 15: *Clinical Hypertension* (ed. JIS Robertson). Amsterdam: Elsevier, 1992: 604–16.

# 46
# Porphyria and hypertension

The acute hepatic porphyrias are rare metabolic diseases comprising enzymic defects at various stages of the haem biosynthetic pathway.[1] All are inherited in a Mendelian dominant fashion. There are three forms, characterized by the site of the enzymic defect; these are acute intermittent porphyria, hereditary coproporphyria, and variegate porphyria. The least uncommon of these rarities is acute intermittent porphyria.

Precipitation of an acute porphyric attack can frequently be a consequence of ingestion of one of a wide range of drugs (Table 46.1). Amongst these are several antihypertensive agents, including captopril, clonidine, enalapril, frusemide, hydralazine, methyldopa, nifedipine, phenoxybenzamine, spironolactone and verapamil. Less certainly indictable, but under suspicion, are bendrofluazide, chlorothiazide, cyclopenthiazide, hydrochlorothiazide, diltiazem and prazosin. The dangers associated with the administration of these drugs impose considerable constraints in treating hypertension in a patient with porphyria.

## Acute hypertension

Transient and usually labile hypertension can accompany an acute attack of any of the three forms of acute hepatic porphyria, and can be severe enough to lead to the malignant phase. Left ventricular function can be markedly impaired, in part as a consequence of the sudden severe rise in arterial pressure, but possibly also because of a

**Table 46.1.** Antihypertensive drugs in the acute porphyrias

| Unsafe | Probably safe | Contentious |
|---|---|---|
| Captopril | Amiloride | Bendrofluazide |
| Clonidine | Atenolol | Chlorothiazide |
| Enalapril | Bumetanide | Cyclopenthiazide |
| Furosemide | Diazoxide | Diltiazem |
| Hydralazine | Ethacrynic acid | Hydrochlorothiazide |
| Methyldopa | Guanethidine | Prazosin |
| Nifedipine | Guanfacine | |
| Phenoxybenzamine | Labetalol | |
| Spironolactone | Metoprolol | |
| Verapamil | Propranolol | |
| | Reserpine | |
| | Timolol | |
| | Triamterene | |

*Source:* From Ref. 1.

defect of intermediary myocardial metabolism, or of catecholamine-induced myocardial necrosis.

The possible reasons for the acute rise in arterial pressure include neurogenic mechanisms secondary to autonomic neuropathy, with interruption, probably of the afferent limb, of the baroreceptor reflex arc. Another possibility is a marked rise in catecholamine secretion, which can, in an acute attack, equal that of a paroxysm of phaeochromocytoma (see also Chapter 38). Obviously, such cases closely mimic phaeochromocytoma, and diagnostic confusion can follow. Further, a porphyric crisis can be accompanied by impaired renal function and oliguria. Porphyrins and their precursors moreover have an acute arterial constrictor action.

--------- Chronic hypertension ---------

Probably largely because of the effects of repeated acute hypertensive episodes on resistance arterial structure and on renal function, perhaps accompanied by baroreflex disorder (page 54), porphyric patients suffering repeated episodes of acute hypertension often progress to chronic, sustained elevation of arterial pressure.

Moreover, many patients with porphyria who have never consciously sustained an acute episode have been found to have chronic hypertension. It is possible that repeated minor attacks could have gone unremarked in some of these cases.

The acute hepatic porphyrias are rare diseases, and hence a most unusual cause of hypertension. However, with porphyria, both acute (often very severe) and chronic hypertension can be complications, and the limited repertoire of antihypertensive drugs suitable for use in porphyria, with the capability of precipitating or worsening an attack if an incorrect choice is made, can present formidable therapeutic problems. Moreover, the very rarity of the porphyrias, with their capacity to mimic other diseases, sets and springs several diagnostic traps.

--------- Reference ---------

1. McInnes GT, Moore MR, McCall KEL. Porphyria and hypertension. In *Handbook of Hypertension*, Vol. 15: *Clinical Hypertension* (ed. JIS Robertson). Amsterdam: Elsevier, 1992: 594–603.

# Section 5
## Hypertension in pregnancy

# 47
# Hypertension in pregnancy

## Definition of hypertension in pregnancy

The definition of hypertension in pregnancy is arbitrary, but is usually taken as a systolic pressure in excess of 140 mmHg and/or a fourth phase diastolic over 90 mmHg.[1-3]

Hypertension in the syndrome of pre-eclampsia/eclampsia can be defined as above, or alternatively as a rise in blood pressure of more than 30 mmHg systolic and/or more than 15 mmHg diastolic during the course of pregnancy[1] (Table 47.1).

## Blood pressure measurement in pregnancy

A particular problem concerns blood pressure measurement in pregnancy. Phase five diastolic pressure (the point of disappearance of sounds) may not be apparent, with these sounds remaining audible down to zero throughout deflation of the cuff.[1,2] Phase four, the point of muffling of sounds, and perhaps a less reliable indicator of true diastolic pressure (page 134), has therefore often to be used. This can obviously hinder comparison with pre-pregnancy measurements of pressure, which would normally be taken at phase five. As always, the phase actually measured, that is, four or five, should be indicated in the case records. Furthermore, whilst blood pressure is conveniently taken with the patient sitting, adoption of the left lateral lying position may in pregnancy allow the measurement of a more reliable 'basal' pressure. Self-measured home blood pressure monitoring has also been advocated in pregnancy.[4,5]

## Differential diagnosis of hypertension in pregnancy: classification

Table 47.1 shows the slightly different classifications of hypertension in pregnancy as recommended by Rubin[1] and by Gifford et al.[2]

Chronic hypertension refers to blood pressure elevation existing from before the onset of gestation. This is most often essential (primary) hypertension; less frequently a secondary form.

Pre-eclampsia is diagnosed when hypertension appears for the first time in pregnancy, and is accompanied by proteinuria, oedema and hyperuricaemia; pregnancy-induced hypertension ('PIH') is an alternative term. Eclampsia denotes the appearance of tonic or clonic seizures in addition to the features of pre-eclampsia. Eclampsia usually, but not always, occurs in a woman with pre-existing pre-eclampsia.

Transient hypertension, which can usually be established only retrospectively, refers to benign elevation of blood pressure late in pregnancy, with a fall post-partum.

High blood pressure induced by pregnancy, i.e. pre-eclampsia/eclampsia, has potentially serious implications for both the mother[6] and the fetus.[7-9] Moreover, the interests of mother and fetus can be conflicting, because although early delivery enhances maternal safety, low gestational age lessens the offspring's chance of survival.

Essential hypertension existing from before pregnancy, or transient hypertension seen for the first time in pregnancy, are of much less immediate clinical importance. Nevertheless, differential diagnosis can pose problems, especially if blood pressure readings made before pregnancy are not available.

**Table 47.1.** Current classifications of hypertension during pregnancy

| Rubin 1988[1] | Gifford *et al.* 1991[2] |
| --- | --- |
| *Chronic hypertension* <br> Hypertension existing from before pregnancy. This is most often essential (primary) hypertension, but can be a secondary form. | *Chronic hypertension* <br> Hypertension existing from before pregnancy; or diagnosed before the 20th week of gestation; or persisting beyond the 42nd day post-partum. |
| *Pregnancy-induced hypertension (PIH)* <br> Hypertension developing during pregnancy, receding after delivery. | *Pre-eclampsia/eclampsia* <br> Hypertension developing during pregnancy and accompanied by proteinuria or oedema or both. |
| *Pre-eclampsia* <br> The combination of PIH with proteinuria. | *Eclampsia* <br> Denotes the occurrence of seizures in a pre-eclamptic patient, not attributable to alternative causes. |
| *Eclampsia* <br> Comprises generalized tonic/clonic seizures usually, but not invariably, occurring in a woman with pre-existing pre-eclampsia. | *Pre-eclampsia superimposed on chronic hypertension* <br> Can be diagnosed by rises of 15 mmHg diastolic or 30 mmHg systolic or 20 mmHg mean arterial pressure, with proteinuria or oedema in a woman with chronic hypertension. |
|  | *Transient hypertension* <br> Hypertension appearing during pregnancy or in the first 24 h post-partum without other features of pre-eclampsia or pre-existing hypertension. |

*Definition:* Hypertension in pregnancy is defined as a blood pressure in excess of 140/90 mmHg; or by an increase during pregnancy of 15 mmHg diastolic and/or 30 mmHg systolic.

## Problems concerning blood pressure evaluation in pregnancy

Information on blood pressure prior to pregnancy is unfortunately missing in many patients, though the problem is diminishing with the wide use of oral contraceptives and the accompanying recommended monitoring of blood pressure (page 160). Moreover, there is now increasingly prevalent opportunistic screening of blood pressure through, for example, 'well women' clinics in the UK.

The earliest blood pressure reading of pregnancy may be at the first antenatal clinic visit some 12 or more weeks after the last menstrual period, although sometimes, unfortunately, much later, especially in women who are socially deprived. The crucial task of the physician is to recognize the patient progressing to pre-eclampsia/eclampsia.[10–14]

## Blood pressure changes in normal pregnancy

Unlike blood pressure in the non-pregnant woman, which changes gradually over many years, and therefore tends to be examined in 'cross-sectional' rather than 'longitudinal' studies, the changes in blood pressure which occur in pregnancy, and especially with hypertension in pregnancy, occur over a relatively short time. Moreover, pregnancy has a brief, finite duration.

It is essential to recognize the pattern of blood pressure changes in normal pregnancy (Figure 47.1).[16–18] Pressure (especially diastolic) usually falls by some 7–10 mmHg in the first trimester, and then rises in the second half of the pregnancy, approaching non-pregnancy levels in the third trimester. The initial fall and subsequent rise of pressure through pregnancy may be particularly marked in those subjects with long-standing prior elevation of blood pressure. Such trends mask considerable individual variation, since blood pressure in pregnancy is subject to similar fluctuations to those found in the normal non-pregnant subject. Multiple measurements made in quiet and relaxed surroundings are likely to best reflect true prevailing pressures.

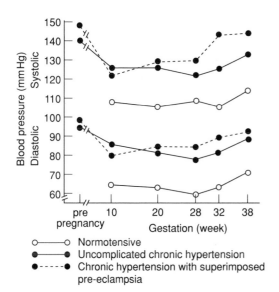

**Figure 47.1.** Serial changes in average systolic and diastolic blood pressure throughout pregnancy in 14 normal women, 17 with uncomplicated chronic hypertension, and 13 women with chronic hypertension plus superimposed pre-eclampsia. (Reproduced from Ref. 15, with permission.)

## Physiology of blood pressure regulation in normal pregnancy

For obvious ethical reasons the study of several aspects of the physiology of normal pregnancy is not easy, especially in its very early stages.

The presence of the placenta imposes a large arteriovenous shunt. The placenta has, moreover, a rich hormonal capacity and considerable metabolic propensity. The low blood pressure of normal pregnancy is associated with vasodilatation, reduced peripheral resistance, and a partly compensatory increase in cardiac output of 30–40% by 16 weeks of gestation.[16,19,20] Cardiac filling pressures do not rise and the peripheral oedema commonly seen in pregnancy seems likely to result in major part from mechanical compression of pelvic veins by the enlarged uterus. Generalized oedema is said to be present in 15% and pedal oedema in 20% of normal pregnant women.[21]

Plasma volume expands in human pregnancy, and reaches a maximum around 36 weeks.[19,20,22] In normal human pregnancy, blood volume in the last several weeks of gestation is on average 5 litres compared with a normal non-pregnant average of 3.5 litres. In animal studies, plasma volume expansion is not measurable until well into pregnancy, long after cardiac output and stroke volume have risen to restore blood pressure in the face of the marked vasodilatation.[23,24]

Renal blood flow (RBF) and glomerular filtration rate (GFR) increase in pregnant women by 40–50% in the first trimester and remain markedly elevated, although declining towards the end of gestation. These increases, together with the plasma volume expansion, lower the normal ranges of plasma urea and creatinine substantially from the first weeks of pregnancy.[25]

In normal human pregnancy, there is marked activation of the renin–angiotensin system, with circulating concentrations of active renin, prorenin (inactive renin), angiotensinogen (renin substrate), angiotensin II and aldosterone all being raised.[26] It has been emphasized that the rise in angiotensinogen is the fundamental process in this range of phenomena; indeed, plasma active renin concentration may be somewhat lower than expected given the slight hypotension and the raised cardiac output (see above) characteristic of normal human pregnancy.[15] The physiological purpose of the enhanced activity of the circulating (and indeed also of the tissue) renin–angiotensin system in normal pregnancy is not fully elucidated. A main action seems undoubtedly to be to facilitate adaptation to the marked changes of renal function which occur, and thus to modulate especially proximal and distal tubular function and the progressive retention of body water.[26] This very pronounced physiological enhancement of the renin–angiotensin system argues powerfully against the therapeutic use, in pregnancy, of drugs, such as angiotensin-converting enzyme inhibitors, which antagonize the system.[15]

Plasma atrial natriuretic peptide concentrations are increased, perhaps reflecting the increased blood volume. Thus pregnancy provides one of the exceptions to the general rule that plasma renin and atrial natriuretic peptide are inversely related (page 45).

## Interpretation of individual blood pressure readings in pregnancy

Definition of absolute ranges for normal and abnormal blood pressure in pregnancy is beset by the same difficulties as prevail in the non-pregnant subject. In populations of pregnant women there is observed a sigmoid distribution of blood pressure values, but over a relatively narrow and much lower range than in the general population (page 9). The majority of pregnant women, including many whose pressures lie at the upper end of the distribution, will not experience hypertension-related problems in pregnancy.

A rise in pressure, or an absence of the usual fall during early pregnancy, may sometimes be more indicative of impending trouble than the absolute level.

As mentioned earlier (page 237), a blood pressure over 140 mmHg systolic and/or 90 mmHg fourth phase diastolic is usually taken arbitrarily to denote hypertension during pregnancy, alternative criteria being a rise in systolic of more than 30 mmHg or of diastolic of more than 15 mmHg during the pregnancy (Table 47.1). Nevertheless, a diastolic pressure at any time above 85 mmHg and at 17–20 weeks values over 110/75 mmHg, should merit concern.[3,7,27]

## Pregnancy in patients with antecedent hypertension ('chronic hypertension')

### Management prior to pregnancy

Recognition of hypertension, and its investigation, should ideally be accomplished before pregnancy occurs. Management is much more difficult if hypertension is recognized only after conception, in the absence of readings before pregnancy.

The majority of subjects with chronic hypertension will be examples of essential rather than of secondary hypertension. Some of the forms of secondary hypertension which can be encountered in pregnancy, and their management, are considered on pages 254–256. It is particularly important that women of childbearing potential with raised blood pressure should be investigated adequately to exclude remediable causes of secondary hypertension well before pregnancy or the prospect of pregnancy. A rigorous approach to diagnosis would usually be expected in any event in young persons and is dealt with in other sections (page 141).

Establishing that a patient has a normal blood pressure before prescribing oral contraceptives and checking the pressure regularly during such use, a practice that should now be routine, can avoid considerable difficulties later.

Chronic essential hypertension accompanies some 10% of pregnancies with little serious consequence, although it can be associated with fetal death in mid-pregnancy,[28] and there is also a clear link between hypertension and maternal death.[6]

It should be recognized that whilst prior elevation of blood pressure may slightly predispose women to the risk of pre-eclampsia/eclampsia (see later), thus putting both mother and baby at potential hazard, there is no convincing evidence that good blood pressure control with drugs prior to pregnancy prevents such a sequel.[29,30] As Roberts and Redman[31] have emphasized, high blood pressure is probably not the prime mover in the disease pre-eclampsia/eclampsia.

### Non-pharmacological measures

Of particular concern often to a young woman wishing to become pregnant is that treatment with drugs, particularly in the first months, may have teratogenic effects, or may damage the fetus in some more subtle way. Since modest blood pressure elevation leads only slowly to arterial and organ damage over many years, the immediate need for antihypertensive drug treatment to protect the potential mother is not usually compelling. Weight loss, reduction of alcohol intake, and adequate exercise, which should also of course be combined with the avoidance of cigarette smoking, can be useful first measures in the mildly hypertensive young woman contemplating later pregnancy (page 129). Moreover, as described above (page 238), maternal blood pressure usually falls during pregnancy.[15] Only occasionally therefore is drug treatment needed in pregnancy for antecedent essential hypertension.

### Bed rest and restriction of activity

Bed rest, restricted activity and even long periods in hospital are still part of the management both of antecedent essential hypertension in pregnancy and of pre-eclampsia (see later),[7] even though this substantial additional impediment to usual everyday life in pregnancy is of uncertain value.

### Antihypertensive drug treatment

If blood pressure remains at a level at which long-term drug therapy is thought to be advisable, then patient and doctor will be faced with a decision on when to start such treatment; the selection of a particular agent; and concerning the continuation of such treatment in the event of pregnancy. A wide range of drugs has been used without apparent adverse effects through conception and into early pregnancy, and with safety also in the later stages of pregnancy. Doubts still linger, nevertheless, in the mind of physicians about the use of pharmacological agents in the first weeks of pregnancy, and similar concerns can often afflict women wishing to conceive, even though some of the latter may, irrationally, continue to smoke cigarettes or to consume alcohol to excess. Details of the merits and demerits of various antihypertensive drugs in relation to their use in pregnancy, in the particular context of pre-eclampsia, are given on pages 251–254. The antihypertensive agents which have been extensively, and apparently safely, used in pregnancy include the $\beta$-blockers atenolol, acebutolol, labetalol, metoprolol, oxprenolol and propranolol; the centrally acting drug methyldopa; and the vasodilator hydralazine. Thiazide diuretics have likewise been widely used, although their value in pre-eclampsia is controversial (page 252).

Pregnancy can sometimes take several years to achieve, and there can be repeated uncertainty as to whether conception has occurred. It is difficult to give hard and fast therapeutic rules, and therefore it is probably preferable to offer principles which can be applied by individual doctors to individual patients. Again, it is emphasized that a rigid, overcautious attitude should be avoided.

There can be little enthusiasm for allowing patients with untreated pressures consistently greater than 170/110 mmHg to attempt pregnancy until the blood pressure has been controlled, but there should be much less concern with readings below 160/100 mmHg. The most appropriate general advice for initiating drug therapy is to apply the criteria for treatment of essential hypertension as set out in Chapter 25.

It is important not to adopt too restrictive an attitude towards a hypertensive woman wanting a child. Successful pregnancies have even been achieved after drug treatment for malignant hypertension.[32,33]

After stopping antihypertensive drugs it may take some months for pressure to rise to pretreatment levels in many subjects.[34] Similarly, whilst the impact of treatment may be well-established within one month, maximum effects may not be reached for 2 or 3 months. Repeated fluctuations of blood pressure, induced by intermittently stopping and starting drugs whilst conception is achieved, are not desirable.

Although establishing good control with drugs and continuing this through conception, pregnancy, delivery and breast feeding offers a tidy and seemingly safe approach, it is one which may, as already mentioned, be questioned constantly by women of childbearing potential, and problems of compliance with therapy may ensue. Requiring re-emphasis is that mild elevation of blood pressure carries little long-term risk to a woman even in her late thirties. Undue anxiety should not, therefore, be generated in patients wishing to avoid drug treatment, and exaggerated claims for benefits of such therapy should be eschewed.

## Management during pregnancy

If hypertension is recognized for the first time after conception has occurred, in the absence of blood pressure measurements from before pregnancy, an initial, and often difficult, problem is diagnosis.

The presence of hypertension before the 20th week of gestation favours the diagnosis of chronic hypertension, as does a history of an earlier, normal pregnancy (Table 47.2). With chronic hypertension, blood pressure usually falls over the first half of pregnancy, as in normal subjects (page 239). Other features indicative of chronic hypertension rather than pre-eclampsia are the absence of proteinuria, oedema or a rise in plasma uric acid concentration.

With establishment of the diagnosis of essential hypertension in pregnancy, treatment, including the use of antihypertensive drugs, follows the pattern discussed above under the heading 'Management prior to pregnancy' above.

**Table 47.2.** Clinical features indicative or contraindicative of pre-eclampsia

| Favouring pre-eclampsia | Against pre-eclampsia |
| --- | --- |
| Almost exclusively first pregnancy[a] | Known hypertension[b] |
| Young (<30 years)[c] | Normal previous pregnancy |
| Race (black persons predisposed) | with or without hypertension |
| Multiple fetuses (tenfold increase independently of whether patient is primigravid or multiparous) | |
| Hydatidiform mole[d] | |
| Diabetes mellitus[e] | |
| Not apparent by end of 2nd trimester | Onset before 20 weeks[d] |
| Heredity tendency | |
| Generalized oedema (weight gain more than 1 kg per week) | No oedema |
| Appearance of proteinuria at 37 weeks | No proteinuria |
| Elevated plasma urate | |

*Sources:* From Refs 35 and 36.
[a] Pre-eclampsia in previous pregnancy especially with same partner greatly enhances risk.
[b] Hypertension especially in older females is much more common than serious pre-eclampsia but those with pre-existing hypertension/renal/heart disease may be more predisposed.
[c] Risk may increase after age > 35.
[d] Blood pressure rise associated with hydatidiform mole occurs early.
[e] Diabetes causes many problems in pregnancy.[37,38]

Again, it should be emphasized that attitudes should not be unduly pessimistic or restrictive. The great majority of these women can proceed, with appropriate medical care, to successful delivery. Termination of pregnancy is rarely necessary.

Chronic antecedent hypertension in women (see Table 47.1) is, even so, probably associated in pregnancy with an increase in middle trimester intra-uterine fetal deaths. Some studies suggest benefit from pressure reduction using antihypertensive drugs.[39,40] These patients with chronic blood pressure elevation also have a slightly increased chance of superimposed pre-eclampsia, which may well account for most of the risk in this group. There is little convincing evidence, however, that the treatment of hypertension has any influence on the supervention of pre-eclampsia.

## Pre-eclampsia: pregnancy-induced hypertension (PIH)

Pre-eclampsia/eclampsia remains one of the commonest forms of secondary hypertension, even though the raised blood pressure may be just one of the many features of this disorder.[31] Pre-eclampsia predominantly afflicts primigravid women.[1]

As Roberts and Redman[31] have pointed out, hypertension is neither invariable nor the fundamental pathophysiological feature of the disease. Thus the therapeutic approach to pre-eclampsia/eclampsia differs from that of essential hypertension. Even so, when hypertension is part of the syndrome of pre-eclampsia/eclampsia, perinatal fetal mortality is doubled.[6,8,9] Pre-eclampsia and eclampsia remain moreover the most important causes of maternal death in many countries, including the UK and the USA.[31]

The appearance of proteinuria in a patient who becomes hypertensive after the 20th week, usually defines pre-eclampsia. However, a trophoblastic disorder, for example hydatidiform mole, can lead to the syndrome before 21 weeks.[41–43]

Progression to full-blown eclampsia can be fulminating and take place within hours to days.[44–46] However, since even eclamptic fits (see later) can sometimes develop in patients without evidence of prior blood pressure elevation, the diagnostic requirement for the pressure to reach particular arbitrary levels should not be enforced rigidly. Similarly, high blood pressures and proteinuria do not in themselves necessarily signify a serious outcome for fetus or mother since, like oedema, each may have an explanation unrelated to pre-eclampsia, especially in a multiparous woman. Furthermore, in hypertensive primigravid women, progression to full eclampsia ensues only in a minority.

### Pathophysiology of pre-eclampsia/eclampsia and of the associated raised blood pressure

It is clear that the syndrome of pre-eclampsia/eclampsia, including the abnormal blood pressure, is induced by the pregnancy, because delivery of fetus and placenta[10,11,37,45,47–49] invariably induces a rapid return to normal blood pressure and to well-being of the mother.[7] Cure similarly follows delivery even when there is no fetus and the condition is due to hydatidiform mole.

Whilst much is known of the hormonal and haemodynamic changes, it is difficult to discern which are causes and which consequences of an abnormal pregnancy. As mentioned above, it has been argued forcefully that hypertension is an accompanying, but not an initiating, component. The failure of blood pressure control to prevent pre-eclampsia relegates hypertension to the lesser role of being simply a marker of this potentially serious disease rather than a causative factor.[11,46] The syndrome of pre-eclampsia can indeed sometimes occur without any apparent blood pressure elevation as defined above.

Whatever the underlying abnormality, the range of sequelae includes a change from a low blood pressure, high cardiac output, vasodilated state to one of high blood pressure, low cardiac output, low plasma volume and increased peripheral resistance.[19,47,48,50]

*Placental abnormalities*

The occurrence of pre-eclampsia in the absence of a fetus, as occurs with hydatidiform mole, clearly shows, as mentioned above, that the presence of a placenta is the only prerequisite for the disease.[41]

In normal human pregnancy, the fetal trophoblast infiltrates the placental bed. The trophoblast cells initially invade the decidua, then, from 12–18 weeks, the myometrium and the walls of the spiral arteries, which supply blood to the villous space of the placenta. The trophoblast invasion destroys the musculoelastic structure of the arterial walls, rendering them readily dilated, and capable of transmitting a greater flow of blood.

In pre-eclampsia, this process is stunted, and does not proceed beyond the stage normally attained at the 12th week of pregnancy[51] (Figure 47.2). Implantation failure appears to be genetically predisposed.[186] Thus impaired utero-placental perfusion is an early and obvious feature of pre-eclampsia.

### Does pre-eclampsia have an immunological cause?

The familial predisposition to pre-eclampsia and its links to both the father and the primigravid mother indicate a possible immunological basis.[52–54] The fetal–placental unit provides an interesting challenge to the maternal immune system. The fetus is genetically distinct from the mother, and might therefore be expected to be rejected immunologically. However, the mother normally copes without problems.[55] It could be that pre-eclampsia results from some inadequacy of the normal maternofetal immunological accommodation.

The evidence for such an underlying immunological cause has been reviewed in several publications.[54–56] Whilst immunological factors are relevant to the syndrome, their primary role if any remains obscure.[54–59] Claims for benefit from therapy with human immunoglobulin have been made in a report of a patient with severe pre-eclampsia and with circulating lupus anticoagulants and anticardiolipin antibodies.[60]

### The role of endothelial dysfunction

Roberts and Redman[31] have pointed out that vascular endothelium could provide a target for circulating products of reduced placental perfusion, and

that therein might be an explanation of several of the features of pre-eclampsia/eclampsia.

Endothelial cells are now recognized as possessing a wide range of biochemical and biophysical functions, comprising vasodilator and vasoconstrictor responses, the mediation of immune processes, the maintenance of vascular integrity, and, in various circumstances, either inhibition or promotion of blood coagulation.[31,61–64] Thus endothelial injury consequent upon events following impaired perfusion could lead to enhanced pressor sensitivity, a tendency towards intravascular coagulation, and leakage from the intravascular compartment, all features seen in pre-eclampsia/eclampsia.[31] Such processes accord with various clinical features of the disease, notably the oedema, proteinuria and vasospasm.

Taylor et al.[65] showed that plasma concentrations of cellular fibronectin, a marker of endothelial activation, were distinctly elevated in the third trimester in women with pre-eclampsia, as compared with similar measurements in normal pregnant women and in women with transient hypertension in pregnancy.

Endothelin, a vasoconstrictor peptide found in endothelial cells (page 47), has been reported variously to be increased[66–68,183,184] or normal[69] in pre-eclampsia. Branch et al.[70] found evidence that serum of pre-eclamptic women could suppress the production of endothelin by endothelial cells, although Brown et al.,[71] could not confirm this (see also Refs 68 and 72).

Additionally or alternatively, deficient or disordered release of nitric oxide (page 48), now recognized to be the endothelial-derived relaxing factor (EDRF), could well have an important pathogenic role.[64,73] It has been suggested that increased free haemoglobin in pre-eclampsia may inhibit EDRF and so be linked to pathogenesis.[74]

Further evidence of widespread endothelial dysfunction in pre-eclampsia is the diminished endothelial production of vasodilator prostaglandins, including prostacyclin.[62,63,75,76] Even so, while there have been reports of benefit with aspirin treatment,[77–79] this has not been seen in all studies,[80,127] and the risk of *abruptio placentae* is

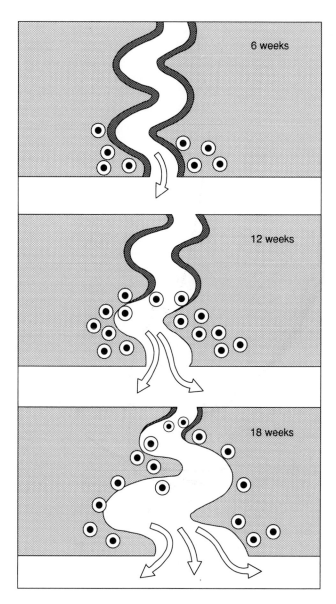

**Figure 47.2.** Diagram of fetal trophoblast infiltration of the placental bed and subsequent invasion of the wall of maternal spiral arteries supplying the intervillous space of the placenta. Trophoblast cells initially invade the decidua (shaded area), then the myometrium (from 12–18 weeks) and infiltrate the wall of the spiral artery. This destroys the musculo-elastic structure, rendering the artery thin-walled, dilated and capable of transmitting a greater flow of blood. In pre-eclampsia, the process does not proceed beyond the state normally reached at 12 weeks. (Modified from Ref. 51, with permission.)

increased (see page 251).[79] Arbogast *et al.*[185] have proposed that very low-density lipoproteins (VLDL) injure the endothelium in pre-eclampsia.

### Is there a disorder of coagulation?

Further evidence of endothelial dysfunction in pre-eclampsia derives from the several accompanying derangements of coagulation. Platelet counts are reduced in patients with pre-eclampsia.[81–84] The above-mentioned evidence for benefit from aspirin treatment, albeit controversial, supports the possibility of a role for platelet aggregation in this syndrome.[77,78,80,127,184] Moreover, platelet adherence and aggregation, with associated fibrin formation, probably play important roles in the consistent impairment of placental function.[187] A number of accompanying abnormalities of coagulation are reported.[85–88] Circulating concentrations of von Willebrand factor are raised.[31,62]

Thrombocytopenia with haemolysis and raised plasma levels of liver enzymes in severe pre-eclampsia constitute the 'HELLP' syndrome.[89,90]

### Role of serotonin

It has been proposed that serotonin has a pivotal role in the genesis of pre-eclampsia/eclampsia.[76] In a milieu characterized by a reduction in EDRF and prostacyclin, serotonin is held to augment the response of smooth muscle to normally occurring concentrations of vasopressor substances. Serotonin is delivered to the microvasculature by platelets, whose aggregation and disruption, with release of free serotonin (page 47) is promoted by dysfunctional endothelium. These concepts provide a rationale for the therapeutic use of aspirin and/or ketanserin in the treatment of pre-eclampsia/eclampsia.

### The renin–angiotensin system

In pre-eclampsia, in contrast to normal pregnancy (page 239), the renin–angiotensin system is relatively suppressed (Figure 47.3). Plasma renin activity, and plasma concentrations of angiotensinogen, active renin, prorenin, angiotensin II

and aldosterone are all lower than in normal pregnant women.[15,26] Thus pre-eclampsia does not appear to be caused by enhanced activity of the renin–angiotensin system. However, it might be argued that circulating concentrations of angiotensin II, although suppressed, are still inappropriately high, and thus could contribute to the hypertension.[15] As mentioned, free serotonin could augment the pressor action of angiotensin II.

The pressor effect of administered angiotensin II is, predictably, inversely proportional to the prevailing plasma concentration of angiotensin II.[91] Thus the rise in blood pressure with infused angiotensin II is diminished in normal pregnancy, and by contrast relatively enhanced in pre-eclampsia. This has formed the basis of a diagnostic procedure for pre-eclampsia, although the value of this procedure has been much disputed.[15,51,92] An increased pressor response to administered angiotensin II in early pregnancy has been taken by some investigators to predict the appearance of frank pre-

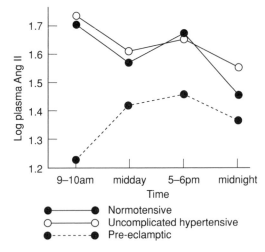

**Figure 47.3.** Group mean log plasma angiotensin II (Ang II) values at various diurnal sampling times and after 26 weeks gestation in 10 normotensive women, 13 with chronic hypertension and 8 with preeclampsia. Angiotensin II values were significantly lower in pre-eclampsia and also showed a significantly different diurnal pattern from the others. (Reproduced from Ref. 15, with permission.)

eclampsia later.[15] It therefore requires re-emphasis that such pressor responses simply reflect the prevailing plasma angiotensin II concentration. If this approach has any diagnostic value, and this is doubtful, a quicker, safer and more accurate method would be the assay of plasma angiotensin II or of plasma renin activity. Infusions of angiotensin II are time-consuming for both investigator and subject, and are accompanied by some risk.

Platelet binding of angiotensin II is lower in normal pregnancy than in the non-pregnant state, paralleling changes in the vascular responsiveness to angiotensin II. Platelet binding of angiotensin II is higher in pre-eclampsia than in normal pregnancy. It has been suggested that enhanced binding of angiotensin II to platelets predicts pre-eclampsia more reliably than any variable derived from angiotensin II infusion studies.[15,92]

### Renal changes

Glomerular capillary endothelial cells are enlarged, and show electron dense cytoplasmic inclusions.[10,31] The capillary lumen can be occluded. These renal lesions are apparently unique to this form of hypertension.[11,12,27,31,93]

Proteinuria, which is unselective, is characteristic.

The large increases in both renal blood flow and glomerular filtration rate characteristic of normal human pregnancy are reversed in pre-eclampsia. Thus there is relative elevation of plasma creatinine, urea and uric acid concentrations. However, these changes evolve from a background of the normal fall in the plasma concentrations of these substances in early pregnancy, with a subsequent rise towards the end of gestation. Thus interpretation can be difficult, but is facilitated by regular charting of the values, and their display in graphic format.

With increasingly severe pre-eclampsia, marked increases in plasma creatinine, urea and uric acid occur. Endogenous serum ouabain (page 49) may be raised.[94]

Rarely, acute renal tubular necrosis may ensue.

Any renal involvement in pre-eclampsia is obviously more serious if superimposed on antecedent impairment of kidney function.[95-98]

### Liver changes

Hepatic involvement may be recognized by the presence of raised plasma levels of liver enzymes. Intrahepatic haemorrhage and necrosis can occur.

The so-called 'HELLP' syndrome comprises haemolysis, hepatic disturbance and thrombocytopenia (page 246).[89,90,99]

### Cerebral changes

Petechial haemorrhages of the brain have been frequently observed in women dying from eclampsia. In life, computer-assisted tomographic (CT) scanning of the brain can reveal areas of low density, most prevalent in the cortex; these probably reflect petechial haemorrhages or small infarctions.[100] Whilst blood flow to the brain is usually near to normal in these patients, cerebral oxygen consumption can be diminished, presumably because of focal changes in blood flow, with brain areas variously being overperfused or underperfused, or with haemorrhage or infarction.

### Cardiac changes

The heart can show subendocardial necrosis.[31]

## Clinical features of pre-eclampsia

Pre-eclampsia is recognized (Tables 47.2 and 47.3) by the presence of hypertension as defined earlier, together with proteinuria of more than 300 mg per 24 h and/or peripheral oedema. Plasma uric acid can be raised. Pre-eclampsia is, as mentioned, most likely in a first pregnancy. In some patients, hypertension or proteinuria can appear only after delivery. Whatever the time of onset, both hypertension and proteinuria disappear within a week of delivery.

As discussed above (page 244), a placental disorder, with hypoperfusion and probable consequent generalized endothelial abnormality, is consistently found. Surprisingly, Doppler ultra-

**Table 47.3.**   Ominous features in pre-eclampsia

BP $> 160/110$ mmHg[a]
Heavy proteinuria $(2+/3+; > 2$ g$/24$ h$)$[a]
Increased serum creatinine $(> 120$ $\mu$mol/litre;
    1.36 mg/dl$)$[a]
Reduced platelet count $(< 100\,000/$mm$^3)$[a]
Elevated liver enzymes[a]
Headache; visual disturbances; epigastric pain
Breathlessness; pulmonary oedema

[a] Changes can be more relevant than absolute values.

sonography, employed to study placental blood flow velocity, has proved less helpful than was expected.[101-104]

### Hypertension

In pre-eclampsia/eclampsia the blood pressure alone has limited relevance to the clinical care of the pregnant patient. Blood pressure readings, and particularly changes in pressure, must be considered in the overall clinical context.[7,11,14]

Whilst hypertension is usually deemed, arbitrarily, to be present in pregnancy if the systolic pressure is above 140 mmHg and/or the fourth phase diastolic is over 90 mmHg, an often more relevant alternative definition in the context of pre-eclampsia/eclampsia takes an increase in systolic pressure of more than 30 mmHg and/or an increase in diastolic pressure of more than 15 mmHg, when readings after the 20th week are compared with values obtained before that time (pages 237–238). Such dynamic assessments are especially valuable when no information is available on non-pregnant values.[3,7] In most obstetric practice a chart, which readily allows trends in pressure to be displayed, may usefully combine plots of blood pressure changes with those of other clinical and biochemical measures.

### Oedema

Oedema, especially of the feet and ankles, is common in normal pregnancy (page 243). More useful diagnostically in pre-eclampsia is the observation of a weight gain of more than 1 kg in one week, especially if there is accompanying generalized oedema.[3,7,14]

### Proteinuria

The appearance of proteinuria in pre-eclampsia usually occurs later than increases in blood pressure and weight.[3,14] Its supervention is of serious prognostic import. The diagnosis of abnormal proteinuria should depend upon the demonstration of more than 300 mg protein in 24 h or 30 mg/dl (dipstick reading of 'one plus') in two cleanly voided specimens obtained at least 4 h apart.

### Uric acid

An elevated plasma concentration of uric acid favours a diagnosis of pre-eclampsia.[105,106]

Any or all of the above features appearing at or later than the 37th week make prior renal or chronic hypertension less likely to be responsible, and indicate pre-eclampsia (see Table 47.2).

## Eclampsia

The supervention of true eclampsia, with repeated tonic and/or clonic convulsions and clouding of consciousness or coma, is a devastating consequence of pre-eclampsia.[36,41] Despite improved management, there remains a distinct associated mortality.[6,46,107-109] The pathological stigmata, outlined above for pre-eclampsia, are likely to be exaggerated (Table 47.3). Headache, epigastric pain and visual disturbance are ominous features.[109,110]

Retinal haemorrhages and exudates, retinal oedema, and papilloedema can appear.[110,111] As discussed also on page 65, some authorities regard their presence as indicating simply malignant phase hypertension complicating pregnancy-induced hypertension, albeit appearing at lower absolute levels of arterial pressure than is usual for the malignant phase, because of the rapid onset and progression of the hypertension.[112] Others, by contrast,[51] emphasizing the generalized vascular disorder of pre-eclampsia/eclampsia, prefer to distinguish the ocular lesions in that condition from true malignant phase hypertension. Most probably, both pathophysiological processes contribute to the retinal manifestations.

### Errors in the diagnosis of pre-eclampsia/eclampsia

The distinction from chronic essential hypertension is discussed on page 242 (see also Tables 47.1 and 47.2). Some other possible sources of confusion require brief mention. Phaeochromocytoma complicating pregnancy should always be considered.[113] Its diagnosis ought now to be straightforward, using biochemical tests which are widely available (page 255). Failure of diagnosis is almost always due to failure to recognize the possibility: the consequences for both mother and fetus are dire.

Pregnant patients, regardless of blood pressure, may alternatively convulse for reasons of previously unrecognized epilepsy, strokes, infectious meningitis or brain tumour. Only in the rarest of situations, however (for example lack of any information on prenatal progress or of knowledge of the patient from friends or relatives), is there any serious diagnostic difficulty with these diseases.

### Management of pre-eclampsia and eclampsia

The principles are clear, but inevitably involve a compromise. They are to protect the mother from the effects of raised blood pressure whilst simultaneously to limit the risks to the fetus by allowing a period of gestation compatible with the best possible chance of fetal survival after birth. Regular medical supervision through pregnancy permits the prompt detection and treatment of problems. Modern neonatal care allows delivery to be contemplated as early as 32 weeks of gestation.[114]

Raised blood pressure found in the critical first 3 months of pregnancy is almost certainly not induced by the pregnancy, unless there is a hydatidiform mole. The evidence that controlling maternal hypertension protects the fetus, is, as already mentioned, scanty, and seems unlikely

to have much effect on the occurrence of pre-eclampsia, of which it is a marker, not a cause. Unless severe, elevated blood pressure does not usually involve short-term consequences for the mother.

There are, therefore, somewhat different objectives and approaches according to the severity of the disease.

With mild pregnancy-induced hypertension, usually appearing late in pregnancy and initially without accompanying proteinuria, the aims are to prevent advance to proteinuria and thence to full convulsive eclampsia, and also to limit the adverse effects on mother and fetus of the impaired maternal renal function and of reduced utero-placental blood flow.

With supervention of severe pre-eclampsia or frank eclampsia, more urgent therapy is needed, directed at control of hypertension and fits, and early delivery.

A management schema is shown in Figure 47.4.

#### Restriction of activity: bed rest

In contrast to advice offered to the non-pregnant hypertensive subject, bed rest is a well-established component of the management of hypertension in pregnancy.[7,22,116] Whilst its value in essential hypertension with pregnancy may be questioned (page 241), it can alone in pre-eclampsia lower pressure adequately, so that drug administration is not required. The corollary is that drug treatment may lessen the need for bed rest in hospital, and this has indeed been used as a marker of therapeutic benefit.

Utero-placental flow is often increased by bed rest, although this does not necessarily reflect vital perfusion.

The risk of premature labour is claimed to be reduced by resting.[22,40]

Daily outpatient care has been strongly and plausibly advocated as an attractive and cheaper alternative to bed rest in hospital.[117]

#### Dietary measures

Correction of obesity is clearly desirable before pregnancy. Moreover, dietary means may help

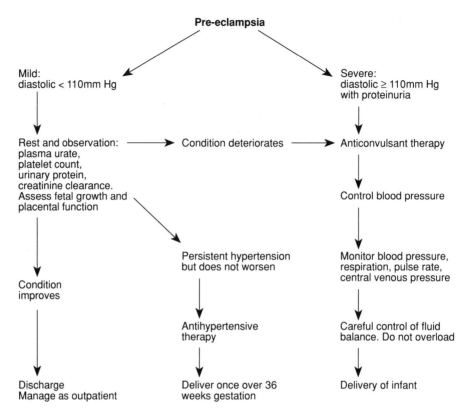

**Figure 47.4.** Scheme for the management of pre-eclampsia. (Adapted from Ref. 115, with permission.)

avoid excessive weight gain during the pregnancy, a time when physical activity is also often less. However, there seems to be no justification in attempting to achieve marked weight loss, such as might be advocated in the non-pregnant woman.[7,22]

Moderation of sodium intake is also sometimes advised. However, pre-eclampsia is associated with plasma volumes which are lower than in normal pregnancy,[118] and sodium restriction has, therefore, not been generally recommended.[19,119]

Other dietary measures of more questionable value have been reviewed by Brown.[22]

The intake of alcohol should be kept to a minimum. Cigarette smoking should be avoided.

*Volume expansion*

The infusion of volume-expanding solutions has also been tried as therapy, albeit with equivocal results.[10,118]

*Aspirin*

This is an area of intense study in major clinical trials.[77,78–80,120–126] Initiated at doses of 150 mg/day or less after 28 weeks of gestation, aspirin has been claimed to diminish the incidence of pre-eclampsia, to prolong gestation and to reduce intra-uterine death in patients at increased risk.[78,79] These are obvious theoretical reasons for its beneficial actions, as detailed on pages 244–246. However, not all studies have shown benefit[77] including one conducted in more than a thousand patients.[80] The risk of *abruptio placentae* is increased.[79] A trial of low-dose aspirin in over 9000 women found no significant reduction in proteinuric pre-eclampsia, intra-uterine growth retardation, stillbirth, or neonatal death, although the likelihood of preterm delivery was less. It was concluded that routine prophylactic or therapeutic antiplatelet therapy to women at risk was not justified.[127]

### Antihypertensive drug treatment: indications and implementation

The lack of convincing evidence of prevention of pre-eclampsia by treating antecedent chronic hypertension has already been discussed (page 241). There is, by contrast, distinct, albeit limited, benefit from antihypertensive drug therapy in mild pre-eclampsia. Perinatal mortality is already low in these women. Nevertheless, controlled trials have shown that antihypertensive drug treatment can reduce the incidence of mid-trimester abortions and of perinatal deaths,[128] limit the development of proteinuria[129–131] and shorten the time spent in hospital.[40,132]

Thus it is now generally recommended that in women who develop diastolic pressures over 95 mmHg, which do not respond to conservative measures (Figure 47.4), antihypertensive drug treatment should be started.

### Antihypertensive drug treatment: evaluation of different agents

The antihypertensive drugs most appropriate for the treatment of pre-eclampsia are methyldopa, or one of a wide range of $\beta$-blockers, including atenolol, acebutolol, oxprenolol, propranolol and labetalol. Hydralazine can be added to the chosen $\beta$-blocker or to methyldopa as necessary to control the blood pressure. There is some, but more limited, experience with the $\alpha$-blocker prazosin and the calcium antagonist nifedipine as supplementary drugs. Diuretics, by contrast, are not generally considered appropriate in this disease. Angiotensin-converting enzyme (ACE) inhibitors are reckoned

to be unsuitable drugs for treating pre-eclampsia. The serotonergic 5-HT$_2$ antagonist ketanserin has given good results[76] and has been advocated as perhaps especially useful in treating the HELLP syndrome.[133] (See also Appendix 1.)

### Methyldopa

Methyldopa has been used extensively in pregnancy,[40,128,134–137] and its safety has been substantiated by follow-up of children for more than 7 years.[138,139] It is the drug of first choice if such therapy is needed before the 28th week of gestation. There is evidence, obtained using methyldopa, for a significant reduction in the incidence of late spontaneous abortion, and of improved overall perinatal mortality.[128,134]

Some other benefits to the mother are based largely on 'surrogate' endpoints. Thus, methyldopa may correct severe hypertension and diminish the number of hospital admissions required for bed rest. However, to claim these as beneficial involves a circular argument, since the decision to undertake bed rest is usually based on arbitrary definitions personal to the physician.

Methyldopa should started at low doses (125 mg twice daily), which are then gradually increased so as to avoid sedation. Depression is unlikely at the lower doses.

### $\beta$-Adrenergic antagonists ($\beta$-blockers)

A range of $\beta$-blockers including atenolol, acebutolol, oxprenolol and propranolol, as well as labetalol, which also possesses $\alpha$-blocking properties, have been widely prescribed in pregnancy with apparent safety to mother and fetus alike. They can limit proteinuria. Their potential benefits are otherwise subject to many of the same caveats as were expressed for methyldopa above.[29,130,131,140–145]

The use of $\beta$-blockers has tended to be predominantly, but not exclusively, in late pregnancy. Before 28 weeks of gestation methyldopa is usually the favoured alternative.[7,40]

Concern has been raised over growth retardation and fetal bradycardia with $\beta$-blockade. Lower doses than were used in many previous studies may be effective and therefore preferable.

There seems little to commend choosing new $\beta$-antagonists in preference to those used in reported studies which have been found to be safe.

Contraindications and side-effects are largely as in non-pregnant subjects (page 118). In particular, $\beta$-blockers should not be employed in patients with reversible airways obstruction.

### Prazosin

Prazosin is an $\alpha$-adrenoreceptor antagonist. Like other drugs of its type, it can cause severe hypotension after the first dose, unless very small amounts are given (page 119). It can be prescribed with a $\beta$-antagonist, and this combination has been reported to improve blood pressure control in patients with severe pregnancy-induced hypertension.[143]

### Ketanserin

Ketanserin, a serotonergic 5-HT$_2$ antagonist also possessing weak $\alpha$-adrenergic antagonism, has been reported to control hypertension in pre-eclampsia.[76] It can also raise platelet count and diminish severe epigastric pain in the HELLP syndrome, a manifestation of severe pre-eclampsia.[133] Oral doses are 20 or 40 mg twice daily.

### Hydralazine

Hydralazine, a direct-acting vasodilating drug, is used long term only in addition to a drug like methyldopa or a $\beta$-antagonist, either of which will control the tendency to reflex tachycardia hydralazine would otherwise cause.[7,39,40] There is now considerable experience with hydralazine in pregnancy. The lupus-like syndrome reported in the non-pregnant state (page 116), has not been seen in pregnancy, perhaps reflecting relative immunological suppression (page 244), but also possibly the dosage limitation. A low starting dose (25 mg twice daily) is advocated, with restriction of the top dose

to 100 mg twice daily. Headache and flushing trouble some patients.

### Calcium antagonists

The vasodilating calcium antagonist of class II, nifedipine, has been used without apparent problem in pregnancy, but experience is very limited.[146–150] It comprises an alternative to hydralazine as treatment additional to methyldopa or a $\beta$-antagonist. Flushing and headache are side-effects, as with hydralazine, and an initial low dose of a slowly absorbed preparation (e.g. adalat retard 10 mg twice daily) should be given. Ankle oedema is often quite marked, and can confuse the assessment of oedema of more ominous origin.

Orally administered (ostensibly 'sublingual') nifedipine has been used in situations requiring urgent blood pressure reduction in pregnancy. However, the notion of sublingual absorption is a misconception; nifedipine has to be swallowed to be absorbed (page 122).[112,151]

Potentiation of neuromuscular blockade has been reported when high doses of class II calcium antagonists are combined with magnesium sulphate (page 31).

### Diuretics

The value of thiazides and loop-acting diuretics in pregnancy remains controversial.[7,152–154] The relative reduction of plasma volume in pre-eclampsia comprises a theoretical contraindication.[153] One trial found significant reduction of birth weight with their use.[155] An overview of randomized trials by contrast supported their safety and efficacy in reducing blood pressure and lessening oedema without incurring either adverse or beneficial effects on perinatal mortality.[154] Diuretics increase plasma urate, which may confuse use of this as a marker of pre-eclampsia.

Potassium-conserving diuretics are rarely required, although they can be useful in the uncommon circumstance of aldosterone-secreting tumour coinciding with pregnancy (page 255). Spironolactone has hormonal effects, evidenced in other situations by its propensity to cause menstrual disturbances and gynaecomastia, and is best avoided in pregnancy. Amiloride is probably preferable.

### Angiotensin-converting enzyme (ACE) inhibitors

Angiotensin-converting enzyme (ACE) inhibitors can cause intra-uterine death in pregnant animals. There also are reports with their use in human pregnancy of fetal abnormalities.[156–159] Whilst successful pregnancies have been observed in patients taking these agents even throughout gestation, their prescription in pregnancy is not advised.[15]

### Parenteral antihypertensive and anticonvulsant therapy

With the development of severe hypertension, and/or the appearance of eclamptic fits, more urgent, often parenteral, treatment can be needed. Oral therapy may alternatively be precluded by vomiting or by impaired consciousness, and in these situations parenteral treatment is also clearly necessary.

As with hypertension in the non-pregnant state (page 151), parenteral treatment for hypertension in pregnancy can be dangerous. Precipitous falls in pressure can seriously compromise the circulation to vital organs (pages 64, 71 and 72), to the detriment severally of the mother, placenta and fetus, especially when placental perfusion is already compromised.

### Hydralazine

Hydralazine can be given by repeated intramuscular or intravenous bolus injections starting with 5 mg and waiting for the maximal antihypertensive effect to appear about 20–30 min later. Failure of response to 20 mg should lead to consideration of alternatives.

### Diazoxide

Diazoxide, now rarely used in other circumstances (page 117), can be effective as an antihypertensive drug, given as 30 mg intravenous boluses.[160]

### Labetalol

Labetalol, given either by intravenous infusions of 1–2 mg/kg over 10 min, or as repeated intravenous bolus injections of 25 or 50 mg at 10-min intervals, can control crises of hypertension.[161,162]

### Ketanserin

Ketanserin can be given as intravenous bolus injections over 5 min at doses of 20 mg three times daily.[133]

### Sodium nitroprusside

Given intravenously by continuous and regulated infusion, sodium nitroprusside allows the most effective and precise minute by minute control of blood pressure,[163,164] and is justified where the mother's life is in serious jeopardy. However, prolonged usage can lead to cyanide accumulation in both mother and fetus.[165,166] Some authorities have advised against the administration of nitroprusside.[2]

### Magnesium sulphate

Magnesium sulphate is employed widely in the USA, but rarely in the UK, to prevent convulsions in severe pre-eclampsia.[167–171] A standard regime is 4 g intravenously followed by 5 g intramuscularly every 4 h. Its value is controversial.[2]

### Other anticonvulsant drugs

Phenytoin and diazepam are used;[170] the former prophylactically.[172,173]

### Timing of delivery

Considerations of fetal well-being usually dictate the timing of delivery. Caesarean section is to be avoided if possible and an aggressive approach to early induction is usually taken.[7]

In the critical 25–30 week gestational period, delivery is unlikely to be contemplated except for maternal reasons. Fetal salvage is excellent after 36 weeks.

Hepatic enlargement, tenderness and abnormal function comprise an obvious indication for induction of labour, irrespective of fetal maturity, because of the risk to the mother.

Rapid maternal weight gain, a fall in GFR, the appearance of significant proteinuria and clinical or ultrasound evidence of fetal growth retardation would usually also lead to a decision for pre-term delivery.

Eclampsia may ensue during delivery or within 24 h of parturition. It is extremely rare beyond this time; it is almost always superimposed on overt pre-eclampsia. The convulsions may begin with little or no warning. When these occur before delivery, delivery is delayed pending their control, adequate lowering of blood pressure and the maintenance of fluid and electrolyte balance.

### Post-partum

All antihypertensive drugs appear to enter breast milk, but there has been little evaluation of their effect for obvious logistic reasons.[174–176] Hypertension induced by pregnancy will always resolve even though it may worsen transiently in the first few days after delivery.[177–179] Indeed, blood pressure may sometimes be elevated after normal delivery. Many physicians would be comfortable to leave mild blood pressure elevation untreated for some weeks during breast feeding. Because of a lack of knowledge in this area, in the rare situation of patients requiring multiple antihypertensive treatment, breast feeding is not advised.

### Subsequent pregnancies

Recurrence of pre-eclampsia in subsequent pregnancy is unusual, and eclampsia very rare. Thus there is no major bar on these grounds to the undertaking of further pregnancies.

## Other syndromes of secondary ——— hypertension in pregnancy ———

Some varieties of secondary hypertension (page 5, Table 1.1) are incompatible with the achievement of conception, and are therefore not relevant in the present context. However, other forms can elude prior detection, coexist with pregnancy and present problems of diagnosis and treatment.

### Drug-induced hypertension: ingestion of pressor substances

These forms of secondary hypertension are not rare, and are dealt with in detail in Chapter 27. Their presence complicating pregnancy should be revealed if a careful history is elicited. The ingestion of pressor amounts of liquorice-containing compounds (page 162) can be more elusive, and the physician should always be wary of this possibility.

### Renovascular disease

Fibromuscular dysplasia involving the renal arteries is not uncommon as a cause of hypertension in women of reproductive age, and is, like atheromatous renal artery disease, more prevalent in smokers (page 179). Even atheromatous renal arterial disease can be encountered in pregnancy.[33,180]

Koskela and Kaski[180] performed renal arteriography post-partum in a series of women who developed severe hypertension in pregnancy. They found renal artery stenosis in 12% of these cases, suggesting that renal artery disease contributing to hypertension in pregnancy can often be overlooked.

Weir and Willocks[33] described a 40-year-old heavy smoker with widespread atherosclerotic disease, renal artery stenosis, angina pectoris and intermittent claudication, who had also suffered previous congestive heart failure and malignant phase hypertension. Nevertheless, despite these problems and her age, she achieved a successful pregnancy under therapy with methyldopa plus bendrofluazide. She continued to smoke heavily, however, and died aged 43 following myocardial infarction.

The behaviour of the renin–angiotensin system in pregnant subjects with renovascular disease is of considerable interest, although observations are sparse. August[15] measured plasma renin activity serially throughout pregnancy in a woman with hypertension and renal artery stenosis. Her plasma renin values rose early in pregnancy and remained near the upper limit of the normal pregnant range throughout most of gestation. She then developed features of superimposed pre-eclampsia, when plasma renin activity fell steeply to below values seen before she became pregnant. These limited data indicate normal responses to pregnancy, renal artery stenosis and pre-eclampsia respectively in this woman.

It appears therefore that renal artery stenosis is not rare in pregnancy with hypertension, probably frequently going undetected. It does not preclude a successful outcome. In most cases, drug therapy is indicated at least until parturition, with any operative intervention deferred. However, drugs which interfere with the renin–angiotensin system, such as ACE inhibitors, should be avoided in pregnancy (page 123). If operation is needed in pregnancy, the less invasive procedure transluminal renal angioplasty is probably preferable to surgery, although experience is very limited and any radiation hazard would need to be taken into account.

### Aldosterone-secreting adenoma (Conn's syndrome)

There are several reports of aldosterone-secreting adenoma in pregnancy.[15] In most instances, hypertension and the characteristic hypokalaemia (Chapter 35) have persisted through gestation. Despite the pregnancy, in which the renin–angiotensin system is normally stimulated, in these patients plasma renin has usually remained low. Thus the renin response is apparently dominated by the aldosterone-secreting tumour rather than the pregnancy; this relationship can be useful diagnostically.

If possible, operation is deferred until after delivery. The hypertension and hypokalaemia are probably best treated in pregnancy with the potassium-conserving diuretic amiloride (page 116). Intuitively, spironolactone, which can disturb the pattern of sex hormones (page 116), seems less suitable, although comparative studies are lacking.

### Phaeochromocytoma

The coexistence of phaeochromocytoma and pregnancy is well-recognized.[15,181] The clinical and biochemical features closely resemble those of phaeochromocytoma in non-pregnant subjects (page 214), although the diagnosis is easily missed if its possibility is not considered. Confusion with pre-eclampsia is especially likely (page 249). Failure to recognize phaeochromocytoma in a pregnant patient before delivery seriously endangers mother and fetus alike, the mortality rate for both being over 50%.

Pregnancy does not preclude the usual biochemical diagnostic tests (page 214), although data on the normal ranges in pregnancy are limited.

Localization of a tumour can be more difficult, because radiological procedures are a hazard to the fetus, especially in early pregnancy. However, magnetic resonance imaging or ultrasonography provide safe alternatives to scintigraphy, arteriography and computerized tomographic scanning.

The presence of a phaeochromocytoma in pregnancy poses severe therapeutic problems. The best interests of mother and fetus can well conflict. As in patients who are not pregnant, hypertension should always be controlled with drugs before proceeding to surgery. α-Adrenoceptor antagonists should be introduced first, and the blood pressure adequately lowered. A non-selective β-adrenoceptor blocker is then added so as to limit the risk of cardiac arrhythmias. Both α- and β-blockers (the latter extensively) have been used in pregnancy without incurring adverse effects on mother or fetus (page 218).

It has been recommended[182] that once drug therapy has been established, in the first and second trimesters the tumour should be removed. At operation, in pregnancy as in the non-pregnant patient, sodium nitroprusside should be available for intravenous infusion in the event of severe elevation of blood pressure (pages 151 and 219). In the third trimester, it is usually recommended that pregnancy be allowed to proceed until the fetus is sufficiently mature to permit delivery by Caesarian section. If possible, the phaeochromocytoma should be removed at the same operation.

It must be recognized that these recommendations, though plausible, are largely *ex cathedra*, since experience is limited.

——————————— Case study ———————————

See Case study 8, Appendix 2.

——————————— References ———————————

1. Rubin PC. Hypertension in pregnancy: clinical features. In *Handbook of Hypertension*, Vol. 10: *Hypertension in Pregnancy* (ed. PC Rubin). Amsterdam, Elsevier, 1988: 10–15.

2. Gifford RW, August PA, Chesley LC *et al*. Working group report on high blood pressure in pregnancy. *US Dept of Health and Public Services*. NIH Publication No. 91-3029, 1991.

3. The 1988 Joint National Committee. The 1988 report of the Joint Committee on Detection, Evaluation and Treatment of High Blood Pressure. *Arch. Intern. Med.* 1988; **148**: 1023–38.

4. Rayburn WF, Zuspan FP, Piehl EJ. Self-monitoring of blood pressure during pregnancy. *Am. J. Obstet. Gynecol.* 1984; **148**: 159–62.

5. Zuspan FP, Rayburn WF. Blood pressure self-monitoring during pregnancy: practical considerations. *Am. J. Obstet. Gynecol.* 1991; **164**: 2–6.

6. Atrash HK, Koonin LM, Lawson HW, Franks AL, Smith JC. Maternal mortality in the United States. 1979–1986. *Obstet. Gynecol.* 1990; **76**: 1955–60.

7. National High Blood Pressure Education Program working group report on high blood pressure in pregnancy. *Am. J. Obstet. Gynecol.* 1990; **163**: 1689–712.

8. Dunlop JCH. Chronic hypertension and perinatal mortality. *Proc. Roy. Soc. Med.* 1966; **59**: 838–41.

9. Lin C, Lindheimer MD, River P, Moawad AH. Fetal outcome in hypertensive disorders of pregnancy. *Am. J. Obstet. Gynecol.* 1982; **142**: 255–60.

10. Lindheimer MD. Hypertension in pregnancy. *Hypertension* 1993; **22**: 127–37.

11. Chesley LC. Diagnosis of pre-eclampsia. *Obstet. Gynecol.* 1985; **65**: 423–5.

12. Lindheimer MD, Katz AI. Pre-eclampsia: pathophysiology, diagnosis and management. *Annu. Rev. Med.* 1989; **40**: 233–50.

13. Loudon L. Some historical aspects of toxaemia of pregnancy: a review. *Br. J. Obstet. Gynaecol.* 1991; **98**: 853–8.

14. Dekker GA, Sibai BM. Early detection of pre-eclampsia. *Am. J. Obstet. Gynecol.* 1991; **165**: 160–72.

15. August P. The renin–angiotensin–aldosterone system in hypertension in human pregnancy. In *The Renin–Angiotensin System* (eds JIS Robertson and MG Nicholls). London: Gower Medical 1993: chapter 52.

16. Chamberlain G. The changing body in pregnancy. *Br. Med. J.* 1991; **302**: 719–22.

17. Christianson MA, Roberta E. Studies on blood pressure during pregnancy. 1. Influence of parity and age. *Am. J. Obstet. Gynecol.* 1976; **125**: 509–13.

18. MacGillivray I, Rose GA, Rowe D. Blood pressure survey in pregnancy. *Clin. Sci.* 1969; **37**: 395–407.

19. Hays PM, Cruikshank DP, Dunn LJ. Plasma volume determination in normal and pre-eclamptic pregnancies. *Am. J. Obstet. Gynecol.* 1985; **151**: 958–66.

20. Robson SC, Hunter S, Boys RJ. Serial study of factors influencing changes in cardiac output during human pregnancy. *Am. J. Physiol.* 1989; **256**: H1060–5.

21. Thomson AM, Hytten FE, Billewicz WZ. The epidemiology of oedema during pregnancy. *J. Obstet. Gynaecol.* 1967; **74**: 1–10.

22. Brown MA. Non-pharmacological management of pregnancy-induced hypertension. *J. Hypertens.* 1990; **8**: 295–301.

23. Phippard AF, Horvath JS, Glyn EM. Circulation adaptation to pregnancy—Serial studies of haemodynamics, blood volume, renin and aldosterone in the baboon (*Papio hamadryas*). *J. Hypertens.* 1986; **4**: 773–8.

24. Easterling TR, Benedetti TJ, Schmucker BC, Millard SP. Maternal haemodynamics in normal and pre-eclamptic pregnancies: a longitudinal study. *Obstet. Gynecol.* 1990; **76**: 1061–9.

25. Davison JM. Renal haemodynamics and volume homeostasis in pregnancy. *Scand. J. Clin. Lab. Invest.* 1984; **44** (suppl. 169): 15–27.

26. Skinner SL. The renin system in fertility and normal human pregnancy. In *The Renin–Angiotensin System* (eds JIS Robertson and MG Nicholls). London: Gower Medical 1993: chapter 50.

27. Davey DA, MacGillivray I. the classification and definition of the hypertensive disorders of pregnancy. *Clin. Exp. Hypertens.* 1986; **B5**: 97–133.

28. Silverstone A, Trudinger BJ, Lewis PJ, Bulpitt CJ. Maternal hypertension and intrauterine foetal death in mid-pregnancy. *Br. J. Obstet. Gynaecol.* 1980; **87**: 457–61.

29. Sibai BM, Mabie WC, Villar M, Shamsa F, Anderson GD. A comparison of no medication versus methyldopa or labetalol in chronic hypertension during pregnancy. *Am. J. Obstet. Gynecol.* 1990; **162**: 960–6.

30. Arias F, Zamora J. Antihypertensive treatment and pregnancy outcome in patients with mild chronic hypertension. *Obstet. Gynecol.* 1979; **53**: 489–94.

31. Roberts JM, Redman CWG. Pre-eclampsia: more than pregnancy-induced hypertension. *Lancet* 1993; **341**: 1447–51.

32. Kincaid-Smith P, Somers K, Browne JCM. Successful pregnancy under treatment for malignant hypertension. *Lancet* 1958; **i**: 508–9.

33. Weir RJ, Willocks J. A successful pregnancy following malignant phase hypertension. *Br. J. Obstet. Gynaecol.* 1976; **83**: 584–6.

34. Schmieder RE, Rockstroh JK. When is discontinuation of antihypertensive therapy indicated? *Cardiovasc. Drugs Ther.* 1990; **4**: 1487–94.

35. Eskenazi B, Fenster L, Sidney S. A multivariate analysis of risk factors for pre-eclampsia. *J. Am. Med. Assoc.* 1991; **266**: 237–41.

36. Saftlas AF, Olson DR, Franks AL, Atrash HK, Pokras R. Epidemiology of pre-eclampsia and eclampsia in the United States. 1979–1986. *Am. J. Obstet. Gynecol.* 1990; **163**: 460–5.

37. Garner PR, Dalton ME, Dudley DK, Huard P, Hardie M. Pre-eclampsia in diabetic pregnancies. *Am. J. Obstet. Gynecol.* 1990; **163**: 505–8.

38. Siddiqi T, Rosenn B, Mimouni F, Khoury J, Miodovnik M. Hypertension during pregnancy in insulin-dependent diabetic women. *Obstet. Gynecol.* 1991; **77**: 514–19.

39. Redman CW. Treatment of hypertension in pregnancy. *Kidney Int.* 1980; **18**: 267–78.

40. Lowe SA, Rubin PC. The pharmacological management of hypertension in pregnancy. *J. Hypertens.* 1992; **10**: 201–7.

41. Redman CWG. Current topic: Pre-eclampsia and the placenta. *Placenta* 1991; **12**: 301–8.

42. Page EW. The relation between hydatid moles, relative ischemia of the gravid uterus, and the placental origin of eclampsia. *Am. J. Obstet. Gynecol.* 1939; **37**: 291–3.

43. Scott JS. Pregnancy toxaemia associated with hydrops foetalis, hydatidiform mole, and hydramnios. *J. Obstet. Gynaecol. Br. Empire.* 1958; **65**: 689–701.

44. Sibai BM, McCubbin JH, Anderson GD, Lipshitz J, Dilts PV jr. Eclampsia I. Observations from sixty-seven recent cases. *Obstet. Gynecol.* 1981; **58**: 609–13.

45. Pritchard JA, Cunningham FG, Pritchard SA. The Parkland Memorial Hospital protocol for treatment of eclampsia: evaluation of 245 cases. *Am. J. Obstet Gynecol.* 1984; **148**: 951–63.

46. Redman CW. Eclampsia still kills. *Br. Med. J.* 1988; **296**: 1209–10.

47. Hankins GD, Wendel GD Jr, Cunningham FG, Leveno KJ. Longitudinal evaluation of haemodynamic changes in eclampsia. *Am. J. Obstet. Gynecol.* 1984; **150**: 506–12.

48. Groenendijk R, Trimbros JB, Wallenburg HC, Hemodynamic measurements in pre-eclampsia: preliminary observations. *Am. J. Obstet. Gynecol.* 1984; **150**: 506–12.

49. Adams EM, MacGillivray I. Long-term effect of pre-eclampsia on blood pressure. *Lancet* 1961; **ii**: 1373–5.

50. Sibai BM, Abdella TN, Spinnato JA, Shower DC. Plasma volume findings in patients with mild pregnancy-induced hypertension. *Am. J. Obstet. Gynecol.* 1983; **147**: 16–20.

51. Redman C. Hypertension in pregnancy. In *The Circulation in the Female: From the Cradle to the Grave* (ed. J Ginsburg). New Jersey: Parthenon, 1989: 63–76.

52. Chesley LC, Cooper DW. Genetics of hypertension in pregnancy: possible single gene control of pre-eclampsia and eclampsia in the descendants of eclamptic women. *Br. J. Obstet. Gynaecol.* 1986; **93**: 898–908.

53. Arngrimsson R, Bjornsson S, Geirsson RT, Bjornsson H, Walker JJ, Snaedal G. Genetic and familial predisposition to eclampsia and pre-eclampsia in a defined population. *Br. J. Obstet. Gynaecol.* 1990; **97**: 762–9.

54. Sibai BM. Immunologic aspects of pre-eclampsia. *Clin. Obstet. Gynecol.* 1991; **34**: 27–34.

55. Redman CWG. The fetal allograft. *Fetal Med. Rev.* 1990; **2**: 21–43.

56. Redman CWG. Immunology of pre-eclampsia. *Semin. Perinatol.* 1991; **15**: 257–62.

57. Milliez J, Lelong F, Bayani N, Jannet D, El Mediadii M, Latrous H, Hammami M, Paniel BJ. The prevalence of autoantibodies during third trimester pregnancy complicated by hypertension of idiopathic fetal growth retardation. *Am. J. Obstet. Gynecol.* 1991; **165**: 51–6.

58. El-Roeiy A, Myers SA, Gleicher N. The relationship between autoantibodies and intrauterine growth retardation in hypertensive disorders of pregnancy. *Am. J. Obstet. Gynecol.* 1991; **164**: 1253–61.

59. Foidart JM, Hunt J, Lapiere CM *et al.* Antibodies to laminin in pre-eclampsia. *Kidney Int.* 1986; **29**: 1050–7.

60. Katz VL, Thorp JM, Watson WJ, Fowler L, Heine RP. Human immunoglobulin therapy for pre-eclampsia associated with lupus anticoagulant and anticardiolipin antibodies. *Obstet. Gynecol.* 1990; **76**: 986–8.

61. Vanhoutte PM (ed.). *Endothelium-Derived Vasoactive Substances.* Clifton, New Jersey: Humana Press, 1988.

62. Roberts JM, Taylor RN, Musci TJ, Rodgers GM, Hubel CA, McLaughlin MK. Pre-eclampsia: an endothelial cell disorder. *Am. J. Obstet. Gynecol.* 1989; **161**: 1200–4.

63. Walsh SW. Pre-eclampsia: an imbalance in placental prostacylin and thromboxane production. *Am. J. Obstet. Gynecol.* 1985; **152**: 335–40.

64. Pinto A, Sorrentino R, Sorrentino P *et al.* Endothelial-derived relaxing factor released by endothelial cells of human umbilical vessels and its impairment in pregnancy-induced hypertension. *Am. J. Obstet. Gynecol.* 1991; **164**: 507–13.

65. Taylor RN, Crombleholm WR, Friedman SA *et al.* High plasma fibronectin levels correlate with biochemical and clinical features of pre-eclampsia but cannot be attributed to hypertension alone. *Am. J. Obstet. Gynecol.* 1991; **165**: 895–901.

66. Kamoi K, Sudo N, Ishibashi M, Yamaji T. Plasma endothelin-1 levels in patients with pregnancy-induced hypertension. *N. Engl. J. Med.* 1990; **323**: 1486–7.

67. Green IA, Leask R, Hodson BA *et al.* Endothelin, elastase, and endothelial dysfunction in pre-eclampsia. *Lancet* 1991; **337**: 558.

68. Dekker GA, Kraayenbrink AA, Zeeman GG, Van Kemp GJ. Increased plasma levels of the novel vasoconstrictor peptide endothelin in severe pre-eclampsia. *Rur. J. Obstet. Gynaecol. Reprod. Biol.* 1991; **40**: 215–20.

69. Furuhashi N, Tsujiei M, Kimura H *et al.* Plasma endothelin level, plasma renin activity and plasma aldosterone concentration in normal pregnancy and pre-eclampsia. *Proceedings, 7th World Congress on Hypertension in Pregnancy,* 1990; 298.

70. Branch DW, Dudley DJ, Mitchell MD. Preliminary evidence for homeostatic mechanism regulating endothelin production in pre-eclampsia. *Lancet* 1991; **337**: 943–5.

71. Brown MA, Zammit VC, Whitworth JA *et al.* Endothelin production in pre-eclampsia. *Lancet* 1991; **338**: 261.

72. Nova A, Sibai BM, Barton JR, Mercer BM, Mitchell MD. Maternal plasma level of endothelin is increased in pre-eclampsia. *Am. J. Obstet. Gynecol.* 1991; **165**: 724–7.

73. Ignarro LJ. Physiological significance of nitric oxide. *Semin. Perinatol.* 1991; **15**: 20–6.

74. Sarrel PM, Lindsay DC, Poole-Wilson PA *et al.* Hypothesis: inhibition of endothelium-derived relaxing factor by haemoglobin in the pathogenesis of pre-eclampsia. *Lancet* 1990; **336**: 1030–2.

75. Friedman SA. Pre-eclampsia: a review of the role of prostaglandins. *Obstet. Gynecol.* 1988, **71**: 122–37.

76. Weiner CP. The role of serotonin in the pre-eclampsia-eclampsia syndrome. *Cardiovasc. Drugs Ther.* 1990; **4**: 37–43.

77. Beaufils M, Uzan S, Donsimoni R, Colau JC. Prevention of pre-eclampsia by early antiplatelet therapy. *Lancet* 1985; **i**: 840–2.

78. Uzan S, Beaufils M, Breart G, Bazin B, Capitant C, Paris J. Prevention of fetal growth retardation with low-dose aspirin: findings of the EPREDA trial. *Lancet* 1991; **337**: 1427–31.

79. Sibai BM, Caritis SN, Thom E *et al.* Prevention of pre-eclampsia with low-dose aspirin in healthy, nulliparous pregnant women. *N. Engl. J. Med.* 1993; **329**: 1213–18.

80. Italian Study of Aspirin in Pregnancy. Low dose aspirin in prevention and treatment of intrauterine growth retardation and pregnancy-induced hypertension. *Lancet* 1993; **341**: 396–400.

81. Redman CWG. Platelets and the beginning of pre-eclampsia. *N. Engl. J. Med.* 1991; **323**: 478–80.

82. Katz VL, Thorp JM, Rozas L, Bowes WA. Natural history of thrombocytopenia associated with pre-eclampsia. *Am. J. Obstet. Gynecol.* 1990; **163**: 1142–3.

83. Burrows RF, Hunter DJ, Andrew M, Kelton JG. A prospective study investigating the mechanism of thrombocytopenia in pre-eclampsia. *Obstet. Gynecol.* 1987; **70**: 334–8.

84. Neiger R, Contag SA, Coustan DR. The resolution of pre-eclampsia-related thrombocytopenia. *Obstet. Gynecol.* 1991; **77**: 692–5.

85. Pritchard JA, Cunningham FG, Mason RA. Coagulation changes in eclampsia: their frequency and pathogenesis. *Am. J. Obstet. Gynecol.* 1976; **124**: 855–9.

86. Estelles A, Gilabert J, Espana F, Aznar J, Galbis M. Fibrinolytic parameters in normotensive pregnancy with intrauterine fetal growth retardation and in severe pre-eclampsia. *Am. J. Obstet. Gynecol.* 1991; **165**: 138–42.

87. De Boer K, Buller HR, Ten Cate JW, Treffers PE. Coagulation studies in the syndrome of haemolysis, elevated liver enzymes and low platelets. *Br. J. Obstet. Gynaecol.* 1991; **98**: 42–7.

88. Terao T, Maki M, Ikenoue T *et al.* The relationship between clinical signs and hypercoagulable state in toxemia of pregnancy. *Gynecol. Obstet. Invest.* 1991; **31**: 74–85.

89. Weinstein L. Syndrome of hemolysis, elevated liver enzymes, and low platelet count: a severe consequence of hypertension in pregnancy. *Am. J. Obstet. Gynecol.* 1982; **142**: 159–68.

90. Martin JN, Blake PG, Lowry SL, Perry KG, Files JC, Morrison JC. Pregnancy complicated by pre-eclampsia-eclampsia with the syndrome of hemolysis, elevated liver enzymes, and low platelet count: how rapid is postpartum recovery? *Obstet. Gynecol.* 1990; **76**: 737–41.

91. Chinn RH, Düsterdieck GO. The response of blood pressure to infusion of angiotensin II: relation to plasma concentrations of renin and angiotensin II. *Clin. Sci.* 1972; **42**: 489–504.

92. Baker PN, Broughton Pipkin F, Symonds EM. Comparative study of platelet angiotensin II binding and the angiotensin II sensitivity test as predictors of pregnancy-induced hypertension. *Clin. Sci.* 1992; **83**: 89–95.

93. Gaber LW, Spargo BH, Lindheimer MD. Renal pathology in pre-eclampsia. *Clin. Obstet. Gynecol.* 1987; **1**: 971–95.

94. Poston L, Morris JF, Wolfe CD, Hilton PJ. Serum digoxin-like substances in pregnancy-induced hypertension. *Clin. Sci.* 1989; **77**: 189–94.

95. Hou SH, Grossman SD, Madias NE. Pregnancy in women with renal disease and moderate renal insufficiency. *Am. J. Med.* 1985; **78**: 185–94.

96. Lindheimer MD, Katz AI. Gestation in women with kidney disease: prognosis and management. *Clin. Obstet. Gynecol.* 1987; **1**: 921–37.

97. Cunningham FG, Cox SM, Harstad TW, Mason RA, Pritchard JA. Chronic renal disease and pregnancy outcome. *Am. J. Obstet. Gynecol.* 1990; **163**: 453–9.

98. Packham DK, Fairley KF, Ihle BU, Whitworth JA, Kincaid-Smith P. Comparison of pregnancy outcome between normotensive and hypertensive women with primary glomerulonephritis. *Clin. Exp. Hypertens.* 1987–1988: **B6**: 387–399.

99. Smith LG, Moise KJ, Dildy GA, Carpenter RJ. Spontaneous rupture of liver during pregnancy: current therapy. *Obstet. Gynecol.* 1991; **77**: 171–5.

100. Brown CE, Purdy P, Cunningham FG. Head computed tomographic scans in women with eclampsia. *Am. J. Obstet. Gynecol.* 1988; **159**: 915–20.

101. Bewley S, Copper D, Campbell S. Doppler investigation of uteroplacental blood flow resistance in the second trimester: a screening study for pre-eclampsia and intrauterine growth retardation. *Br. J. Obstet. Gynaecol.* 1991; **98**: 871–9.

102. Fleischer A, Schulman H, Farmakides G *et al.* Uterine artery Doppler velocimetry in pregnant women with hypertension. *Am. J. Obstet. Gynecol.* 1986; **154**: 806–13.

103. Trudinger BJ, Giles WB, Cook CM. Flow velocity wave forms in the maternal uteroplacental and fetal umbilical placental circulations. *Am. J. Obstet. Gynecol.* 1985; **152**: 155–63.

104. Steel SA, Pearce JM, McParland P, Chamberlain GV. Early Doppler ultrasound screening in prediction of hypertensive disorders of pregnancy. *Lancet* 1990; **335**: 1548–51.

105. Redman CWG, Beilin LJ, Bonnar J, Wilkinson RH. Plasma urate measurements in predicting fetal death in hypertensive pregnancy. *Lancet* 1976; **i**: 1370–3.

106. McFadyen IR, Greenhouse P, Price AB, Geirsson RT. The relation between plasma urate and placental bed vascular adaptation to pregnancy. *Br. J. Obstet. Gynaecol.* 1986; **93**: 482–7.

107. Sibai BM, Taslimi M, Abdella TN, Brooks TF, Spinnato JA, Anderson GD. Maternal and perinatal outcome of conservative management of severe

pre-eclampsia in midtrimester. *Am. J. Obstet. Gynecol.* 1985; **152**: 32–7.

108. Sibai BM. Eclampsia: VI. Maternal-perinatal outcome in 154 consecutive cases. *Am. J. Obstet. Gynecol.* 1990; **163**: 1049–55.

109. Sibai BM, Sherif A, Fairlie F, Moretti M. A protocol for managing severe pre-eclampsia in the second trimester. *Am. J. Obstet. Gynecol.* 1990; **163**: 733–8.

110. Sibai BM, Spinnato JA, Watson DL, Lewis JA, Anderson GD. Eclampsia. IV. Neurological findings and future outcome. *Am. J. Obstet. Gynecol.* 1985; **152**: 184–92.

111. Seidman DS, Serr DM, Ben-Rafael Z. Renal and ocular manifestations of hypertensive diseases of pregnancy. *Obstet. Gynecol. Sum.* 1991; **46**: 71–5.

112. Spence JD, Arnold JMO, Gilbert JJ. Vascular consequences of hypertension and effects of antihypertensive therapy. In *Handbook of Hypertension*, Vol. 15: *Clinical Hypertension* (ed. JIS Robertson). Amsterdam: Elsevier, 1992: 621–54.

113. Schenker JG, Chowers I. Pheochromocytoma and pregnancy: review of eighty-nine cases. *Obstet. Gynecol. Surv.* 1971; **26**: 739–47.

114. Oddendaal HJ, Pattinson RC, Bam R, Grove D, Kotze TJ. Aggressive or expectant management for patients with severe pre-eclampsia between 28 and 34 weeks gestation: a randomized controlled trial. *Obstet. Gynecol.* 1990; **76**: 1070–5.

115. Symonds EM. Pregnancy hypertension. In *Diseases of the Heart*, 1st edn. (eds DG Julian, AJ Camm, KM Fox *et al.*). London: Baillière Tindall, 1989: 1372–83.

116. Symonds EM. Bed rest in pregnancy. *Br. J. Obstet. Gynaecol.* 1982; **89**: 593–5.

117. Tuffnell DJ, Lilford RJ, Buchan PC *et al.* Randomised controlled trial of day care for hypertension in pregnancy. *Lancet* 1992; **339**: 224–7.

118. Brown MA, Zammit VC, Mitar DM. Extracellular fluid volumes in pregnancy-induced hypertension. *J. Hypertens.* 1992; **10**: 61–8.

119. Gallery ED, Hunyor SN, Gyory AZ. Plasma volume contraction: a significant factor in both pregnancy associated hypertension (pre-eclampsia) and chronic hypertension in pregnancy. *Q. J. Med.* 1979; **48**: 593–602.

120. Stuart MJ, Gross SJ, Elrad H, Graeber JE. Effects of acetylsalicylic-acid ingestion on maternal and neonatal hemostasis. *N. Engl. J. Med.* 1982; **307**: 909–12.

121. Wallenburg HC, Dekker GA, Makovitz JW, Rotmans P. Low-dose aspirin prevents pregnancy-induced hypertension and pre-eclampsia in angiotensin-sensitive primigravidae. *Lancet* 1986; **i**: 1–3.

122. Schiff E, Pelag E, Goldenberg M *et al.* The use of aspirin to prevent pregnancy-induced hypertension and lower the ratio of thromboxane $A_2$ to prostacyclin in relatively high-risk pregnancies. *N. Engl. J. Med.* 1989; **321**: 351–6.

123. Benigni A, Gregorini G, Frusca T *et al.* Effect of low dose aspirin on fetal and maternal generation of thromboxane by platelets in women at risk for pregnancy-induced hypertension. *N. Engl. J. Med.* 1989; **321**: 357–62.

124. Wallenburg HCS, Dekker GA, Makovitz JW, Rotmans N. Effect of low-dose aspirin on vascular refractoriness in angiotensin-sensitive primigravid women. *Am. J. Obstet. Gynecol.* 1991; **164**: 1169–73.

125. Schiff E, Barkai G, Ben-Baruch G, Mashiach S. Low-dose aspirin does not influence the clinical course of women with mild pregnancy-induced hypertension. *Obstet. Gynecol.* 1990; **76**: 742–4.

126. Clarke RJ, Mayo G, Price P, Fitzgerald GA. Suppression of thromboxane $A_2$ but not of systemic prostacyclin by controlled-release aspirin. *N. Engl. J. Med.* 1991; **325**: 1137–41.

127. CLASP Collaborative Group. A randomised trial of low-dose aspirin for the prevention and treatment of pre-eclampsia among 9364 pregnant women. *Lancet* 1994; **343**: 619–29.

128. Redman CW, Beilin LJ, Bonnar J, Ounsted MK. Fetal outcome in trial of antihypertensive treatment in pregnancy. *Lancet* 1976; **ii**: 753–6.

129. Lamming GD, Symonds EM. Use of labetalol and methyldopa in pregnancy-induced hypertension. *Br. J. Clin. Pharmacol.* 1979; **8** (suppl. 2): 217–22.

130. Gallery EDM, Ross MR, Gyory AZ. Antihypertensive treatment in pregnancy: analysis of different responses to oxprenolol and methyldopa. *Br. Med. J.* 1985; **291**: 563–6.

131. Rubin PC, Butters L, Clark DM *et al.* Placebo-controlled trial of atenolol in treatment of pregnancy-associated hypertension. *Lancet* 1983; **i**: 431–4.

132. Redman CWG, Roberts JM. Management of pre-eclampsia. *Lancet* 1993; **341**: 1451–4.

133. Spitz B, Witters K, Hanssens M *et al.* Ketanserin, a $5HT_2$ serotonergic receptor antagonist, could be

useful in the HELLP syndrome. *Hypertens. Pregnancy* 1993; **12**: 183–190.

134. Redman CWG, Beilin LJ, Bonnar J. Treatment of hypertension in pregnancy with methyldopa: blood pressure control and side effects. *Br. J. Obstet. Gynaecol.* 1977; **84**: 419–26.

135. Leather HM, Humphreys DM, Baker P, Chadd MA. A controlled trial of hypotensive agents in hypertension in pregnancy. *Lancet* 1968; **ii**: 488–90.

136. Fidler J, Smith V, Fayers P, DeSwiet M. Randomized controlled comparative study of methyldopa and oxprenolol in treatment of hypertension in pregnancy. *Br. Med. J.* 1983; **286**: 1927–30.

137. Kincaid-Smith P, Bullen M, Mills J. Prolonged use of methyldopa in severe hypertension in pregnancy. *Br. Med. J.* 1966; **1**: 274–6.

138. Ounsted M, Cockburn J, Moar VA, Redman CWG. Maternal hypertension with superimposed pre-eclampsia: effects on child development at 7.5 years. *Br. J. Obstet. Gynaecol.* 1983; **90**: 644–9.

139. Cockburn J, Moar VA, Ounsted M, Redman CWG. Final report of the study on hypertension during pregnancy: the effects of specific treatment on the growth and development of the children. *Lancet* 1982; **i**: 647–9.

140. Rubin PC. Beta-blockers in pregnancy. *N. Engl. J. Med.* 1981; **305**: 1323–6.

141. Wichman K, Ryden G, Karlberg BE. A placebo controlled trial of metoprolol in the treatment of hypertension in pregnancy. *Scand. J. Clin. Lab. Invest.* 1984; **94** (suppl. 169): 90–5.

142. Lardoux H, Gerard J, Blazquez G, Chouty F, Flouva B. Hypertension in pregnancy: evaluation of two beta blockers atenolol and labetalol. *Eur. Heart J.* 1983; **4** (suppl. A): 35–40.

143. Lubbe WF, Hodge JV. Combined alpha and beta receptor antagonism with prazosin and oxprenolol in control of severe hypertension in pregnancy. *N. Z. Med. J.* 1981; **94**: 169–72.

144. Sibai BM, Gonzalez AR, Mabie WC, Moretti M. A comparison of labetalol plus hospitalization versus hospitalization alone in the management of pre-eclampsia remote from term. *Obstet. Gynecol.* 1987; **70**: 323–7.

145. Livingstone I, Craswell PW, Bevan EB. Propranolol in pregnancy three year prospective study. *Clin. Exp. Hypertens.* 1983; **B2**: 341–50.

146. Walters BN, Redman CW. Treatment of severe pregnancy-associated hypertension with the calcium antagonist nifedipine. *Br. J. Obstet. Gynaecol.* 1984; **91**: 330–6.

147. Ulmsten U. Treatment of normotensive and hypertensive patients with preterm labor using oral nifedipine, a calcium antagonist. *Arch. Gynecol.* 1984; **236**: 69–72.

148. Constantine G, Beevers DG, Reynolds AL, Luesley DM. Nifedipine as a second-line antihypertensive drug in pregnancy. *Br. J. Obstet. Gynaecol.* 1987; **94**: 1136–42.

149. Rubin PC, Butters L, McCabe R. Nifedipine and platelets in pre-eclampsia. *Am. J. Hypertens.* 1988; **1**: 175–7.

150. Barton JR, Hiett AK, Conover WB. The use of nifedipine during the postpartum period in patients with severe pre-eclampsia. *Am. J. Obstet. Gynecol.* 1990; **162**: 788–92.

151. Van Harten J, Burggraaf K, Danhof M *et al*. Negligible sublingual absorption of nifedipine. *Lancet* 1987; **ii**: 1363–5.

152. Kraus GW, Marchese JR, Yen SSC. Prophylactic use of hydrochlorothiazide in pregnancy. *J. Am. Med. Assoc.* 1966; **198**: 1150–4.

153. Sibai BM, Grossman, RA, Grossman HG. Effects of diuretics on plasma volume in pregnancies with long-term hypertension. *Am. J. Obstet. Gynecol.* 1984; **150**: 831–5.

154. Collins R, Yusuf S, Peto R. Overview of randomised trials of diuretics in pregnancy. *Br. Med. J.* 1985; **290**: 17–23.

155. MacGillivray I, Hytten FE, Taggart N. *et al*. The effects of a sodium diuretic on total exchangeable sodium and total body water in pre-eclamptic toxaemia. *J. Obs. Gyn. Br. Cmwlth.* 1962; **69**: 548–53.

156. Ferris TF, Weir EK. Effect of captopril on uterine blood flow and prostaglandin E synthesis in the pregnant rabbit. *J. Clin. Invest.* 1983; **71**: 809–15.

157. Knott PD, Thorpe SS, Lamont CAR. Congenital renal dysgenesis possibly due to captopril. *Lancet* 1989; **i**: 451.

158. Rosa FW, Bosco LA, Graham CF, Milstein JB, Dreis M, Creamer J. Neonatal anuria with maternal angiotensin-converting enzyme inhibition. *Obstet. Gynecol.* 1989; **74**: 371–4.

159. Schubiger G, Flury G, Nussberger J. Enalapril for pregnancy-induced hypertension: acute renal failure in a neonate. *Ann. Intern. Med.* 1988; **108**: 215–16. (Published erratum appears in *Ann. Intern. Med.* 1988; **108**: 777.)

160. Dudley DKL. Minibolus diazoxide in the management of severe hypertension in pregnancy. *Am. J. Obstet. Gynecol.* 1985; **151**: 196–200.

161. Trust PM, Rosei EA, Brown JJ *et al.* Effect on blood pressure, angiotensin II and aldosterone concentrations during treatment of severe hypertension with intravenous labetalol: comparison with propranolol. *Br. J. Clin. Pharmacol.* 1976; **3** (suppl. 3): 799–803.

162. Cumming AMM, Brown JJ, Lever AF *et al.* Treatment of severe hypertension by repeated bolus injections of labetalol. *Br. J. Clin. Pharmacol* 1979; **8** (suppl. 2): 199–204.

163. Stempel JE, O'Grady PJ, Morton MJ, Johnston KA. Use of sodium nitroprusside in complications of gestation hypertension. *Obstet. Gynecol.* 1982; **60**: 533–8.

164. Shoemaker CT, Meyers M. Sodium nitroprusside for control of severe hypertensive disease of pregnancy: a case report and discussion of potential toxicity. *Am. J. Obstet. Gynecol.* 1984; **149**: 171–3.

165. Naulty J, Cefalo RC, Lewis PE. Fetal toxicity of nitroprusside in the pregnant ewe. *Am. J. Obstet. Gynecol.* 1981; **139**: 708–11.

166. Lewis PE, Cefalo RC, Naulty JS, Rookley FL. Placental transfer and fetal toxicity of sodium nitroprusside. *Gynecol. Obstet. Invest.* 1977; **8**: 46–7.

167. Dinsdale HB. Does magnesium sulfate treat eclamptic seizures? Yes. *Arch. Neurol.* 1988; **45**: 1360–1.

168. Kaplan PW, Lesser RP, Fisher RS, Repke JT, Hanley DF. No, magnesium sulfate should not be used in treating eclamptic seizures. *Arch. Neurol.* 1988; **45**: 1361–4.

169. Watson KV, Moldow CF, Ogburn PL, Jacob HS. Magnesium sulfate: rationale for its use in preeclampsia. *Proc. Natl Acad. Sci. USA* 1986; **83**: 1075–8.

170. Crowther C. Magnesium sulfate versus diazepam in the management of eclampsia: a randomized clinical trial. *Br. J. Obstet. Gynaecol.* 1990; 97–110.

171. Lindheimer MD. Magnesium sulphate and preeclampsia or eclampsia. *Arch. Neurol.* 1989; **46**: 1360–1.

172. Domisse J. Phenytoin sodium and magnesium sulphate in the management of eclampsia. *Br. J. Obstet. Gynaecol.* 1990; **97**: 104–9.

173. Conyaji KJ, Otiv SR. Single high dose of intravenous phenytoin sodium for the treatment of eclampsia. *Acta Obstet. Gynecol.* 1990; **69**: 115–18.

174. White WB, Andreoli JW, Cohn RD. Alpha-methyldopa disposition in mothers with hypertension and in their breast fed infants. *Clin. Pharmacol. Ther.* 1985; **37**: 387–90.

175. Miller ME, Cohn RD, Burghart PH. Hydrochlorothiazide disposition in a mother and her breast-fed infant. *J. Pediatr.* 1982; **101**: 789–91.

176. Krause W, Stoppelli I, Milia S, Rainer E. Transfer of mepindolol to newborns by breast-feeding mothers after single and repeated daily doses. *Eur. J. Clin. Pharmacol.* 1982; **22**: 53–5.

177. Bryans CI Jr. The remote prognosis in toxemia of pregnancy. *Clin. Obstet. Gynecol.* 1966; **9**: 973–90.

178. Chesley LC, Annitto JE, Cosgrove RA. The remote prognosis of eclamptic women: sixth periodic report. *Am. J. Obstet. Gynecol.* 1976; **124**: 446–59.

179. Sibai BM, Mercer BM, Dahmus MA. Severe pre-eclampsia in the second trimester: recurrence risk and long term prognosis. *Am. J. Obstet. Gynecol.* 1991; **164** (suppl.): 244.

180. Koskela O, Kaski P. Renal angiography in the follow-up examination of toxemia of late pregnancy. *Acta Obstet. Gynecol. Scand.* 1971; **40**: 41–43.

181. Hall AS, Ball SG. Pheochromocytoma and pregnancy. In *Handbook of Hypertension*, Vol. 15: *Clinical Hypertension* (ed. JIS Robertson). Amsterdam: Elsevier, 1992: 530–1.

182. Burgess GE. alpha blockade and surgical intervention in phenochromocytoma in pregnancy. *Obstet. Gynecol.* 1979; **53**: 266–70.

183. Wang M-X, Brown MA, Buddle ML *et al.* Endothelin excretion in hypertensive pregnancy. *Am. J. Hyp.* 1994; **7**: 308–13.

184. Barden A, Beilin LJ, Ritchie J *et al.* Plasma and urinary endothelin 1, prostacyclin metabolites, and platelet consumption in pre-eclampsia and essential hypertensive pregnancy. *Blood Pressure* 1994; **3**: 38–46.

185. Arbogast BW, Leeper SC, Merrick RD *et al.* Which plasma factors bring about disturbance of endothelial function in pre-eclampsia? *Lancet* 1994; **343**: 340–1.

186. Arngrimssan R, Connor JM, Geirsson RT *et al.* Is genetic susceptibility for pre-eclampsia and eclampsia associated with implantation failure and fetal demise? *Lancet* 1994; **33**: 1643–4.

187. Janes SL, Goodall AH. Flow cytometric detection of circulating activated platelets and platelet hyper-responsiveness in pre-eclampsia and pregnancy. *Clin. Sci.* 1994; **86**: 731–9.

# Appendix 1
# Drugs used in hypertension

This appendix offers a ready guide to commonly used antihypertensive agents and their classification. The list of drugs is not exhaustive and only limited information on individual agents is given. A more detailed account of antihypertensive drugs and their use is given in Chapters 22 and 47. Readers must refer to the data from manufacturers and drug regulatory authorities in different countries for further appropriate information. Lower doses are usually advisable in elderly patients, while larger doses of diuretics can be valuable with renal failure. Some drugs, which are excreted by the kidney, should be given in lower doses with renal impairment.

| Agent | Dose | Side-effects | Comments |
|---|---|---|---|
| **CENTRALLY ACTING DRUGS** | | | |
| Methyldopa | 250 mg twice or thrice daily. Increase by 250–500 mg daily at intervals of more than 2 days. Maximum 3 g. Start 125 mg twice daily in elderly or in pregnancy. | Drowsiness, dry mouth, metallic taste, nasal stuffiness, postural hypotension, initial fluid retention (use with diuretic),rashes, diarrhoea, rarely toxic hepatitis, positive Coombs' test 20% but haemolytic anaemia rare. | Widely prescribed in past but now used as reserve agent, e.g. when $\beta$-blockers contraindicated or in patients 'difficult to control'. Extensive experience of its use in pregnancy but newer drugs often favoured. Intravenous preparation rarely used. |
| Clonidine | 50 $\mu$g thrice daily, increase at intervals of more than 2 days, maximum 600–1200 $\mu$g daily although sometimes 1800 $\mu$g needed (250 $\mu$g slow release capsules, transdermal preparation available). | Drowsiness, dry mouth, 'rebound' hypertension, less postural hypotension than methyldopa, constipation, skin reactions to patch. | Drowsiness and 'rebound hypertension' if drug stopped has limited its use in UK. |
| Rilmenidine | Definitive dose not yet settled. 1 mg once daily has been effective. | See clonidine and comments opposite. | Claimed less drowsiness and dry mouth than clonidine. Not yet established. |
| Reserpine | 0.25 mg daily for 1 week reducing to 0.1 mg daily. | Nasal stuffiness, drowsiness, lethargy, depression with large doses. | Inexpensive and widely prescribed in USA, Germany, Switzerland, but little use in UK because of perceived risk of depression. |
| **DIURETICS** | | | |
| *Thiazides (common examples include):* | | | |
| Bendrofluazide | 2.5–5.0 mg daily. | Biochemical abnormalities, more apparent at high doses, hypokalaemia, impairment of glucose tolerance, increase uric acid, may precipitate gout, raise serum cholesterol, rarely cause severe | Very commonly used drugs with established safety profile, but avoided in pregnancy hypertension. Keep dose in range shown to give maximal pressure effect against minimal biochemical disturbance. |
| Hydrochloro-thiazide | 12.5–50 mg daily; occasional maximum 100 mg daily. | | |
| Chlorothiazide | 125–500 mg daily; occasional maximum 1 g daily. | | |

| Agent | Dose | Side-effects | Comments |
|---|---|---|---|
| Chlorthalidone[1] | 25–50 mg daily. | decrease of serum sodium. Provoke male sexual impotence, cause muscle cramps, constipation, lethargy, dizziness, very rarely serious sulphonamide type reaction (jaundice, rash, pancreatitis, blood dyscrasias, angiitis, pneumonitis, interstitial nephritis). | Awareness of hypokalaemia important especially because of concern of ventricular arrhythmias. Avoid combination with proarrhythmic drugs. Consider 'loop diuretic' when GFR < 15/20 ml/min.<br>[1] Chlorthalidone has very long half life.<br>[2] Derived chemically from thiazides but lowers pressure at doses below those causing diuresis. |
| Indapamide[2] | 2.5 mg daily. | | |
| Xipamide | 10–20 mg daily. | | |
| *Loop-acting:* | | | |
| Frusemide | 20–40 mg daily (up to 2 g daily in severe renal impairment). | Marked diuresis may trouble some patients, hypokalaemia, hypovolaemia. May have less hyperglycaemic and uricaemic effects than thiazides. Skin eruptions, blood dyscrasias, ototoxicity (especially with large dose rapid i.v. injection in renal failure). Myalgia with high dose bumetanide. All can provoke urinary retention with prostate enlargement | Contraindicated if hypersensitive to sulphonamides. Used particularly when GFR low in high doses or as adjunct to therapy with ACE-inhibitor or minoxidil in hypertension difficult to control. Thiazides usually used in preference in hypertension but see side-effects. Various claims for clinically useful differences between agents listed. Ethacrynic acid is little used in UK probably because of problems with gastro-intestinal disturbance and deafness. |
| Bumetanide | 0.5–2 mg daily (up to 10 mg daily in severe renal impairment). | | |
| Piretanide | 6–12 mg with breakfast. | | |
| Ethacrynic acid | 50–150 mg daily. | | |
| *Potassium conserving diuretics:* | | | |
| Amiloride | 2.5–20 mg daily. Up to 75–80 mg may be used in Conn's syndrome. | Hyperkalaemia especially if impaired renal function or patient on indomethacin-like drug or ACE-inhibitor. Amiloride may act for 4–5 days so hyperkalaemia can be prolonged. Gastrointestinal disturbance. | Amiloride and triamterene act on the sodium/potassium exchange of the distal tubule and are usually combined with a thiazide diuretic. They are an effective way of maintaining serum potassium. They have blood pressure lowering effect and do not appear to worsen blood glucose or uric acid levels. Triamterene, unlike amiloride, is protein bound (60%) and highly metabolised in the liver. High dose amiloride has been used extensively for the treatment of Conn's syndrome. |
| Triamterene | 150–250 mg in divided dose. | | |
| Spironolactone[1] | 50–100 mg once daily. (Up to 400 mg in divided doses with meals in Conn's syndrome.) | Hyperkalaemia, oestrogen-like gynaecomastia, impotence, menstrual irregularity, gastro-intestinal disturbance, peptic ulceration. | Unlike amiloride and triamterene spironolactone blocks aldosterone receptors.<br>[1] Spironolactone is no longer recommended in the UK for long-term treatment of essential hypertension. Its usefulness in Conn's syndrome is limited by its side-effects in high dose; amiloride may be preferable. |

| Agent | Dose | Side-effects | Comments |
|---|---|---|---|

## $\beta$-ADRENOCEPTOR ANTAGONISTS ($\beta$-BLOCKERS)

Numerous drugs are available and are broadly categorized here into non-selective (block both $\beta_1$- and $\beta_2$-adrenoceptors), selective ($\beta_1$-selective) and those with vasodilating properties. Some have more intrinsic sympathomimetic activity (ISA) than others, e.g. pindolol, with different degrees of lipid solubility and potential for central effects. These different properties may have more impact on side-effects profile than blood pressure reduction.

| Agent | Dose | Side-effects | Comments |
|---|---|---|---|
| See individual drugs below | | Bradycardia, myocardial depression, broncho-constriction, heart block, cold peripheries, lipid soluble $\beta$-blockers, e.g. propranolol, may cause dreams/insomnia. Raise lipids, raise blood glucose, care on withdrawal especially if ischaemic heart disease because of increase in heart rate. | Various claims are made concerning potential advantages/disadvantages of different properties of $\beta$-antagonists. All can cause bronchoconstriction (should be avoided in asthma) and depress myocardial function so extreme care is required for their use in patients with poor ventricular function. Cold extremities, common in hypertension, may be worsened and caution is needed in patients with peripheral vascular disease. |
| *Non-selective agents:* | | | |
| Propranolol | 40 mg daily to 160 mg twice daily. Long-acting preparation 80–320 mg daily. i.v. 1 mg up to 10 mg over 1 minute (maximum 5 mg under anaesthesia). | | Half-life 1–6 h. Lipid soluble, non-selective (i.e. blocks $\beta_1$ and $\beta_2$). First pass effect. No ISA. Metabolized in the liver. Lower dose in liver or renal failure. 90% protein bound. |
| Nadolol | 80–240 mg once daily. | | Long half-life 16–24 h. Not lipid soluble. No first-pass effect. No ISA. 20% protein bound. Renal excretion—lower dose in renal failure. |
| Oxprenolol | 40–160 mg twice to three times daily. Slow release 160–480 mg daily. | | Short half-life 2 h. Lipid soluble. First-pass effect. Modest ISA. 80% protein bound. Liver metabolism similar to propranolol. |
| Penbutolol | 10–40 mg once daily. | | Long half-life 27 h. Lipid soluble. First-pass effect. 98% protein bound. Liver metabolism. |
| Pindolol | 5–15 mg twice or thrice daily. | | Half-life 4 h. Low lipid solubility. Small first-pass effect. ISA. 50–70% protein bound. Liver and kidney metabolism. |
| Sotalol | 80–480 mg once daily. i.v. 20–60 mg over 2–3 min. | | Has class III antiarrhythmic effect at higher doses. Risk of torsades de pointes with diuretics, hypokalaemia or drugs prolonging QT interval. Long half-life. Not lipid soluble. No first-pass effect. No ISA. 5% protein bound. Excreted by kidneys. |

| Agent | Dose | Side-effects | Comments |
|-------|------|--------------|----------|
| β-ADRENOCEPTOR ANTAGONISTS—β-BLOCKERS—*continued* | | | |
| *Non-selective agents:* | | | |
| Timolol | 5–45 mg once daily. | | Half-life 4–5 h. Low lipid solubility. First-pass effect. No ISA. Some protein binding—limited data. Metabolized liver and kidney. |
| *Cardioselective β-blockers:* | | | Cardioselective drugs may potentially cause less bronchospasm and fewer problems with cold extremities but selectivity is lost as dose increases. |
| Atenolol | 25–100 mg once daily. i.v. 5–10 mg slowly (1 mg per minute). | | Half-life 6–9 hours. Not lipid soluble. No first-pass effect. No ISA. 5% protein bound. Renal excretion. |
| Acebutolol | 200–400 mg once daily. | | Half-life 7 h. Not lipid soluble. First-pass metabolism. Major metabolite diacetolol contributes to its activity. Both acebutolol and diacetolol have some ISA. 10–15% protein bound. Liver (acebutolol) and renal (diacetolol) excretion. |
| Bisoprolol | 5–20 mg once daily. | | High $\beta_1$ selectivity. Half-life 10–12 hours. Low lipid solubility. No/low first-pass effect. No ISA. 30% protein bound. Liver and renal excretion. |
| Metoprolol | 50–200 mg twice daily. | | Half-life 3–5 h. No ISA. Not highly selective. Metabolised in liver. 12% protein-bound. Lipophilic. |
| Nebivolol | 2.5–5 mg once daily. | | High $\beta_1$ selectivity. Not registered in UK. |
| *β-Blockers with vasodilating properties:* | | | |
| Labetalol | 200–400 mg once daily to 400 mg three times daily. i.v. dose 100–800 mg twice daily. i.v. infusion 1–2 mg/kg over 10 min., or as 25 or 50 mg bolus at 10 min. intervals. Doses usually lower in pregnancy hypertension. | | Some α-blocking properties but otherwise like propranolol but with slight ISA. Extensive use in pregnancy hypertension. Used orally and i.v. for urgent blood pressure reduction. Half-life 3–4 h. High lipid solubility. Some first-pass metabolism. Modest ISA. 50–90% protein bound. Liver metabolism. |
| Carvedilol | 12.5 mg once daily to 50 mg twice daily. | | β-Blocking properties similar to propranolol. Also α-blocking. Half-life 7 h. High first pass metabolism. Metabolites excreted in the bowel. Vasodilating properties may result in fewer vasoconstrictor or cardioinhibitory side-effects. |

| Agent | Dose | Side-effects | Comments |
|---|---|---|---|

### α-ADRENOCEPTOR ANTAGONISTS (α-BLOCKERS)

See text for phentolamine and phenoxybenzamine used for phaeochromocytoma. Prazosin was the first selective $\alpha_1$-blocking agent to find widespread clinical use. Unpredictable first-dose hypotension led to initial difficulties. Newer longer acting doxazosin and terazosin claimed to have less (but still distinct) first-dose problems and convenience of once daily dosing. Neutral or beneficial effect on lipids (may increase HDL) perceived as benefit.

| Agent | Dose | Side-effects | Comments |
|---|---|---|---|
| Prazosin | Test dose 0.5 mg. 0.5–10 mg twice daily. | First dose effect. Postural hypotension. Drowsiness. | Used more as supportive rather than initial therapy. First-pass metabolism. Renal excretion. |
| Doxazosin | 1–16 mg daily increasing at 2 weekly intervals. | Headache, dizziness, lethargy. | No first-pass metabolism. Perceived beneficial effects on lipids by increasing HDL/LDL cholesterol ratio and lowering triglycerides. |
| Terazosin | 1 mg at bedtime. 2–10 mg daily increasing each week. | Dizziness, lethargy. | |
| Indoramin | 25–100 mg twice daily. | | At higher doses drowsiness/dry mouth/nasal stuffiness may be more common than with other $\alpha_1$-blockers. Some antihistamine effect—care with alcohol. |

### CALCIUM ANTAGONISTS

Larger heterogeneous group of which the antihypertensive agents are usually classified into class I, verapamil-like; class II, nifedipine-like; class III, properties between I and II, diltiazem-like

| Agent | Dose | Side-effects | Comments |
|---|---|---|---|
| Verapamil | 80–240 mg twice daily. 160–480 mg once daily slow release. | Constipation is a common problem. Headaches, dizziness, facial flushing may occur but much less common than with vasodilating class II calcium antagonists. Hypotension and bradycardia if given with $\beta$-blocker or in left ventricular failure. | Care with $\beta$-blockers. Increases digoxin levels. Useful alternative to $\beta$-blocker, e.g. in asthmatics. Cimetidine increases half-life. |
| Nifedipine | a) Adalat retard tablets 10–40 mg twice daily. b) Adalat long-acting (LA) tablets 30–90 mg once daily. c) Adalat capsules 5–20 mg thrice daily. d) Coracten capsules 10–40 mg twice daily. | Headache, facial flushing, tachycardia, ankle swelling. | Start low dose especially in elderly to avoid side-effects. Extended release system may give better tolerance. These can be bitten and *swallowed* to give rapid hypotensive effect. Rapid lowering of blood pressure is however rarely needed (see text). |
| Nicardipine | 20–40 mg thrice daily. | | Similar to nifedipine—may have less myocardial depression. |
| Amlodipine | 5–10 mg daily. | | Long half-life and slow absorption. Less tachycardia and headache claimed. Fewer drug interactions than nifedipine. |
| Felodipine | 5–10 mg once daily usually; 20 mg maximum. | | May be less risk of myocardial depression and currently under investigation in treatment of heart failure. |

| Agent | Dose | Side-effects | Comments |
|---|---|---|---|
| *Class III:* | | | |
| Diltiazem | 60–180 mg twice daily usually. Maximum 480 mg total daily dose. Numerous slow-release/long acting/ retard preparations 90–180 mg once to twice daily. | Nifedipine/verapamil-like side-effects but less extreme of both. Rarely severe skin reaction. | Problems in use similar to those of verapamil. |

## ANGIOTENSIN CONVERTING ENZYME (ACE) INHIBITORS

A number of drugs are now widely available which act by inhibiting the enzyme which converts angiotensin I to the active peptide angiotensin II. This enzyme also breaks down bradykinin and other peptides which may account for beneficial actions of this group of drugs but also may relate to some of the class-related side-effects. The drugs differ in whether or not they require conversion in the liver for activity (pro-drug), their length of action, route of excretion, experience of use in patients and large scale trials.

*Side effects:*

All may cause severe falls in blood pressure in patients who are salt deplete through for example high dose diuretics or who have treated heart failure. For the majority of patients starting treatment for raised blood pressure this is not relevant. Renal failure can be induced in patients with bilateral renal artery stenosis, or stenosis of a solitary renal artery, or if prolonged hypotension occurs. A dry irritating cough prevents their use in some patients. Angio-oedema is very rare but associated with their use. Rash and headache have been reported.

*Comments:*

*Not* used in pregnancy but otherwise now widely prescribed and considered 'first line' therapy by many clinicians. Major concern is their use in the presence of renal artery stenosis (which may not be apparent) since pressure control may improve but measurement of overall renal function will not detect deterioration in function (leading to possible loss through arterial occlusion) of kidney beyond stenosis. Low starting doses, especially in elderly, are recommended with careful monitoring of renal function especially if renal impairment. Serious hyperkalaemia can be induced in those with renal impairment or taking potassium-sparing diuretic. Avoid salt depletion, e.g. temporarily stop diuretics prior to administration to avoid first-dose hypotension. Care needed with introduction in treated heart failure. Reduce maintenance doses in those with renal impairment.

| Agent | Dose | Side-effects | Comments |
|---|---|---|---|
| Captopril | 12.5–50 mg twice daily. | Taste loss and proteinuria associated only with high doses in selected patient groups. | Wide experience of use. Not a pro-drug. Has rapid absorption giving 'full' ACE-inhibition (and potential first-dose hypotension) within 20–60 min but short lived unless repeat dose or with higher initial dose. Usual maintenance dose 25–50 mg twice daily. |
| Cilazapril | 1–5 mg once daily (0.25 mg available). | | Requires conversion to cilazaprilat (see enalapril). Usual maintenance 2.5–5 mg daily. |
| Enalapril | 2.5–40 mg once daily. | | Requires conversion to enalaprilat for activity taking 2–4 hours after ingestion but depending on dose to achieve full ACE-inhibition (i.e. delayed first-dose hypotension if occurs). Longer half-life than captopril so often used once daily. Usual maintenance dose 10–20 mg daily. |
| Fosinopril | 10–40 mg once daily. | | Liver, gut and renal elimination. |

| Agent | Dose | Side effects | Comments |
|---|---|---|---|
| Lisinopril | 2.5–40 mg once daily. | | Long half-life and active without conversion. Slow absorption causes delay of 4–6 hours to achieve full ACE-inhibition after first dose. Usual maintenance dose 10–20 mg daily. |
| Perindopril | 2–8 mg once daily. | | Requires conversion to perindoprilat (see enalapril). Usual maintenance 4–6 mg daily. |
| Quinapril | 2.5–80 mg once daily. | | Requires conversion to quinaprilat. Usual maintenance dose 20–40 mg daily. |
| Ramipril | 1.25–10 mg once daily. | | Potent drug with very long half-life. Requires conversion to ramiprilat for activity (see enalapril). Usual maintenance dose 2.5–5 mg daily. |

## VASODILATING DRUGS

These drugs cause vasodilation through a presumed direct relaxation of vascular smooth muscle, the mechanism of which is unclear. They can cause reflex tachycardia and fluid retention and are used in conjunction with other agents to offset these effects, often as a 'third line' treatment.

| Agent | Dose | Side effects | Comments |
|---|---|---|---|
| Hydralazine | 25–100 mg twice to three times daily (but see side effects). 10 mg starting dose available. Intravenous and intra muscular preparations available for rare use in urgent pressure reduction. Low dosage 5–10 mg should be used (as drug taken orally undergoes considerable pre-systemic metabolism) and can be increased and repeated at 20–30 minute intervals. | The main concern has been the development of 'lupus syndrome'. This is unusual if total daily dose below 200 mg but women may be more susceptible than men. Arthralgia may be an early (often neglected) start of the syndrome. Headache and tachycardia are prominent side-effects in some patients and can be avoided by using low starting dosage. Fluid retention may recur. | In the past widely used as a 'third line' agent added to, for example, β-blockers and diuretics. Problems with 'lupus syndrome' have restricted its use and many would advocate only doses below 100 mg total daily. Vasodilating calcium antagonists often now chosen in preference. |
| Minoxidil | Total daily dose 5 to 50 mg, usually given in two doses. Start 2.5 mg daily increasing every 3 or more days to 5 mg twice daily to usual maximum of 25 mg twice daily. | Marked fluid retention and reflex tachycardia. Hypertrichosis makes drug unacceptable to women. | Reserved for treatment of severe hypertension resistant to other drugs. Large doses of frusemide, e.g. 250–500 mg daily may sometimes be required to counteract fluid retention. Used with β-blockers or other drugs which can block the reflex tachycardia. |
| Sodium nitroprusside | Intravenous use for hypertensive crises. i.v. infusion. 0.3 micrograms/kg/minute adjusted to 0.5–6 micrograms/kg/minute. Maximum 8 micrograms/kg/min. | Rapid reduction in BP, headache, nausea. 'Cyanide side effects': <br>• tachycardia <br>• sweating <br>• hyperventilation <br>• arrhythmias <br>• metabolic acidosis <br>• cyanosis. | Rarely required but very effective agent to reduce BP rapidly but predictably by constant minute by minute adjustment of infusion rate as required according to pressure. Short term (intravenous) use only. Protect from light. Cyanide antidotes are available (dicobalt edetate, sodium nitrite, sodium thiosulphate). |

# Appendix 2
## Test cases

There follow brief accounts of 23 illustrative cases of hypertension. Where the text is interrupted by: ————◆———— the reader is intended to pause and to consider what next step he or she would take. At the end of each description we give our own comments.

The cases progress sequentially from commonplace but important examples through to rarities. All the accounts are based on patients known personally to the authors, although some have been shortened and otherwise modified for didactic purposes.

## Case study 1

A 40-year-old salesman is found on routine insurance medical examination to have a blood pressure of 200/118 mmHg. He neither smokes nor drinks alcohol, and there is nothing of relevance found in the personal or family history or on clinical examination.

Repeated measurements over the next 4 weeks confirm pressures always in the range of 200–220/110–120 mmHg. In this period various investigations including urine testing; measurement of plasma electrolytes, urea, creatinine, lipids and aldosterone; intravenous urography; abdominal ultrasonography; and ECG are all normal. An echocardiogram shows mild left ventricular hypertrophy.

————————◆————————

Treatment is started with atenolol 100 mg daily. This is well-tolerated, but only partially effective; after 2 months blood pressure is 160/100 mmHg. Hydrochlorothiazide 25 mg plus amiloride 2.5 mg is therefore added. Three months later values of 150/90 mmHg indicate that further control is advisable, and amlodipine 5 mg once daily is also prescribed.

The patient is subsequently reviewed 6-monthly and has pressures in the range 120–130/80–90 mmHg. Echocardiography at one year of therapy, which is well-tolerated, shows regression of left ventricular hypertrophy.

### Comment

This is an example of uncomplicated essential hypertension, of sufficient severity to warrant early therapy, a view reinforced by evidence of left ventricular hypertrophy. Not unusually, a triple combination of drugs is needed to achieve good control. Convenience is facilitated by giving these in once-daily doses.

For further reading see Chapters 22 and 25.

# Case study 2

A 44-year-old non-smoking male company executive is found on routine examination to have a blood pressure of 180/120 mmHg. He is physically fit and only a moderate drinker of wine. His own history is unremarkable, although his mother, now 80, has mild diabetes mellitus; his father died at 76 after a myocardial infarction.

Clinical examination is also unremarkable. Detailed investigation, urged by his company, includes urine testing; measurement of plasma electrolytes, urea, creatinine, uric acid, lipids, renin and aldosterone; chest X-ray; renal arteriography; ECG and echocardiogram. All are normal; notably there is no suggestion of left ventricular hypertrophy.

◆

Repeated clinic pressures are nearly always raised, although not so markedly as at the initial visit (range 140–160/104–110 over 6 weeks). However, measurements made by the subject himself at his home are much lower (range 110–120/70–80 mmHg), and a 24-h ambulatory record shows no blood pressure elevation.

◆

The subject is reassured, no treatment is prescribed, and he is kept simply under 4-monthly routine clinic review. Interestingly, these later pressures taken by the doctor are never higher than 120/80 mmHg.

## Comment

This is probably an example of the so-called 'white-coat' effect, where the excitement of a clinic visit, with the presence of the doctor, can transiently raise blood pressure to atypical levels. This example illustrates the use of 24-h blood pressure recording, and emphasizes that drug therapy should not be started impetuously in such instances.

That said, requiring mention is that 'white-coat' hypertension is not known certainly to be benign; it is a reasonable precaution in the present instance to maintain regular, but not over-frequent, review.

For further reading, see Chapter 3 and page 136.

# Case study 3

A 35-year-old male travel agent is found by his primary care physician to have a blood pressure of 146/100 mmHg. A non-smoker, he drinks beer heavily at weekends and is overweight at 92 kg (he is 1.68 m tall). No relevant history is obtained other than that his father died at 68 of a stroke.

◆

He is advised to moderate his drinking, to exercise regularly and to reduce weight.

The advice is taken; the patient takes up badminton twice weekly, limits his eating and drinking, and within 6 months has a weight of 76 kg. Monthly checks of blood pressure over this time show a steady decline, to a reading of 118/78 mmHg at 6 months. He is, however, kept under regular review by his doctor.

### Comment

This case exemplifies the attention to commonsense aspects of lifestyle which can avoid the need for drug therapy in mild hypertension. In any event, antihypertensive drugs should never be introduced prematurely in mild hypertension.

Not all overweight beer drinkers are as readily compliant as this man; the practitioner is wise to review the patient regularly so as to detect or prevent relapse.

For further reading see Chapters 22 and 25.

# Case study 4

A 40-year-old female accountant is found to have, on routine examination for insurance purposes, a blood pressure of 140/100 mmHg. She is a non-smoker, a very moderate drinker and has never taken oral contraceptives. Her weight is normal. Nothing of relevance is discovered in her past history; however, her 62-year-old mother has diabetes mellitus, and her 72-year-old father is under therapy for hypertension and has suffered two strokes.

Clinical examination of the patient is unremarkable. On detailed investigation she is found only to have mild glucose intolerance with transient glycosuria on glucose tolerance testing (high blood glucose levels at 1 h, but with a return to normal levels by 2 h).

◆

Repeated blood pressure measurements over 3 months consistently give values in the range 130–140/96–100 mmHg. Mild hypertension is confirmed on 24-h recording at 3 months.

◆

The mild but distinct hypertension, together with incipient diabetes mellitus and poor family history lead to a decision for drug therapy. Diuretics and β-blockers are to be avoided, if possible, because of the diabetes.

Enalapril is therefore started and the patient tolerates this well, with good blood pressure control (118/70 mmHg at a dose of 5 mg once daily after 6 months). She is seen 3-monthly.

## Comment

This is a good illustration of the type of patient with mild hypertension in whom drug treatment is advisable, but should not be introduced precipitately. The family history, especially her mother's diabetes mellitus, and the subject's own marginal glucose intolerance prompt drug therapy despite the mildness of the hypertension. This example should be compared with Case studies 2 and 3.

For further reading see Chapters 9, 22 and 25.

# Case study 5

A 66-year-old retired bank manager is noted by his primary care physician to have blood pressures around 180/80 mmHg on repeated measurements over one year. The only other item of possible relevance is that the patient's serum total cholesterol concentration is raised at 7.0 mmol/litre (272 mg/dl).

◆

Treatment is begun with enalapril 5 mg once daily. No other measures are instituted. This drug is well-tolerated, and subsequent blood pressures are around 130/80 mmHg.

### Comment

This appears to be the correct approach. Isolated systolic hypertension in elderly subjects, as here, has been shown to carry a distinct morbidity, and controlled trials have clearly shown the ability of antihypertensive treatment to limit that morbidity.

The physician is probably also correct to ignore the hypercholesterolaemia. In hypertensive subjects over 60, elevated total serum cholesterol has been found to carry a good, not adverse, prognosis.

For further reading see Chapters 20 and 21.

# Case study 6

A 68-year-old retired widower is found by his primary care physician to have a blood pressure of 190/106 mmHg. Several subsequent readings over the following 2 months are similarly found to lie in the range 190–210/106–116 mmHg.

◆

Treatment is initiated with bendrofluazide 5 mg daily, increasing after 2 months to 10 mg daily; atenolol 100 mg daily is then added; and subsequently nifedipine retard 10 mg twice daily. Even so, after 1 year blood pressure remains at 210/110 mmHg.

◆

The physician reviews the problem: the patient denies alcohol consumption; he is not on non-steroidal anti-inflammatory drugs or indeed any other medication; the doses of antihypertensive agents, particularly of the diuretic, seem adequate; there is no evidence of secondary hypertension; and there is no suggestion of concomitant disease. However, his pulse rate is 76 per min, and plasma potassium 4.2 mmol/litre, despite his ostensibly taking substantial doses of atenolol and bendrofluazide, thus questioning compliance.

◆

The situation is discussed with the patient's daughter, who lives nearby. She states that he is sometimes confused and forgetful; a subsequent search of his house reveals large quantities of unconsumed antihypertensive drugs.

◆

She undertakes to supervise his drug intake daily. After this, on only atenolol 100 mg daily, blood pressures are well-controlled at 130–140/86–94 mmHg. Pulse rate is around 60 per min.

### Comment

This case illustrates a very common problem—poor compliance with therapy—a fault frequently found, but by no means exclusively so, in old patients. The physician correctly reviewed the likely causes of drug-resistant hypertension in this instance. A very frequent reason for drug resistance, which was excluded in the present patient, is concurrent administration of a non-steroidal anti-inflammatory drug.

Also noteworthy is that often, as here, reversion to a simple dosage schedule can be more effective than the attempt to pursue a complex one.

For further reading see Chapter 25.

# Case study 7

A 36-year-old married female nurse consults an optometrist because of increasing difficulty in reading print over the past month. He notices the presence of bilateral retinal haemorrhages and exudates plus papilloedema, and refers her for an urgent medical opinion.

On examination the extensive retinopathy is confirmed. Blood pressure is 260/150 mmHg. There is heavy proteinuria. She now mentions also increasing shortness of breath on exertion for the past month.

This woman therefore has malignant phase hypertension.

$\blacklozenge$

She is admitted to hospital forthwith. Detailed questioning reveals that she has had three pregnancies, respectively 12, 10 and 6 years earlier; all were uneventful and blood pressure was said to be normal throughout all three. For the past 5 years she has been taking an oral contraceptive containing 30 $\mu$g oestrogen plus 2 mg of progestogen; no measurements of blood pressure have been made in this time.

Nothing else of relevance is revealed; serum creatinine and urea concentrations are within the normal range.

$\blacklozenge$

The oral contraceptive is discontinued forthwith and mechanical contraception adopted. Blood pressure falls to 180/120 mmHg within 24 h of a single 50 mg oral dose of atenolol. This is increased to 100 mg daily, and pressure decreases further in the next few days. She is discharged taking a combination of atenolol 100 mg plus hydrochlorothiazide 25 mg plus amiloride 2.5 mg daily. No cause for hypertension other than the pill is found on detailed investigation. Six months later blood pressures are around 110/80 mmHg, the retinal lesions have cleared, and she has neither proteinuria nor exertional dyspnoea.

$\blacklozenge$

The antihypertensive drugs are withdrawn, whereupon blood pressure rises slightly, to around 130/80 mmHg.

$\blacklozenge$

She remains off therapy and is warned not to restart oral contraception.

### Comment

This case re-emphasizes the need for regular blood pressure measurements in all women who take oral contraceptives. The oestrogen–progestogen pill, even when containing as little as 30 $\mu$g oestrogen, causes at least a slight rise in blood pressure in nearly every woman; occasionally, as here, the increase is marked.

Advance to the malignant phase is well-recorded, albeit rare. Fortunately, in this case the condition was diagnosed before renal function became impaired and before any medical catastrophe occurred. The omission of blood pressure checks during oral contraceptive treatment was nevertheless especially reprehensible in a senior nurse who was, at the time, working in the gynaecological department of a teaching hospital.

Further discussion is given in Chapter 27, page 158.

# Case study 8

A 38-year-old woman is referred by her obstetrician for a medical opinion. She has been under drug treatment for essential hypertension for the past 5 years and is at present on atenolol 100 mg plus bendrofluazide 5 mg daily. She is now 4 months pregnant. She has had two previous pregnancies, respectively 19 and 17 years ago. Both were uneventful and went to full term without problems; so far as she knows there was no mention then of hypertension. She has never taken oral contraceptives. She is anxious to proceed with the present pregnancy if possible. Her blood pressure now is 126/78 mmHg; there is no proteinuria.

◆

She is advised that she should continue with the pregnancy under regular 2–3 weekly supervision. Bendrofluazide is discontinued and atenolol 100 mg daily is sole therapy.

Through the second trimester blood pressure falls slightly to values around 110/70 mmHg, then rises to a maximum of 136/88 mmHg in the final week. Delivery is uneventful. Subsequently good control of her hypertension is maintained, as before, on atenolol 100 mg plus bendrofluazide 5 mg daily.

**Comment**

This case illustrates that it is unnecessary to be alarmist concerning pregnancy with treated essential hypertension, even in women in their late thirties. Blood pressure usually falls somewhat in the middle trimester of normal pregnancy and a similar pattern, as here, can obtain also with antecedent hypertension. Whilst a close watch should be kept, the development of pre-eclampsia is unlikely.

Diuretics are not advised in pregnancy; in the present instance the diuretic was withdrawn without problem.

It is re-emphasized that pre-existent hypertension should not engender an unduly restrictive attitude towards pregnancy. Successful pregnancies have been achieved in women who have had previous malignant hypertension.

For further information see Chapter 47.

# Case study 9

A 35-year-old male housepainter presents with a 5-week history of increasing exertional dyspnoea, especially obvious on climbing ladders, and morning headaches. He smokes 30–40 cigarettes daily and drinks heavily (beer and whisky) at weekends.

He is found to have a blood pressure of 260/130 mmHg, distinct proteinuria and extensive bilateral retinal haemorrhages and exudates, but no obvious papilloedema. There is no overt cardiac failure, although there are a few inspiratory crepitations on auscultation of the lung bases.

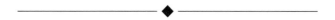

This is a case of malignant hypertension, requiring urgent treatment and investigation, even in the absence of papilloedema. He is referred for immediate hospital admission that day, where treatment is at once started with oral atenolol 100 mg daily. Blood pressure has fallen to around 150/100 mmHg within 3 days. Hydrochlorothiazide 25 mg plus amiloride 2.5 mg is then added; he remains on this combination over the next 3 years with outpatient blood pressures around 130/80 mmHg.

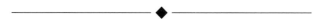

Detailed investigation fails to reveal an underlying cause for his malignant hypertension; plasma electrolytes are consistently normal, renal function is unimpaired, and renal ultrasound, intravenous urography and renal arteriography are all unremarkable. Left ventricular hypertrophy is however evident initially on both ECG and echocardiogram.

In addition to his antihypertensive drugs, he is advised, successfully, to cease smoking and to moderate his alcohol consumption.

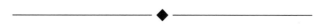

Six months after presentation, the retinal lesions have cleared, left ventricular hypertrophy has regressed and there is no proteinuria. He continues symptom-free at full-time work.

## Comment

This case illustrates that malignant hypertension is an immediate medical emergency; the diagnosis no longer requires the criterion of papilloedema. Parenteral treatment is, however, not usually needed. Once blood pressure is controlled, full search (which in this case was negative) for a possible cause of hypertension must be undertaken. Drug treatment may interfere with some investigations, such as measurement of plasma renin and aldosterone. However, it is paramount to control blood pressure in this situation and not to delay for investigation. Renal arteriography can be undertaken more safely with good pressure control and modern biochemical techniques can exclude phaeochromocytoma, even with drug administration. The malignant phase is more frequent in cigarette smokers.

For further reading see Chapters 7, 8, 13, 14 and 25.

# Case study 10

A 50-year-old male solicitor presents to his primary care physician with increasing, although mild, exertional dyspnoea over 4–6 months. He smokes 15–20 cigarettes daily but does not drink alcohol. He is found to have a blood pressure of around 220/120 mmHg, mild proteinuria and bilateral retinal haemorrhages and exudates plus papilloedema.

A correct diagnosis of malignant hypertension is made but no immediate treatment is given; an appointment is made for the patient to be seen by a consultant physician some 3 weeks hence.

Ten days later, before the hospital visit, the primary care physician is summoned over the telephone by the patient's wife, anxious because for 2 days he has had severe headaches and increasing dyspnoea, now provoked by only mild exertion.

On the physician's arrival 2 h later, the patient is found to be mentally confused, with very severe headache, and with a blood pressure of 270/150 mmHg.

---◆---

The hospital consultant is now summoned for an urgent domiciliary visit.

The consultant arrives 3 h later to find the patient having a generalized convulsion. Blood pressure, measured with difficulty, is around 300/160 mmHg.

---◆---

This is hypertensive encephalopathy, and is treated by giving an intravenous bolus of 25 mg labetalol, followed by a second 25 mg bolus 10 min later. Blood pressure is now around 180/110 mmHg and there are no further convulsions. The patient is transferred immediately to hospital where his blood pressure is controlled with oral atenolol 100 mg daily; no further parenteral treatment is needed. Four days later he is no longer confused, does not have a headache, and blood pressure is around 140/100 mmHg.

---◆---

In hospital he is found to have a plasma sodium concentration of 134 mmol/litre and potassium of 3.2 mmol/litre. There is also mild renal impairment, with plasma creatinine 140 mmol/litre.

---◆---

The mild hypokalaemia and hyponatraemia could indicate secondary aldosterone excess, and this is confirmed by the later demonstration of elevated plasma renin (despite his having received i.v. labetalol) and aldosterone concentrations. Other investigations are essentially negative, renal arteriography being normal and there being no evidence biochemically of phaeochromocytoma.

---◆---

The patient is subsequently discharged on atenolol 100 mg daily plus a combination of hydrochlorothiazide 25 mg with amiloride 2.5 mg daily. Blood pressure remains in the range 120–140/80–90 mmHg. He is told to stop smoking.

He remains well and symptom-free. One year later the retinal lesions have fully resolved, there is no proteinuria, renal function has improved (plasma creatinine 115 mmol/litre) and plasma electrolyte levels are normal (sodium 140, potassium 4.1 mmol/litre).

## Comment

The management of this case should be contrasted, unfavourably, with that of Case study 9. Malignant hypertension requires admission to hospital forthwith for urgent treatment and subsequent investigation. Despite the correct diagnosis, management was initially incorrectly tardy here. Prompt action would have prevented the progression to hypertensive encephalopathy, and would probably also have limited the renal impairment.

The later acute hypertensive encephalopathy was correctly dealt with by immediate parenteral treatment. Especially commendable is that too great a reduction in blood pressure, which can be dangerous, was avoided.

Note that hyponatraemia can help to differentiate secondary aldosterone excess (i.e. hyperaldosteronism stimulated by enhancement of the renin–angiotensin system) from primary aldosterone excess, where the renin system is suppressed and hypernatraemia is typical (see Case study 20). Malignant phase is unusual but well-documented in patients with Conn's syndrome.

Whilst secondary aldosteronism could have been due to renal artery stenosis, this possibility was examined and excluded here. The cause was undoubtedly stimulation of the renin system because of renal arterial lesions of malignant hypertension. The manifestations of secondary aldosterone excess disappeared on adequate antihypertensive treatment and healing of the arterial lesions of malignant hypertension. Renal function also improved concurrently.

Again, note that the malignant phase is more likely with cigarette smoking.

For further reading see Chapters 8, 13, 14 and 25.

# Case study 11

A 56-year-old bus driver notices what he thinks is blood in his urine. He seeks an urgent appointment with his own doctor. The doctor confirms blood in the urine on sample 'stick' testing and arranges an 'urgent' outpatient appointment at the genito-urinary clinic. The patient continues to work until he is seen 3 weeks later and admitted as a day case for intravenous urography and cystoscopy. Both tests are normal. Two weeks later, the patient, who wears glasses only for reading, feels his vision is 'not right' and attends his local optometrist. Severe retinopathy, with bilateral haemorrhages and exudates is diagnosed, and his own doctor, to whom he is promptly referred back, then finds a blood pressure reading of 208/126 mmHg. A diagnosis of malignant phase hypertension is made and he is sent that evening for hospital admission and urgent treatment.

## Comment

Routine blood pressure measurement by the patient's own doctor, by the nursing staff, by doctors at the clinic, or on admission for investigation would have avoided unnecessary tests and would have led to appropriate treatment much earlier. Malignant phase hypertension is a rare but well-documented cause of haematuria.

For further reading, see Chapters 13, 16, 23, 24 and 25.

# Case study 12

A 59-year-old man has felt vaguely unwell all day at his job as a fork-lift truck driver. On retiring to bed he becomes extremely breathless and his primary care physician is called. An emergency doctor arrives who has no records of the patient. Examination confirms acute left ventricular failure with a blood pressure of 210/126 mmHg. The optic fundi are normal. There has been no chest pain to suggest myocardial infarction. The patient gives no history of hypertension and cannot recall having his pressure measured. The doctor is not sure what treatment should be given.

### Comment

Acute pulmonary oedema complicating severe hypertension is rare, and the absence of serious retinopathy on fundoscopy argues against this as the cause of his acute breathlessness. It is very common for high blood pressure to be associated acutely and transiently with such pulmonary oedema and appropriate treatment is intravenous frusemide; or immediate sublingual nitrate as a vasodilator, together with a diuretic. In this case, an ECG confirmed previous myocardial infarction but this was considered to be 'old', from an unrecognized past event, and thrombolysis was not undertaken.

For further reading, see Chapter 17.

# Case study 13

A 45-year-old newsagent/tobacconist is seen at his home by his primary care physician, complaining of worsening exertional breathlessness for one month and ankle swelling for 2 weeks. The history also reveals that he has been getting up frequently at night to pass urine and had paroxysmal nocturnal dyspnoea during the previous night. He is a heavy cigarette smoker (60/day) who has never had his blood pressure measured previously. There is no previous renal history.

He is found to be in cardiac failure, with elevated central venous pressure, an enlarged distended liver, and both peripheral and pulmonary oedema. Blood pressure is 240/130 mmHg and he has bilateral retinal haemorrhages and exudates plus papilloedema.

◆

This man has malignant phase hypertension and is rightly admitted to hospital forthwith. At hospital he is found also to have heavy proteinuria plus haematuria, and to be in renal failure with plasma creatinine of 840 mmol/litre and potassium 6.5 mmol/litre. Abdominal ultrasound shows the kidneys to be of normal size.

◆

Regular haemodialysis is promptly undertaken, with relief of the cardiac failure as well as of the azotaemia and hyperkalaemia. Additionally with dialysis there is a fall in blood pressure to around 160/110 mmHg.

◆

Even so, antihypertensive drug treatment is introduced after 4 days; enalapril 5 mg daily is begun and continued.

With this and continued twice weekly dialysis, blood pressure settles around 130/80 mmHg. Although strongly enjoined to stop smoking, he ignores the advice. Arteriography shows no abnormality of the main renal arteries.

Six months later the retinal lesions have resolved and the patient awaits renal transplantation.

## Comment

This is a case of malignant hypertension, apparently, but not certainly, on a basis of essential hypertension. The main renal arteries are demonstrably normal, and the kidneys are of normal size, indicating that the renal failure is probably due to arterial lesions of malignant hypertension within the kidneys. If so, had the diagnosis been made earlier, and had antihypertensive treatment been started sooner, renal function could have been preserved.

It is also noteworthy that the removal of sodium and water by haemodialysis can substantially correct hypertension. Again, the more ready development of the malignant phase in smokers is to be emphasized.

This case should be compared with Case studies 9 and 10.

For further reading see Chapters 8, 13, 14, 16, 25 and 33.

# Case study 14

A 50-year-old woman presents to her primary care physician complaining of severe nocturia (up to four times nightly) together with headaches, particularly severe on rising in the mornings. Her blood pressure is found to be 220/110 mmHg.

◆

On referral to hospital these findings are confirmed, with one important additional historical item. That is that for many years the woman has been addicted to liquorice-containing sweets. Her exact consumption is difficult to ascertain but is undoubtedly grossly excessive, comprising at least two boxes daily.

◆

Liquorice excess as the probable cause of her problems is confirmed by the pattern of plasma electrolytes (sodium 144 mmol/litre, potassium 2.0 mmol/litre, bicarbonate 32 mmol/litre). Plasma concentrations of aldosterone, renin and angiotensin II are all subnormal.

◆

The patient is persuaded with difficulty to abandon her long-established predilection for liquorice. However, the efforts are successful, following which blood pressure falls to around 140/80 mmHg, the pattern of plasma electrolytes becomes normal, and the nocturia disappears.

## Comment

This case again shows the importance of careful elicitation of the history. The nocturia here reflected the renal effects of the liquorice-induced potassium deficiency. Note also that with liquorice excess, both aldosterone and renin are low in plasma (compare with Case study 20).

Further details of liquorice-induced hypertension are given in Chapter 27, page 162.

# Case study 15

A 55-year-old farm labourer who has suffered two myocardial infarctions and has been a known hypertensive for over 10 years has had a well-controlled blood pressure (range 120–130//80–90 mmHg) on an unchanged dose of β-blocker plus thiazide diuretic over the past 5 years. Despite advice, he continues to smoke 10–15 cigarettes daily. Plasma lipid levels are normal. At routine 3-monthly review his pressure is found unexpectedly to have risen to 200/126 mmHg. There are no new symptoms, compliance with therapy is claimed to be good, and the optic fundi show no haemorrhages or exudates. Renal function remains good as shown by normal levels of plasma urea and creatinine. However, plasma sodium and potassium have both fallen slightly, respectively to 134 and 3.7 mmol/litre.

A repeat intravenous urogram now shows features suggestive of left renal artery stenosis. There is a 2-min delay after the appearance of the right urogram before the left side is seen, whilst by 15 and 20 min the affected left urogram is markedly denser than on the normal right side. These signs were not present on the urogram of 10 years earlier. Both this intravenous urogram and ultrasonography show that the left kidney is 2.5 cm shorter than the right.

Renal arteriogram confirms the presence of an atheromatous stenosis at the origin of the left main renal artery.

The lesion is successfully dilated one week later by transluminal angioplasty. Good blood pressure control is then re-established on the previous drug regime.

## Comment

This case illustrates several important points. The supervention of renal artery stenosis can be a reason for the appearance of drug-resistant hypertension in a previously well-controlled compliant patient.

Renal artery stenosis is especially to be suspected in a patient already with overt atheromatous disease, in this case in the coronary circulation. The association of arterial atheromatous disease, including renal artery stenosis, with smoking is also emphasized.

The slight hyponatraemia and hypokalaemia could well indicate secondary aldosterone excess due to increased renin secretion because of the renal artery stenosis. However, this would be difficult to evaluate in a patient already receiving a β-blocker and a diuretic and, probably correctly therefore, measurements of plasma renin and aldosterone were not pursued here.

It should be re-emphasized that with unilateral renal artery stenosis the established urogram is denser on the affected side. Neglect or ignorance of this important point can lead to a disastrous surgical attack on the contralateral normal kidney (compare this with Case studies 6 and 16).

For further reading see Chapters 25, 29 and 31.

# Case study 16

A 50-year-old lorry driver, a heavy smoker, develops sudden severe left loin pain, followed by haematuria for 2 days. Three days later he develops polyuria, nocturia, thirst, polydipsia, weight loss, severe headaches and visual impairment. His primary care physician finds his blood pressure to be 230/130 mmHg and that he has bilateral retinal haemorrhages and exudates with papilloedema.

◆

Immediate hospital admission is arranged. On arrival at hospital additional findings are pronounced hyponatraemia and hypokalaemia (respectively 124 and 2.8 mmol/litre); both plasma renin and aldosterone are found to be markedly elevated.

◆

The history and findings, and especially the mode of onset, indicate that this is a case of hyponatraemic hypertensive syndrome, probably due to left renal artery thrombosis. Renal arteriogram confirms left renal artery occlusion.

◆

Hypovolaemia is partially corrected by the infusion of 1 litre of normal saline, when a small dose (6.25 mg) of captopril is given by mouth. Within 30 min blood pressure falls steeply, from 220/120 to 110/70 mmHg; with continued captopril 50 mg by mouth three times daily over the next 10 days the gross electrolyte abnormalities are corrected, and the blood pressure settles to around 120–130/80–90 mmHg.

◆

Left nephrectomy is then performed, the operation specimen being confirmed as a shrunken ischaemic kidney having an atheromatous renal artery with superimposed thrombosis.

◆

Drug treatment is stopped at the time of operation. The patient subsequently remains well and symptom-free. One year later blood pressure is recorded as 124/70 mmHg, and plasma electrolytes and renal function remain normal. Optic fundi are now also normal.

### Comment

This illustrates one of the most striking ways in which renal artery stenosis can present, as the hyponatraemic hypertensive syndromee. The severe renal artery lesion (in this instance occlusion) causes intense renin secretion with secondary aldosterone excess and potassium loss. Simultaneously the combination of severe hypertension with very high plasma angiotensin II levels promotes a natriuresis from the contralateral normal kidney, sodium loss and hence even further elevation of renin, angiotensin II and aldosterone.

The syndrome, as here, can be treated by the lowering of plasma angiotensin II with the giving of an ACE inhibitor. However, the combination of sodium depletion, hypovolaemia and very high plasma angiotensin II means that there is then a risk of severe initial hypotension; this was partly limited in the present case by prior saline infusion, and by using a small first dose of captopril. Even so, the steep fall in pressure raised concern.

Renal surgery or renal artery surgery, as here, provides definitive treatment.

The association of renal artery atheroma with cigarette smoking is again seen. This case should be compared with Case studies 15 and 21.

For further reading see Chapters 29 and 31.

# Case study 17

A 55-year-old widow has been observed by her primary care physician to have blood pressures around 190/110 mmHg over some 4 months. Treatment is therefore begun with nifedipine retard 10 mg twice daily. Four weeks later she attends the doctor stating that for the initial 8 days of therapy she experienced headache and facial flushing, which symptoms then subsided despite her continuing treatment. She has also, however, developed marked, persistent swelling of the ankles.

On examination pitting oedema of both ankles is confirmed. Blood pressure has fallen to 140/90 mmHg. Body weight is not recorded.

◆

The doctor prescribes additional bendrofluazide 5 mg daily. Nifedipine continues unchanged. Two weeks later the ankle oedema has cleared and blood pressure has fallen further to 116/74 mmHg.

### Comment

This case illustrates a very frequent problem and a controversial issue. The development of ankle or pedal oedema is a common complication of therapy with class II (dihydropyridine) calcium antagonists such as nifedipine. However, it is widely held that this oedema is not associated with measurable sodium retention or weight gain, and is not responsive to diuretic treatment. Further, it is suggested that the addition of diuretic effects little or no more blood pressure fall.

Nevertheless, some workers have reported nifedipine treatment to cause sodium retention and weight gain, and that the addition of diuretic will correct these features, relieve pedal oedema and cause further lowering of blood pressure (see Table 22.1). At any rate, in cases such as the present, the addition of a diuretic appears well worth trying.

For further reading see Chapter 22.

# Case study 18

A 21-year-old soldier is found at routine examination to have a blood pressure of 190/100 mmHg. He has never been unwell and denies any symptoms. He has already performed 2 years of military service without problems; he plays soccer weekly, does regular physical training and has completed several assault courses uneventfully. No abnormalities had been found on medical examination before he joined the army 2 years earlier; his blood pressure then was said to be 'normal'.

◆

This problem is promptly solved. The raised blood pressure is confirmed. He is found to have feeble femoral pulses which are later than the radial pulse. Prominent collateral arteries are observed, especially over the back of the chest.

◆

Coarctation of the aorta is confirmed on chest radiography, when left ventricular enlargement is seen to be accompanied by erosion at the lower borders of several ribs, the latter a consequence of the collateral arterial circulation which has developed to bypass the coarctation.

The abnormality is defined on aortography and is dealt with by surgical reconstruction. Six months after operation the brachial blood pressure is 130/76 mmHg.

**Comment**

This embarrassing case fortunately had a happy outcome. The patient did not develop any complications of aortic coarctation, and surgical correction was unevenful as well as being successful in restoring the blood pressure to normal levels.

The lesion should have been detected at routine paediatric examination in infancy, but was missed. Further, the brachial hypertension which was probably present at the time of his medical examination on recruitment was overlooked, presumably because assessment was too cursory.

The very rarity of aortic coarctation renders it readily missed. However, it can be detected clinically within minutes if the femoral and radial pulses are palpated simultaneously and compared. This simple examination should be performed in all hypertensive subjects, irrespective of their age, and the findings recorded. Sometimes, even with coarctation, the femoral pulses are easily felt and it is emphasized that it is the *delay* that is the paramount sign.

For further details see Chapter 28.

# Case study 19

A 22-year-old unmarried male university student is referred because of five attacks which have occurred during the past 10 months, three whilst playing squash, one when straining at stool, and one apparently unprovoked. All have been similar, lasting some 20–45 min. In attacks he is pale, sweating profusely, with a slow, regular pulse rate, and with a headache throbbing in time with the slow pulse. In two of the attacks a companion has also noticed swelling in the front of the neck, in the region of the thyroid gland.

On examination no abnormalities are found; blood pressure (which has not been measured in an attack) is around 120/70 mmHg.

◆

The history is almost pathognomonic of paroxysmal attacks accompanying phaeochromocytoma, the slow pulse indicating that here noradrenaline rather than adrenaline is being predominantly released in the attacks. The thyroid swelling, although not commonly reported, is very characteristic. Subsequently an attack is witnessed in which thyroid swelling is confirmed, the heart rate is recorded as 34 per min, and the blood pressure is 210/120 mmHg.

◆

An excess of noradrenaline is demonstrated in both plasma and urine. Computer-assisted tomography demonstrates a roughly spherical tumour some 6-cm in diameter lying above the right kidney.

◆

Pre-operative treatment is begun with the α-blocker phenoxybenzamine, initially 10 mg daily, rising to 30 mg daily. The non-selective β-blocker propranolol is then added at 40 mg twice daily, increasing to 160 mg twice daily.

◆

The phaeochromocytoma is removed uneventfully via a loin incision, and drug therapy is subsequently withdrawn.

The patient remains normotensive, well and symptom-free.

**Comment**

This is a classical example, in which virtually all the relevant data were revealed in the history. Biochemical testing and CT scan were essentially confirmatory. Diagnosis can be much more difficult in the absence of paroxysms, without symptoms of phaeochromocytoma, and with sustained rather than intermittent hypertension.

Drug therapy here was to minimize risk should a further paroxysm occur, a circumstance especially likely at operation. The need to establish α-adrenergic blockade before introducing β-blockade is emphasized.

Details of phaeochromocytoma are given in Chapter 38.

# Case study 20

A 19-year-old female medical student is found by a colleague during a physiology class to have a blood pressure of 220/120 mmHg. On referral the severe hypertension is confirmed, but no abnormality is revealed on detailed physical examination; the only possibly relevant item in the history is of nocturia over the past 3 months.

◆

Routine testing shows the plasma sodium to be 146 mmol/litre, potassium 2.1 mmol/litre and bicarbonate 34 mmol/litre. Renal function is normal.

◆

This biochemical pattern is consistent with primary aldosterone excess and the nocturia could well reflect the potassium depletion.

◆

The diagnosis is confirmed by demonstrating plasma aldosterone to be consistently elevated, whilst plasma renin and angiotensin II are subnormal.

◆

CT scan shows a spherical tumour 2 cm in diameter in the left adrenal cortex. Plasma taken at sampling from the left adrenal vein contains very high aldosterone, with cortisol concentrations appropriate for the sampling site.

◆

Blood pressure and the plasma electrolyte abnormalities are controlled with oral amiloride 60 mg daily.

◆

Through a left loin incision, the left adrenal gland, containing a typical aldosterone-secreting adenoma, is excised.

This woman subsequently remains well and normotensive without treatment.

**Comment**

This is a typical instance of Conn's syndrome. The case illustrates well that secondary forms of hypertension, though rare, are well worth seeking, especially in young persons, and that very simple initial investigations even, as here, in the absence of remarkable signs or symptoms, can be revealing. The hypernatraemia provides a point of distinction from secondary forms of aldosterone excess, in which hyponatraemia typically accompanies potassium deficiency (compare with Case studies 10, 14 and 21). Note that very large doses of potassium-conserving diuretic may be needed pre-operatively in patients with primary aldosterone excess to control hypertension and the electrolyte abnormalities.

Further details of Conn's syndrome are given in Chapter 35.

# Case study 21

An 8-year-old girl, previously well, develops nocturnal enuresis. Her primary care physician finds her blood pressure to be 170/110 mmHg.

She is referred to hospital. There, hypertension is confirmed. The optic fundi are clear. Overall renal function is normal, there is no proteinuria and abdominal ultrasound is normal. However, both plasma sodium (132 mmol/litre) and potassium (3.0 mmol/litre) are low, indicating secondary aldosterone excess, and this is confirmed by the demonstration of very high plasma concentrations of renin and aldosterone.

◆

Despite its rarity, renin-secreting tumour is a distinct possibility, especially in a very young subject.

◆

Arteriography shows both main renal arteries to be normal, but does demonstrate a tumour some 2 cm diameter in the cortex of the left kidney. Renal venous samples contain high concentrations of renin in plasma drawn from the left kidney.

◆

Pre-operative ACE inhibition, by giving oral captopril 100 mg twice daily lowers blood pressure to 110/70 mmHg and corrects the plasma electrolytes. At operation an attempt is made to shell out the tumour, but this proves impossible and a left nephrectomy is performed. The specimen is confirmed as containing a typical juxtaglomerular-cell tumour rich in extractable renin.

Post-operatively the patient remains well and normotensive.

**Comment**

This is a classic example of a considerable hypertensive rarity. Less than a hundred examples have so far been reported.

For further reading see Chapter 30.

# Case study 22

A 65-year-old woman is found to have myxoedema. She also has a raised blood pressure of around 200/110 mmHg. It is suggested that, in addition to thyroid hormone replacement, she should have antihypertensive treatment.

◆

However, her primary care physician decides that she should receive only thyroxine, and this is done. Four months later she is euthyroid and the blood pressure has fallen to 130/80 mmHg.

### Comment

The physician was correct. Although not widely recognized, thyroid deficiency is freqently accompanied by hypertension, which can be corrected by thyroid replacement therapy.

For further details see Chapter 41 and especially Figure 41.1.

# Case study 23

A 53-year-old workman is admitted to hospital for an operation, under general anaesthetic, for varicose veins. At routine pre-operative examination the anaesthesiologist finds a blood pressure of 170/104 mmHg and seeks an urgent medical opinion. The patient is not on any therapy and is a non-smoker.

◆

Three hours later the physician finds a blood presure of around 160/100 mmHg. There are no relevant signs or symptoms; in particular there is no evidence of secondary hypertension.

◆

The physician advises that the operation proceeds as planned. No special precautions are recommended, but it is arranged that the patient attends the medical clinic 2 months after surgery for routine assessment.

### Comment

This is a common, usually, as here, minor problem. The patient may have mild hypertension but not severe enough to merit early therapy or to delay surgery. As likely a possibility is that the unaccustomed hospital environment has transiently elevated the blood pressure.

The most pressing need is the application of reassurance to patient and anaesthesiologist.

For further reading see Chapter 25.

# Appendix 3
# Therapeutic guidelines—
# a critical appraisal

## — International Therapeutic Guidelines —

A plethora of guidelines for the treatment of hypertension has appeared. Despite the presence of several authorities on more than one of the relevant committees, divergent recommendations are frequently made. Moreover, the guidelines reported contain numerous erroneous and misleading assertions. Thus an attempt to present these guidelines in full would not, in our opinion, be helpful to the reader. Our own recommendations are given in Chapter 25.

Some idea of the divergencies and disagreements between the various guidelines may be gained from Tables A3.1–A3.4, which are adapted from Swales.[1]

A detailed critique of the reports by one of the present authors is reprinted here.

## Guidelines for the treatment of
## — hypertension: a critical review —

The following text is reproduced from *Cardiovascular Drugs and Therapy* (1994; **8**: 91–8), with permission.

### Introduction

The year 1993 witnessed extensive activity on the part of those physicians, statisticians and epidemiologists concerned with the proffering of advice on the treatment of hypertension. The US Joint National Committee,[4] the British Hypertension Society,[3] a combined committee of the WHO/ISH,[7] and the Canadian Hypertension Society[2] all published revised accounts of their earlier recommendations; and a New Zealand advisory committee contributed a discussion paper on the topic.[6] Further instructions directed to doctors in Australia[5] remain young. The crop has been enriched by several strictures upon, and summaries and round table discussions of, the guidelines themselves.[1,9–12]

The need for further criticisms of, and elucidation of, the multiform offerings of guidance may therefore be questioned; the present essay certainly requires justification. Whilst there can be no doubt of the sincerity and dedication of the members of these diverse committees, or of the value of their publications in fostering interest in clinical hyper-

**Table A3.1** Points of agreement in published guidelines for treating hypertension

Early urgent treatment of severe or malignant hypertension
Need for period of assessment before treating mild-to-moderate hypertension with drugs
Non-pharmacological management as first approach to treating mild-to-moderate hypertension
Lower blood pressure threshold for drug treatment in the presence of other cardiovascular risk factors
Value of treating elderly hypertensives
Systolic as well as diastolic criteria for treatment

**Table A3.2** Diastolic and systolic blood pressure thresholds for drug treatment of hypertension

| | Diastolic blood pressure (mmHg) | Systolic blood pressure (mmHg) | Period of observation (months) | Treatment level in presence of other risk factors (mmHg) |
|---|---|---|---|---|
| Canada[2] | 100 | | | 90 |
| UK[3] | 100 | 160 | 3–6 | 90 (diastolic) |
| USA[4] | 90[a] | 140 | 3–6 | |
| | 95[a] | 150 | 3–6 | 90 (diastolic) |
| Australia[5] | 100 | 160 | 1 | 95 (diastolic) |
| New Zealand[6][b] | 100 | 170 | 6 | 90 (diastolic) |
| WHO/ISH[7] | 95 | 160 | 3–6 | 140/90 |

[a]'Difference of opinion.'
[b]70% 10-year risk reduction.
WHO, World Health Organization; ISH, International Society of Hypertension.

**Table A3.3** Recommendations for initial treatment

| | Diuretics and β-blockers only | All classes |
|---|---|---|
| Canada[2] | + | 0 |
| UK | | |
| (1989)[8] | + | 0 |
| (1993)[3][a] | + | + |
| USA (JNC)[4] | + | 0 |
| Australia[5] | 0 | + |
| New Zealand[6] | + | 0 |
| WHO/ISH[7] | 0 | + |

[a] 'Divided'.

**Table A3.4** Target blood pressure

| | Diastolic blood pressure (mmHg) | Systolic blood pressure (mmHg) |
|---|---|---|
| Canada[2] | | |
| UK[3] | 80–90 | <160 |
| USA[4] | <90 ?85 | <140 ?130 |
| Australia[5] | | |
| New Zealand[6] | <90 | |
| WHO/ISH[7] | | |
| Older | <90 | <140 |
| Younger | 80 | 120–130 |

tension and in the improvement of means for its prevention and treatment, the approach has inherent and well-recognized intellectual defects, albeit these are often ignored.

Even more importantly, and perhaps surprisingly, the various accounts contain some crucial errors of fact. Because these publications are directed specifically to those inexpert in the field, the likely perpetuation of the misconceptions is especially unfortunate.

In the present account I shall concentrate predominantly, but not exclusively, on those publications which appeared in 1993.

### National and racial bias

Five[2-6] of the six sets of guidelines originate in countries with predominant Anglo-Saxon race and culture; only the WHO/ISH report[7,12] has a wider remit, and even that account derives from a committee with a strong Anglo-Saxon element. Inevitably therefore, although the USA Committee[4] does enter at length into the needs of the American black population, and the Canadians discuss this more briefly,[2] the advice given, and the studies from which it is compiled, have limited application. These circumstances reflect, of course, the origins of most of the trials of treatment of hypertension, and the varied extent of national interest in the topic.

The reality, nevertheless, is a major unfortunate, if unavoidable, constraint. Moreover, given the racial and cultural similarities between the origins of the several guidelines, it is questionable why six variants are necessary, or even justified. Considerations of national or of organizational prestige may, however inaptly, be involved. In any event, the outcome is that we now see what has been pejoratively termed a 'guidelines industry'.[76] A single set of guidelines, with dissenting or controversial views included, would have been more helpful. The round table discussion[10] could well have preceded, rather than followed, the individual reports. This might have avoided the anomaly

whereby at least three advisers appear on more than one committee,[3,4,6,7] and have apparently endorsed, simultaneously, somewhat conflicting recommendations. It seems that the environmental atmosphere of different committees, in varying locations, engenders either differing views or acquiescence, a realization not reassuring to the reader. Swales[76] has commented on another aspect; if the guidelines define optimal antihypertensive care, failure to achieve the defined standard must be suboptimal. Effective optimal care necessitates a major increase in medical expenditure.

### The conflict between consensus and science

The obligation upon a committee to produce a paper recommending guidelines calls for a semblance of non-existent accord, even amity.[1] Whilst this approach may have some (perhaps dubious) merit in proferring simple working rules for doctors inexpert in hypertension, it incurs penalties which are often insufficiently appreciated.

The scientific method depends essentially on continued criticism, questioning and debate. The attempt at consensus runs directly contrary, and its defects have been repeatedly emphasized,[13-16] although the warnings have often been unheeded. Consensus reports are especially vulnerable to the vagaries of selection of the members of the relevant committee; moreover, as was noted above, the ambience of different committees can apparently evoke from susceptible individuals vacillating opinions. Perhaps not surprisingly also, members of such committees are sometimes less vigilant than would be the case were they writing and signing scientific papers as individuals.

Again, it requires emphasis that these criticisms do not indict either the motives or the integrity of the members of the committees. The recent comment 'corrupt science moves from mandated conclusion back to selected data in order to reach the mandated conclusion' is extreme, if evidently heartfelt.[17] Even so, the 1993 guidelines exude some alarming scientific complacency.

## Guidance on the initiation of antihypertensive drug treatment

This is the least controversial and probably the most useful aspect of the reports. They are clear and accurate on the indications for and tempo of urgent treatment with drugs in the malignant phase and in severe hypertension; they emphasize rightly the value of treating hypertension in elderly subjects; and of the therapy of 'isolated systolic' hypertension.

There is proper emphasis on repeated measurements of blood pressure over weeks or months before introducing antihypertensive drugs in patients with more mild hypertension.

There are, however, minor but important differences between the reports on the recommended thresholds for the initiation of drug treatment after a period of suitable observation in mild hypertension.[1,76] Albeit with extensive and various qualifications, on which the papers themselves should be read for details, severally the British Hypertension Society[3] advises that antihypertensive drugs be initiated if the fifth phase diastolic pressure persists at or above 100 mmHg; the US Joint National Committee[4] and the New Zealand group[6] take the more aggressive threshold of 90 mmHg; whilst the WHO/ISH Committee[7] espouses the intermediate threshold of 95 mmHg, a value which is not usually indicated exactly on clinical sphygmomanometers.

## Hypertensive organ damage

Four[2-4,12] of the five committees which published in 1993, as well as the round table report,[10] use the unhappy expression 'target organ damage' to indicate lesions caused by hypertension, in the USA case[4] this being abbreviated to the even less felicitous 'TOD'.

The term 'target organ' is more properly applied to an organ which is appropriately, and usually physiologically, the target of a circulating hormone secreted by a distant endocrine gland. The phrase 'target organ' implies in this, its proper context, a purposeful, regulated relationship.[18] The damage caused by hypertension is not strictly either of

these. 'Hypertensive organ damage' would be a more suitable expression.

There is general emphasis in the guidelines on more urgent and aggressive antihypertensive therapy in patients showing hypertensive organ damage, or possessing cardiovascular risk factors additional to hypertension. The New Zealand paper[6] points out that hypertension-related risk depends on the presence of other risk factors, and recommends that the decision to treat should result from an overall assessment rather than from blood pressure measurements alone. The WHO/ISH Committee proceeds further, however, to the incautious claim[7] 'continued cigarette smoking, elevated fasting glucose, elevated serum cholesterol, and low HDL-cholesterol all . . . increase the absolute benefit of blood pressure lowering.' This improbable assertion is not referenced, and seems to have been derived *ex cathedra*. In an evaluation of the Australian treatment trial,[19] Ramsay[20] reached different conclusions; antihypertensive drug therapy appeared to him to be no more beneficial in the presence of other risk factors, and he advised that the decision to treat mild hypertension with drugs should not be influenced by the presence or absence of those factors.

## Benefits from treating hypertension

There are disturbingly inaccurate claims and inexplicable anomalies in the guidelines publications concerning the benefits to be derived from the treatment of hypertension. These stem from the problem of selecting which particular meta-analysis to best illustrate such benefits. Meta-analysis is especially vulnerable to distortion, depending on the trials chosen for inclusion.[17,21,22] In the present context, the much denigrated, but remarkably long-lived USA Hypertension Detection and Follow-up Program (HDFP) study[23] has for many years been predominantly, but not exclusively, contentious. Briefly, the criticisms[24] of HDFP are that, in patients in the intervention group, multiple risk factors in addition to hypertension were addressed (correction of overweight, dietary cholesterol reduction and anti-smoking counselling were attempted); that these patients were seen more often and in generally more favourable circumstances than were those in the 'control' group; that they were given free drugs, investigational tests and transportation to and from the clinic; and that a Program physician was on call for them at all times.

MacMahon et al. published in 1986[25] a meta-analysis of nine trials of treatment of hypertension. Two of these nine, HDFP[23] and MRFIT,[26] involved multiple risk factor interventions; these two trials were accordingly indicated separately and with qualifications.[25] This meta-analysis concuded that antihypertensive treatment was accompanied by a substantial reduction in both fatal and non-fatal stroke, by a modest reduction in all-cause mortality, but by no significant reduction in fatal or non-fatal myocardial infarction.

In 1990 a different meta-analysis,[27] by Collins et al., appeared. This included 13 separate trials (the authors state that there were 14, but this seems to be because they took the two subgroup analyses on the VA study[34,35] to be two separate trials; the figure of 14 is repeated in the USA guidelines[4]). Of the two multiple risk factor intervention studies, MRFIT[26] was now discarded, although, oddly, HDFP[23] was elevated to the status of an unconfounded trial, and without the former caveats. The authors state unambiguously:[27]

Trials of multiple risk factor interventions, including not only blood pressure reduction but also separate interventions to alter some other risk factor(s) were ... not included ... the only confounding that remains is that due to any direct or indirect side-effects of the drugs tested in these trials.

These are laudable precepts, but they are not met by HDFP[23] which should not therefore, according to the authors' own criteria, have been considered.

A further curiosity is that non-fatal coronary events in HDFP in the 1986 analysis[25] were defined by electrocardiographic criteria, whereas in 1990[27] only events suggested on the clinical history were taken. Of interest is that one statistician, MacMahon, appears as an author of both the 1986 and the 1990 meta-analyses.[25,27] In a separate paper,

MacMahon[28] explains that the MRFIT study[26] was excluded from the later publication,[27] because of the potential confounding likely to result from the concurrent interventions for smoking cessation and cholesterol lowering in that trial'. Why HDFP[23] which, inter alia, also attempted these interventions, was not similarly eliminated is not revealed. These issues are important, because HDFP was a large study, with a correspondingly marked capability of distorting a meta-analysis.

Coronary events were, according to this second meta-analysis,[27] reduced significantly by a mean of 14%, although with very wide 95% confidence intervals of 4–22%. The apparent effect on coronary artery morbidity was entirely due to the contentious inclusion of HDFP.[23] As was promptly pointed out,[21] with HDFP omitted, as it should have been, coronary events were almost exactly as frequent in the control and intervention groups.

It was also[27] found that antihypertensive treatment lowered stroke incidence markedly, by an average 42% with 95% confidence intervals of 33–50%. This suggested that virtually all the stroke risk attributable to hypertension was rapidly eliminated by therapy, a finding, however gratifying, which was so improbable medically, not least because of the known inadequacy of much antihypertensive drug therapy,[80] that it ought to have occasioned more consideration than it has apparently done so far.

Three further trials, all conducted in elderly hypertensive patients, have been published[29–31] since the controversial Collins et al. meta-analysis.[27] All three[29–31] confirmed that antihypertensive drug treatment substantially prevented stroke. Moreover, the Swedish STOP trial[30] found that therapy lowered all-cause mortality. The SHEP trial,[29] which considered isolated systolic hypertension in elderly patients, additionally showed that drug treatment lowered the incidence of coronary deaths and that it diminished all morbid coronary events by 27%. By contrast, no significant reduction in coronary events was observed in either STOP[30] or the British MRC trial[31] in elderly subjects.

Once more the vagaries of meta-analysis are

evident concerning the treatment of hypertension in elderly patients. In one such survey,[32] Thijs et al. excluded the SHEP trial[29] on the grounds that isolated systolic hypertension is haemodynamically distinct from other forms of hypertension, although they did, inexplicably, include two British trials[31,33] which involved substantial numbers of patients with isolated systolic hypertension.

These inconsistencies have been considered at some length because they bear crucially on the extent to which drug therapy has succeeded in ameliorating hypertension-related coronary artery disease. Three[4,6,7] of the 1993 papers choose to quote, uncritically, the Collins et al. 1990 meta-analysis[27] in this regard, and consequently present a complacently euphoric view of such benefits. The British Hypertension Society 1993 report[3] is indeterminate in this respect. Whereas the 1989 guidelines from that Society[8] carefully pointed out that both HDFP[25] and MRFIT[26] involved multiple risk factor interventions and that the absence of an untreated control group reduced their relevance, the 1993 paper,[3] quoting SHEP, STOP and the MRC trial in elderly hypertensive patients,[29-31] refers vaguely to 'the emerging evidence that drug treatment may reduce coronary events in addition to preventing strokes'. The British Hypertension Society paper does not, however,[3] proceed explicitly to cite the Collins et al. meta-analysis.[27]

The others are less cautious. The WHO/ISH Committee quotes in one place the Collins et al. meta-analysis[27] as showing with drug treatment a reduction in 'the risk of non-fatal myocardial infarction and death from ischaemic heart disease by about 15–20%', and elsewhere as demonstrating a lowering of 'the risk of coronary events by about a sixth'. As mentioned above, the actual figure[27] is a mean of 14%, with 95% confidence intervals of 4–22%. The Collins et al. meta-analysis[27] has well-advertised deficiencies, but if it is to be quoted, this should be done accurately. The WHO/ISH Committee does not. Whilst the errors are probably inadvertent, their appearance risks the impression of seeking to claim excessive therapeutic benefit.

These are not negligible matters. The shortfall in restricting hypertension-related coronary morbidity with drug treatment comprises a critical area of future research. This remains a major epidemiological and therapeutic problem, in which complacency would be dangerously misplaced.

## Classes of drug to be employed

The various guidelines[2-7,10] rightly emphasize that the benefits from treating hypertension have so far been demonstrated only from drug use; whatever the efficacy of non-pharmacological measures in lowering blood pressure, this has not yet been translated to a reduction in morbidity visible in trials. It is hence useful to enumerate which classes of drug have been employed in trials showing therapeutic benefit.

Neither the present author nor others[77] accept that the trials included in the Collins et al. meta-analysis[27] are necessarily those most suitable for evaluation in this way. As was discussed earlier, the selection of such trials is controversial. Nevertheless, these 13 (not 14)[19,23,33-44] plus the three subsequent studies[29-31] on hypertension in elderly subjects are the most quoted in the guidelines. They therefore merit scrutiny. Of these 16 trials, sundry diuretics, in various doses, and with widely differing attempts at potassium conservation, figure in all. Centrally acting agents (methyldopa, clonidine or rauwolfia derivatives) are next most frequent, featuring in 14 of the 16.[19,23,29,33-44] $\beta$-Blockers appear in less than half (only 7) of the trials.[19,29-31,33,36,38] Requiring emphasis is that $\beta$-blockers were not used in the large controversial HDFP.[23] Hydralazine[19,23,34,35] and guanethidine[23,38,41] each appear in three studies; nifedipine[31,33] and debrisoquine[37,42] each in two; and bethanidine in one.[42] Moreover, combined therapy, with more than one class of drug being given together, was a very usual requirement. No ACE inhibitor or pure $\alpha$-blocker was used in any of the 16 trials.

The authors of the various guidelines are sometimes remarkably ill-informed on these aspects. The USA Committee[4] states: 'diuretics and beta-blockers are the only classes of drugs that have been used in long-term controlled clinical trials and shown to reduce morbidity and mortality.' The Canadians write[2]: 'these are the only classes of drugs that have been shown in long-term controlled clinical trials to reduce rates of illness and death.' These claims are very wide of the truth. Even further away from reality is the New Zealand Committee's assertion[6] that 'Low dose diuretics and low dose beta-blockers should be considered as first line treatment. . . . These are the only classes of drugs which have been shown in randomised clinical trials to reduce the risk of cardiovascular events among patients treated for raised blood pressure.' (Although this solecism may partly reflect unfortunate syntax.) These several spurious notions are then advanced by all three committees,[2,4,6] as reasons for restricting the first choice for therapy to those two drug classes.

The British Hypertension Society report[3] only slightly less rashly states: 'Two classes of drugs have been adequately and extensively tested in long term prospective outcome trials: diuretics (particularly the thiazides) and beta-blockers'.

The WHO/ISH Committee[7] by contrast specifically recognize[5,6] the much wider range of drugs which has been employed; its favouring of diuretics (in low dose) and $\beta$-blockers presumably reflects, as does the first British Hypertension Society report,[8] the fashionable preference for these as first-choice drugs. Strangely, the round table report adds to the confusion by stating 'All five guidelines acknowledged that only diuretic or beta-blocker-based therapeutic regimens had been demonstrated to prevent cardiovascular morbidity and mortality'.[10]

Although all five of the committees whose findings were published in 1993 assert[2–4,6,7] that any benefit from the use of calcium antagonists in restricting morbidity has not been assessed, this is not strictly correct; nifedipine was employed as a supplementary drug in at least two[31,32] of the 16 trials considered above.

The various misconceptions not surprisingly lead some of the committees to adopt strangely inappropriate stances. The US Joint National Committee,[4] reversing an earlier decision,[9] does not recommend calcium antagonists or ACE inhibitors as first-choice drugs, even though the safety of these agents has now been extensively examined in long-term studies. The British Committee was unable to reach agreement on this point.[3]

The evidence currently available suggests to the present reviewer rather that the undoubted benefits from treating hypertension derive from blood pressure reduction *per se*, and have been achieved with a wide range of drugs. This does not gainsay that different drug classes may evince differential benefit in relation to certain complications; however, such evidence as is presently available on this aspect is both limited and controversial.

The curious reluctance on the part of some committees to recommend even well-tried newer drugs contrasts with the willingness of them all[2–4,6,7] to advocate various non-pharmacological means of blood pressure reduction both as precursors to and accompaniments of drug therapy, even though little is known of either the safety or efficacy of such non-pharmacological measures, or of their capacity to lower hypertension-related morbidity. None of the committees comments on this rational inconsistency.

## Renin and prognosis

None of the 1993 reports considers the potentially important issue of plasma renin in relation to prognosis, aside from one vague and unhelpful allusion,[4] an omission already criticized elsewhere.[9]

It was initially proposed[45] that hypertensive patients with elevated plasma levels of renin, and hence, by implication, high plasma angiotensin II, were more prone to develop stroke and myocardial infarction. Later studies failed to confirm the association with stroke but did again show that with myocardial infarction.[46–48] Contrariwise one large prospective survey[49] did not confirm either of the associations claimed. The original notions are nevertheless plausible, because administered angiotensin II has been shown to cause arterial, myocardial and renal lesions.[48] If correct, the ideas have therapeutic relevance, since drugs which lower plasma angiotensin II, such as $\beta$-blockers or ACE inhibitors, should be especially effective in limiting some of the complications of hypertension, whereas diuretics, which elevate angiotensin II, should be partly adverse. There might also be reservations about dietary sodium restriction, which also elevates plasma renin and angiotensin II, as a non-pharmacological measure.

It is noteworthy that Alderman, the first author of a prospective study[47] implicating angiotensin II in this way, was insufficiently impressed with his own results to make any distinction between the use of diuretics or $\beta$-blockers as first-choice drugs.[50] Despite Alderman's apparent lack of conviction,[50] the controversies could nevertheless usefully have been expounded in the guidelines publications.

## Non-pharmacological measures, especially sodium restriction

The guideline reports[2–4,6,7] correctly recognize that non-pharmacological measures, including dietary salt restriction, alcohol restriction, weight reduction and physical exercise, whatever their capability of lowering blood pressure,[51–55,81] remain unassessed in relation to limiting the complications of hypertension. This deficiency does not deter the committees from recommending[2–4,6,7] such measures both as a prelude and an accompaniment to drug therapy. This conflicts oddly with hesitations[2–4,6,10] concerning the use of ACE inhibitors or calcium antagonists. The committees further seem blind to the rational inconsistency involved in assuming that an arbitrarily selected dietary habit may be harmful and that an equally arbitrarily chosen modification of that habit could only be beneficial.

The opportunity is missed to discuss critically the controversies surrounding dietary sodium restriction.[51–55] No distinction is made between sodium restriction as an adjunct to drug treatment in essential hypertension, which can be useful in

lowering blood pressure in some, especially middle-aged to elderly patients,[54,55] and sodium restriction as a broad-scale preventive measure, of which the theoretical basis,[56,57] efficacy[51,54–56] and safety[52,58] are all more doubtful. As mentioned earlier, there is no consideration of sodium restriction in relation to changes in plasma renin.

The effect of sodium restriction in raising serum cholesterol is discussed in the following section.

The US Joint Committee[4] cites the Law et al. meta-analysis[59] on sodium restriction without reference to its well-advertised deficiencies,[60] or to the findings of other meta-analysts[60] who have reached very different conclusions.

## Serum cholesterol and lipid pattern

This is a very unsatisfactory aspect of the guidelines as presented. An elevated serum cholesterol concentration in hypertension is generally taken to be adverse, and this concept is coupled with some vague injunctions that serum cholesterol should be lowered, but little or no clear advice on how this might be achieved.

Whilst an elevated serum cholesterol concentration in young or middle-aged persons is associated with increased cardiovascular risk, the relation to overall prognosis is much less clear.[15,16] In hypertensive persons over the age of 60, the correlation of serum cholesterol concentration with cardiovascular morbidity is loose, and is outweighed by the beneficial effects of a higher serum cholesterol level in relation to other diseases. In a detailed analysis[61] of the EWPHE trial,[43] it was found that hypertensive men and women over the age of 60 had on average a 1-year *longer* survival for an increase in total serum cholesterol of 2.3 mmol/litre. The MRC trial in elderly hypertensives[31] also revealed a better prognosis associated with elevation of serum cholesterol.

These very pertinent aspects are accorded little or no space in the guidelines. For example, the WHO/ISH report[7] states, without qualification, that: 'high serum cholesterol levels . . . unfavourably influence the long-term prognosis in hypertensive people'. This claim would be difficult to defend concerning patients over 60 on the presently available evidence. As this Committee's report is elsewhere concerned, rightly, with treating hypertension in elderly subjects, the statement is unhelpful, if not frankly misleading.

There is little or no discussion on the elevation of serum cholesterol caused by thiazides[62] and β-blockers,[63] the two classes of drug most favoured by the committees. Both the large MRC[64] and HDFP[65] studies showed that thiazides raised serum cholesterol transiently, despite, in the case of HDFP, concurrent dietary attempts at cholesterol lowering.[23] The potential problem has worried some,[28,66] but not all,[67] observers. However, regardless of the presence of those observers on several of the committees,[3,6,7] and the general concern about serum cholesterol elevation, the issue has not merited much attention in the guidelines. Similarly disregarded are reports that dietary sodium restriction can raise serum cholesterol, at least short-term.[52,68–70]

It has been repeatedly noted that dietary attempts to lower serum cholesterol, as implemented in clinical practice, are largely ineffective,[55,71–74] although the regimen adopted by Zen monks[75] can achieve this. Guidelines addressed to practising doctors ought surely to have recognized and discussed the problems.

## Conclusions

The published guidelines are undoubtedly useful in drawing wide attention to the benefits to be obtained from treating hypertension and by indicating how its control can be attained. However, it is questionable whether such a diversity of often, but not always, similar recommendations is necessary or desirable. Moreover, guidelines, by definition, should guide; they are dangerous if they mislead. Lest the iconoclasm of the present critique should risk suggesting nihilism, our own recommendations on antihypertensive therapy are set out in Chapter 28.

As indicated herein, it is disconcerting to find, in the current guidelines, so many unsubstantiated,

inaccurate and occasionally frankly incorrect statements. Inexact science is both aesthetically distasteful and intrinsically debilitating.[24] Moreover, many physicians will look no further than these publications if hypertension is not their specialty—indeed, the guidelines are specifically addressed to such persons. Thus misconceptions and inapt procedures risk perpetuation. Especially unfortunate is the general avoidance in these reports of discussion of important current controversies. Thus in some respects the publications show more affinity with the theological orthodoxy demanded in earlier centuries than with contemporary scientific debate.

Chalmers[78] has impugned insistent, but usually occult, governmental influence, coercing the committees towards apparent consensus and the advising of cheap medicines. Economic constraints may demand parsimony, but this should not be disguised as scientific verity.[79]

Dissemination of awareness of the benefits to be derived from treating hypertension, and instruction on such therapy is meritorious. However, distorted or exaggerated claims of efficacy are meretricious. There is consequently a real danger that genuine achievements, which are in this field considerable, may be discredited. Alternatively, misplaced complacency, which is already evident, risks inhibiting very necessary debate, enquiry and research.

——————— References ———————

1. Swales JD. Guidelines on guidelines. *J. Hypertens.* 1993; **11**: 899–903.
2. Carruthers SG, Larochelle P, Haynes RB *et al.* Report of the Canadian Hypertension Society consensus conference: 1. Introduction. *Can. Med. Assoc.* 1993; **149**: 289–93.
3. Sever P, Beevers G, Bulpitt C *et al.* Management guidelines in essential hypertension: report of the second working party of the British Hypertension Society. *Br. Med. J.* 1993; **306**: 983–7.
4. Fifth Report of the Joint National Committee on Detection, Evaluation, and Treatment of High

Blood Pressure (JNCV). *Arch. Intern. Med.* 1993; **153**: 154–82.

5. Hypertension Guidelines Committee, South Australian Faculty, Royal Australian College of General Practitioners. Hypertenion: diagnosis, treatment and maintenance. Guidelines endorsed by the High Blood Pressure Research Council of Australia. Adelaide: South Australian Faculty, Royal Australian College of General Practitioners, 1991.

6. Jackson R, Barham P, Bills J *et al.* Management of raised blood pressure in New Zealand: a discussion document. *Br. Med. J.* 1993; **307**: 107–10.

7. Guidelines Sub-Committee. 1993 Guidelines for the treatment of mild hypertension: memorandum from a World Health Organization/International Society of Hypertension Meeting. *J. Hypertens.* 1993; **11**: 905–18.

8. Swales JD, Ramsay LE, Coope JR *et al.* Treating mild hypertension: report of the British Hypertension Society working party. *Br. Med. J.* 1989; **298**: 694–8.

9. Weber MA, Laragh JH. Hypertension: steps forwards and steps back. The Joint National Committee Fifth Report. *Arch. Intern. Med.* 1993; **153**: 149–52.

10. Alderman MA, Cushman WC, Hill MN, Krakoff LR. International round table discussion of national guidelines for the detection, evaluation, and treatment of hypertension. *Am. J. Hypertens.* 1993; **6**: 974–81.

11. Alderman MA. A review of the Joint National Committee on Detection, Evaluation, and Treatment of High Blood Pressure. *Am. J. Hypertens.* 1993; **6**: 896–8.

12. Subcommittee of WHO/ISH Mild Hypertension Liaison Committee. Summary of 1993 World Health Organization/International Society of Hypertension guidelines for the management of mild hypertension. *Br. Med. J.* 1993; **307**: 1541–6.

13. Pickering GW. *The Nature of Essential Hypertension.* London: J & A Churchill, 1961.

14. Skrabanek P. Nonsensus consensus. *Lancet* 1990; **335**: 1446–7.

15. Sheldon TA, Smith GD. Consensus conferences as drug promotion. *Lancet* 1993; **341**: 100–2.

16. Oliver MF. National cholesterol policies. *Europ. Heart J.* 1993; **14**: 581–3.

17. Skrabanek P. The epidemiology of errors. *Lancet* 1993; **342**: 1502.

18. Welbourne RB. Endocrine diseases. In *Companion Encyclopedia of the History of Medicine*, Vol. 1 (eds WF Bynum and ·R Porter). London: Routledge, 1993: 484–511.

19. The Australian Therapeutic Trial in Mild Hypertension. Report by the management committee. *Lancet* 1980; **i**: 1261–7.

20. Ramsay LE. Mild hypertension: treat patients, not populations. *J. Hypertens.* 1985; **3**: 449–55.

21. Alderman MH. Meta-analysis of hypertension treatment trials. *Lancet* 1990; **335**: 1092–3.

22. Ravnskov U. Cholesterol lowering trials in coronary heart disease: frequency of citation and outcome. *Br. Med. J.* 1992; **305**: 15–19.

23. Hypertension Detection and Follow-up Program Cooperative Group. Five-year findings of the Hypertension Detection and Follow-up Program. I. Reduction in mortality of persons with high blood pressure, including mild hypertension. *J. Am. Med. Assoc.* 1979; **242**: 2562–71.

24. Robertson JIS. Antihypertensive drug treatment: an appraisal of trials. *Neth. J. Med.* 1993; **43** (suppl.): 3–11.

25. MacMahon SW, Cutler JA, Furberg CD, Payne GH. The effects of drug treatment for hypertension on morbidity and mortality from cardiovascular disease: a review of randomized controlled trials. *Prog. Cardiovasc. Dis.* 1986; **29** (suppl. 1): 99–118.

26. Multiple Risk Factor Intervention Trial Research Group. Multiple risk factor intervention trial: risk factor changes and mortality results. *J. Am. Med. Assoc.* 1982; **248**: 1465–77.

27. Collins R, Peto R, MacMahon S *et al.* Blood pressure, stroke, and coronary heart disease. Part 2, short-term reductions in blood pressure: overview of randomised drug trials in their epidemiological context. *Lancet* 1990; **335**: 827–38.

28. MacMahon S. The effects of antihypertensive drug treatment on the incidence of stroke and of coronary heart disease. *Clin. Exp. Hypertens.* 1989; **A11**: 807–23.

29. SHEP Cooperative Research Group. Prevention of stroke by antihypertensive drug treatment in older persons withisolated systolic hypertension: final results of the Systolic Hypertension in the Elderly Program (SHEP). *J. Am. Med. Assoc.* 1991; **265**: 3255–64.

30. Dahlöf B, Lindholm LF, Hansson L *et al.* Morbidity and mortality in the Swedish Trial of Old Patients

with Hypertension (STOP-Hypertension). *Lancet* 1991; **338**: 1281–5.

31. MRC Working Party. Medical Research Council trial of treatment of hypertension in older adults: principal results. *Br. Med. J.* 1992; **304**: 405–12.

32. Thijs L, Fagard R, Lijnen P *et al.* A meta-analysis of outcome trials in elderly hypertensives. *J. Hypertens.* 1992; **19**: 1103–9.

33. Coope J, Warrender TS. Randomised trial of treatment of hypertension in elderly patients in primary care. *Br. Med. J.* 1986; **293**: 1145–51.

34. Veterans Administration Cooperative Study Group on Antihypertensive Agents. Effects of treatment on morbidity in hypertension: results in patients with diastolic blood pressure averaging 115 through 129 mmHg. *J. Am. Med. Assoc.* 1967; **202**: 1028–34.

35. Veterans Administration Cooperative Study Group on Antihypertensive Agents. Effects of treatment on morbidity in hypertension: II. Results in patients with diastolic blood pressure averaging 90 through 114 mmHg. *J. Am. Med. Assoc.* 1970; **213**: 1143–52.

36. Helgeland A. Treatment of mild hypertension: a five year controlled drug trial. The Oslo study. *Am. J. Med.* 1980; **69**: 725–32.

37. Barraclough MA, Joy MD, MacGregor GA *et al.* Control of moderately raised blood pressure: report of a cooperative randomized controlled trial. *Br. Med. J.* 1973; **3**: 434–6.

38. Medical Research Council Working Party. MRC trial of treatment of mild hypertension: principal results. *Br. Med. J.* 1985; **293**: 97–104.

39. Smith WM. Treatment of mild hypertension: results of a ten-year intervention trial. *Circ. Res.* 1977; **40** (suppl. 1): 98–105.

40. Hypertension–Stroke Cooperative Group. Effect of antihypertensive treatment on stroke recurrence. *J. Am. Med. Assoc.* 1974; **299**: 409–18.

41. Wolff FW, Lindeman RD. Effects of treatment in hypertension: results of a controlled study. *J. Chron. Dis.* 1966; **19**: 227–40.

42. Carter AB. Hypotensive therapy in stroke survivors. *Lancet* 1970; **i**: 485–9.

43. Amery A, Birkenhäger W, Brixko P *et al.* Mortality and morbidity results from the European Working Party on high blood pressure in the elderly trial. *Lancet* 1985; **i**: 1349–54.

44. Perry HM, Goldman AI, Levin MA *et al.* Evaluation of drug treatment in mild hypertension: VA-NHLBI feasibility trial. *Ann. NY Acad. Sci.* 1978; **304**: 267–88.

45. Brunner HR, Laragh JH, Baer L *et al.* Renin and aldosterone, heart attack and stoke. *N. Engl. J. Med.* 1972; **286**: 441–9.

46. Brunner HR, Gavras H, Laragh JH *et al.* The risk of low renin hypertension: an updated analysis. *Eur. Soc. Clin. Invest. 9th Annual Meeting, Rotterdam 1975.* Abstract no. 53.

47. Alderman MH, Madhavan S, Ooi WL *et al.* Association of the renin–sodium profile with the risk of myocardial infarction in patients with hypertension. *N. Engl. J. Med.* 1991; **324**: 1098–104.

48. Gavras I, Gavras H. Angiogensin II—possible adverse effects on arteries, heart, brain, and kidney: experimental, clinical, and epidemiological evidence. In *The Renin–Angiotensin System*, Vol. 1 (eds JIS Robertson and MG Nicholls). London: Gower Medical, 1993: 40.1–40.11.

49. Meade TW, Cooper JA, Peart WS. Plasma renin activity and ischemic heart disease. *N. Engl. J. Med.* 1993; **329**: 616–19.

50. Alderman MH. Which antihypertensive drugs first—and why! *J. Am. Med. Assoc.* 1992; **267**: 2786–7.

51. Swales JD. Salt saga continued: salt has only small importance in hypertension. *Br. Med. J.* 1988; **297**: 307–8.

52. Muntzel M, Drücke T. A comprehensive review of the salt and blood pressure relationship. *Am. J. Hypertens.* 1992; **5** (suppl.): 1–42.

53. De Wardener HE, Kaplan NM. On the assertion that a moderate restriction of sodium intake may have adverse effects. *Am. J. Hypertens.* 1993; **6**: 810–14.

54. Grobbee DE, Hofman A. Does sodium restriction lower blood pressure? *Br. Med. J.* 1986; **293**: 27–9.

55. Ramsay LE, Yeo WW, Chadwick IG, Jackson PR. Non-pharmacological management of hypertension. *Neth. J. Med.* 1993; **43** (suppl.): 44–51.

56. Overlack A, Ruppert M, Kolloch R *et al.* Divergent hemodynamic and hormonal responses to varying salt intake in normotensive subjects. *Hypertension* 1993; **22**: 331–8.

57. Robertson JIS. The renin–aldosterone connection: past, present and future. *J. Hypertens.* 1984; **2** (suppl. 3): 1–14.

58. Alderman MH, Cohen H, Madhaven S. Low urinary sodium and increased myocardial infarction and total cardiovascular disease among treated hypertensives. *J. Hypertens.* 1992; **10** (suppl. 4): 137.

59. Law MR, Frost CD, Wald NJ. Analysis of data from trials of salt reduction. *Br. Med. J.* 1991; **302**: 819–24.

60. Swales JD. Dietary salt and blood pressure: the role of meta-analyses. *J. Hypertens.* 1991; **9** (suppl. 6): 42–6.

61. Staessen J, Amery A, Birkenhäger W *et al.* Is a high serum cholesterol level associated with longer survival in elderly hypertensives? *J. Hypertens.* 1990; **8**: 755–61.

62. Ames RP. The effect of anti-hypertensive drugs on serum lipids and lipoproteins: I. Diuretics. *Drugs* 1986; **32**: 260–78.

63. Ames RP. The effects of antihypertensive drugs on serum lipids and lipoproteins: II. Non-diuretic drugs. *Drugs* 1986; **32**: 335–57.

64. Medical Research Council Working Party on mild-to-moderate hypertension. Adverse reactions to bendrofluazide and propranolol for the treatment of mild hypertension. *Lancet* 1981; **ii**: 679–85.

65. Curb JD, Maxwell MH, Schneider KA *et al.* Adverse effects of antihypertensive medications in the Hypertension Detection and Follow-up Program. *Progr. Cardiovasc. Dis.* 1986; **29** (suppl. 1): 73–88.

66. Poulter N, Sever P, Thom S. Antihypertensive and adverse biochemical effects of bendrofluazide. *Br. Med. J.* 1990; **300**: 1465.

67. Ramsay LE, Yeo WW. Antihypertensive and adverse biochemical effects of bendrofluazide. *Br. Med. J.* 1990; **301**: 240–1.

68. Masugi F, Ogihara T, Hashizume K *et al.* Changes in plasma lipids and uric acid with sodium loading and sodium restriction in patients with essential hypertension. *J. Human Hypertens.* 1988; **1**: 293–8.

69. Egan BM, Weder AB, Petrin J, Hoffman RG. Neurohumoral and metabolic effects of short-term dietary NaCl restriction in men. *Am. J. Hypertens.* 1991; **4**: 416–21.

70. Ruppert M, Overlack A, Kolloch R *et al.* Neurohumoral and metabolic effects of severe and moderate salt restriction in non-obese normotensive adults. *J. Hypertens.* 1993; **11**: 743–9.

71. Ramsay LE, Yeo WW, Jackson PR. Dietary reduction of serum cholesterol: time to think again. *Br. Med. J.* 1991; **303**: 953–7.

72. Hunninghake DB, Stein EA, Dujovne CA *et al.* The efficacy of intensive dietary therapy alone or combined with lovastatin in outpatients with hypercholesterolemia. *N. Engl. J. Med.* 1993; **328**: 1213–19.

73. Sox HC. Screening for lipid disorders under health system reform. *N. Engl. J. Med.* 1993; **328**: 1269–71.

74. Gibbins RL, Riley M, Brimble P. Effectiveness of programme for reducing cardiovascular risk for men in one general practice. *Br. Med. J.* 1993; **305**: 1652–6.

75. Otani H, Kita T, Ueda Y *et al.* Long-term effects of a cholesterol-free diet on serum cholesterol levels in Zen monks. *N. Engl. J. Med.* 1992; **326**: 416.

76. Swales JD. Sticking to guidelines can be expensive. *Br. Med. J.* 1994; **308**: 855.

77. Kaplan NM. Dredging the data on antihypertensive therapy. *Am. J. Hypertens.* 1991; **4**: 195–7.

78. Chalmers JP. The National Consensus Conference: not always what it seems. *Blood Pressure* 1994; **3**: 4–6.

79. Robertson JIS. Should the costs of development inhibit research into new antihypertensive drugs? *Cardiovasc. Drugs Therap.* 1989; **3**: 757–9.

80. Hansson L. Shortcomings of current antihypertensive therapy. *Am. J. Hypertens.* 1991; **4** (suppl.): 84–7.

81. Neaton JD, Grimm RH, Prineas RJ *et al.* Treatment of mild hypertension study: final results. *J. Amer. Med. Ass.* 1993; **270**: 713–24.

# Index

Note: Page numbers in italics refer to illustrations or tables; page numbers in bold refer to case studies.